THE PHYSIOLOGY OF THE JOINTS

Seventh edition

A.I. KAPANDJI

Honorary Member of the French Society of Orthopaedics and Traumatology
Honorary Member and President (1987-1988) of the French Society of Hand Surgeons
Member of the American Society for Surgery of the Hand and of the Italian Society for Surgery of the Hand
Corresponding Foreign Member of the Argentine Society of Orthopaedics and Traumatology

THE PHYSIOLOGY OF THE JOINTS

Foreword by Professor Raoul Tubiana

1

Seventh edition

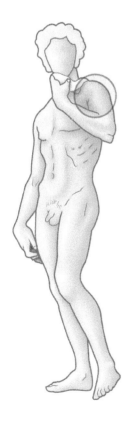

1. The Shoulder
2. The Elbow
3. Pronation-Supination
4. The Wrist
5. The Hand

871 original drawings by the author
Translated by Dr Louis Honoré

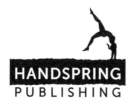

HANDSPRING
PUBLISHING

Handspring Publishing
Carmelite House
50 Victoria Embankment
London EC4Y 0DZ
www.handspringpublishing.com

Seventh edition first published in 2018 in French by Éditions Maloine under the title
Anatomie fonctionnelle: 1. Membre inférieur by A.I. Kapandji.
Copyright © Éditions Maloine 2018 – ISBN: 978-2-224-03541-9

Seventh edition first published in 2019 in English in the United Kingdom by Handspring Publishing (an imprint of Jessica Kingsley Publishers, an imprint of Hodder & Stoughton Ltd, an Hachette UK Company) by arrangement with Éditions Maloine.

ISBN 978-1-912085-59-0

British Library Cataloguing in Publication Data

A catalogue record for this book is available from the British Library

Library of Congress Cataloguing in Publication Data

A catalogue record for this book is available from the Library of Congress

Notice
Neither the Publisher nor the Author assume any responsibility for any loss or injury and/or damage to persons or property arising out of or relating to any use of the material contained in this book. It is the responsibility of the treating practitioner, relying on independent expertise and knowledge of the patient, to determine the best treatment and method of application for the patient.

Cover painting: A.I. Kapandji

Printed in France

To my wife
To my mother, the artist
To my father, the surgeon

Foreword

It is my great privilege to write the foreword for the seventh edition of Adalbert Kapandji's *Physiology of the Joints*, which has already been translated into eleven languages. Of all living French medical authors, Dr Kapandji is probably the most widely read in other countries.

This new edition, greatly expanded and enlivened by the use of colour, is intended for a very wide readership. It will be of the greatest interest to orthopaedic surgeons, but it is also aimed at medical practitioners in general, physiotherapists and students of anatomy, as well as all those who are fascinated by the intricate play of biomechanics in the human body and the harmony of its structure.

I have long admired Dr Kapandji's work; with his vast knowledge of surgery and biomechanics, he has brought traditional anatomy up to date and breathed new life into it by clarifying its functional aspect with scientific precision.

Using his great artistic gifts he has complemented his work with an abundance of illustrations. By facilitating understanding of the text and making the study of biomechanics more pleasurable, these illustrations have everywhere proved to be an excellent teaching tool.

Adalbert Kapandji has produced this book entirely independently, unaided by any support from academic institutions or universities. This goes to show that in research and in teaching, and perhaps in other fields also, the setting, however useful, carries less weight than the intrinsic merit of the work.

Professor Raoul Tubiana

Preface

Since the first publication of this book more than 35 years ago, interest in it has never flagged among physicians and surgeons or physiotherapists, osteopaths and specialists in rehabilitation medicine. Its success abroad has been assured by the publication of eleven translations, not only in the main European languages but also in Japanese and even Korean.

Knowledge advances, however, as do publishing techniques, and for those reasons both author and publisher consider that the time has come to undertake a complete revision of the work.

This edition will be the beginning of a fresh future for the book, because both text and diagrams have been reworked and enriched, and all diagrams and illustrations have been printed in colour, which adds to their clarity and beauty. All this has required a great deal of work, only possible with the aid of the computer.

It is our hope that with the new edition this classic work, universally known and valued, will gain a new lease of life.

Contents

Chapter 1

THE SHOULDER

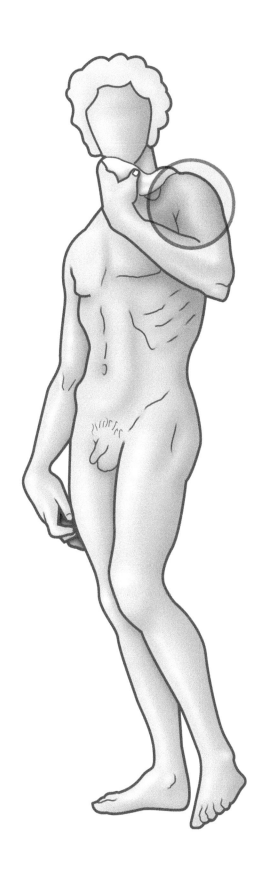

Physiology of the shoulder

The shoulder, the **proximal joint** of the upper limb (see figure on p. 3), is the **most mobile** of all the joints in the human body. It has **three degrees of freedom** (Fig. 2), and this allows orientation of the upper limb in the **three planes of space** that correspond to its **three major axes**:

1) The **transverse axis** (1), lying in the coronal plane, allows the movements of flexion and extension to occur in a sagittal plane (Figs 3 and 4, p. 7).

2) The **antero-posterior axis** (2), lying in a sagittal plane, allows the movements of abduction (the upper limb moves away from the body) and of adduction (the upper limb moves towards the body) to occur in a coronal plane (Figs 7-10, p. 9).

3) The **vertical axis** (3), running through the intersection of the sagittal and coronal planes, controls the movements of flexion and extension, which take place in a horizontal plane with the arm abducted to 90° (Figs 17-19, p. 13).

The **long axis of the humerus** (4) allows two distinct types of lateral and medial rotation to occur:

1) **Voluntary rotation** (also known as 'adjunct rotation' of MacConaill), which depends on the third degree of freedom (Figs 11-13, p. 11) and can only occur in **triaxial joints** (enarthroses). It is produced by contraction of the rotator muscles.

2) **Automatic rotation** (also known as the 'conjunct rotation' of MacConaill), which occurs without voluntary movement in **biaxial joints**, or even in triaxial joints when only two of their axes are in use. We will come back to this point when we discuss Codman's 'paradox' (p. 18).

The **reference position** is defined as the position where the upper limb hangs vertically at the side of the body so that the long axis of the humerus (4) coincides with the vertical axis (3). In abduction at 90° its long axis (4) coincides with the transverse axis (1). In flexion at 90°, it coincides with the antero-posterior axis (2).

Thus the shoulder is a joint with three main axes and three degrees of freedom. The long axis of the humerus can coincide with any of these axes or lie in any intermediate position, thereby permitting the movement of lateral or medial rotation.

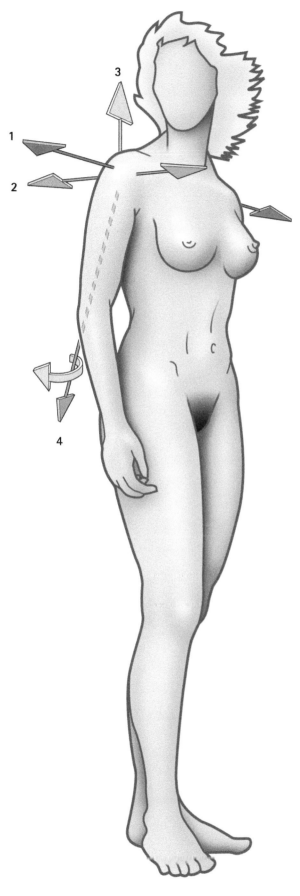

Fig. 2

Flexion-extension and adduction

Movements of **flexion-extension** (Figs 3-6) are performed in a sagittal plane (Plane A, Fig. 20, p. 15), about a transverse axis (Axis 1, Fig. 2):

- **Extension:** a movement of small range, up to 45-50°.
- **Flexion:** a movement of great range, up to 180°. Note that the position of flexion at 180° can also be defined as abduction at 180° associated with axial rotation (see Codman's paradox, p. 18).

The terms antepulsion and retropulsion are often wrongly used to mean flexion and extension respectively. This can lead to confusion with movements of the shoulder girdle in the horizontal plane (Figs 14-16, p. 11), and it is best to avoid these terms in relation to the movements of the upper limb.

The movements of **adduction** (Figs 5 and 6) take place in the coronal plane, starting from the reference position (complete adduction), but they are mechanically impossible because of the presence of the trunk. Adduction is possible, however, from the reference position only when it is combined with:

- **a movement of extension** (Fig. 5; adduction is minimal)
- **a movement of flexion** (Fig. 6; adduction can reach 30-45°).

Starting from any position of abduction, adduction, also called 'relative adduction', is always possible in the coronal plane up to the reference position.

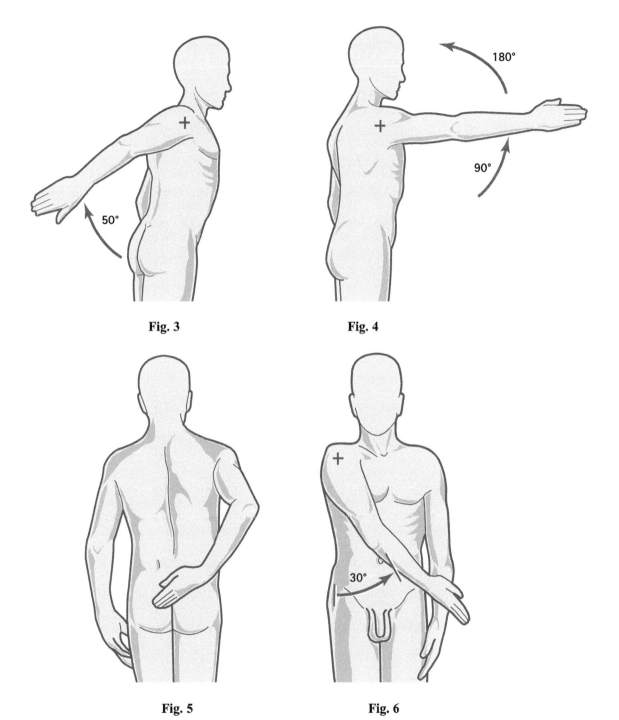

Fig. 3

Fig. 4

Fig. 5

Fig. 6

Abduction

Abduction (Figs 7-10) is the movement of the upper limb away from the trunk and takes place **in a coronal plane** (Plane B, Fig. 20, p. 15) **about an antero-posterior axis** (Axis 2, Fig. 2, p. 5). The range of abduction is 180° when the arm comes to lie vertically above the trunk (Fig. 10).

Two points deserve attention:

* After the 90° position, the movement of abduction brings the upper limb closer to the plane of symmetry of the body and becomes, strictly speaking, a movement of adduction.
* The final position of abduction at 180° can also be reached by flexion to 180°.

In terms of the muscles and joint movements involved, **abduction**, starting from the reference position (Fig. 7), proceeds through **three phases:**

1) abduction from 0° to 60° (Fig. 8), taking place only at the shoulder joint

2) abduction from 60° to 120° (Fig. 9), requiring recruitment of the scapulo-thoracic 'joint'

3) abduction from 120° to 180° (Fig. 10), involving movement at the shoulder joint and the scapulo-thoracic 'joint' combined with flexion of the trunk to the opposite side.

Note that pure abduction, which occurs exclusively in the coronal plane lying parallel to the plane of the back, is rarely used. In contrast, abduction combined with some degree of flexion, i.e. elevation of the arm in the plane of the scapula at an angle of 30° anterior to the coronal plane, is the physiological movement most often used, particularly to bring the hand to the back of the neck or the mouth. This plane of movement corresponds to the position of equilibrium for the shoulder muscles (Fig. 22, p. 15).

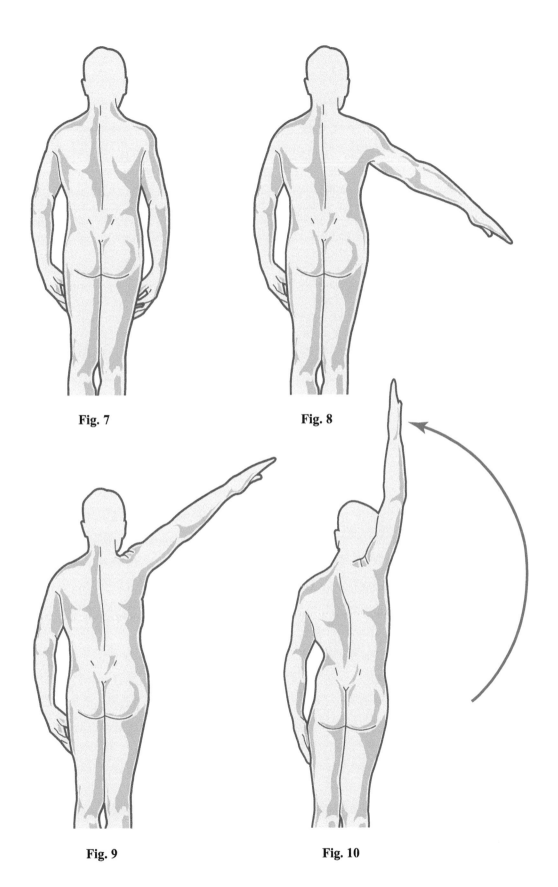

Fig. 7

Fig. 8

Fig. 9

Fig. 10

Axial rotation of the arm

Rotation of the arm at the shoulder joint

Rotation of the arm about its long axis (Axis 3, Fig. 2, p. 5) can occur in any position of the shoulder. It corresponds to the **voluntary or adjunct rotation** that takes place at joints with three axes and three degrees of freedom. This rotation is usually quantitated from the reference position, i.e. with the arm hanging vertically along the body (Figs 11-13, superior view).

Reference position (Fig. 11)

This is also called the position of null rotation. To measure the range of rotatory movements the elbow must be flexed at 90°, with the forearm lying in the sagittal plane. Without this precaution, the range of such rotatory movements of the arm would also include those of lateral and medial rotation of the forearm. This reference position, with the forearm lying in the sagittal plane, is purely arbitrary. In practice, the starting position most commonly used, since it corresponds to the position of equilibrium for the rotator muscles, is that of a 30° medial rotation with respect to the true reference position when the hand lies in front of the trunk. This position could thus be called the **physiological reference position.**

Lateral rotation (Fig. 12)

This extends up to 80° and always falls short of 90°. The full range of 80° is rarely achieved with the arm hanging vertically along the body. In contrast, the type of lateral rotation most often used and so most important functionally takes place in a plane lying between the physiological reference position (medial rotation = 30°) and the classic reference position (rotation = 0°).

Medial rotation (Fig. 13)

This is up to 100-110°. This full range is achieved only **with the forearm passing behind the trunk** and the shoulder slightly extended. This movement must occur freely to allow the hand to reach the back and is essential for posterior perineal hygiene. The first 90° of medial rotation must also be associated with shoulder flexion as long as the hand stays in front of the trunk. The muscles responsible for axial rotation will be discussed later. Axial rotation of the arm in positions outside the reference position can be accurately measured only with the **use of polar coordinates** (Fig. 24, p. 17) or by the meridian test (Fig. 25, p. 17). For each position the rotator muscles behave differently, with some losing and others acquiring rotator function; this is another example of the **law of inversion of muscular action**, which depends on the position of the muscle.

Movements of the shoulder girdle in the horizontal plane

These movements involve the **scapulo-thoracic 'joint'** (Figs 14-16) as follows:

- **reference position** (Fig. 14)
- **retraction of the shoulder girdle** (Fig. 15)
- **protraction of the shoulder girdle** (Fig. 16).

Note that the range of protraction is greater than that of retraction. The muscles brought into play in these movements are as follows:

- Protraction: *pectoralis major, pectoralis minor, serratus anterior*
- Retraction: rhomboids, *trapezius* (the transverse fibres), *latissimus dorsi.*

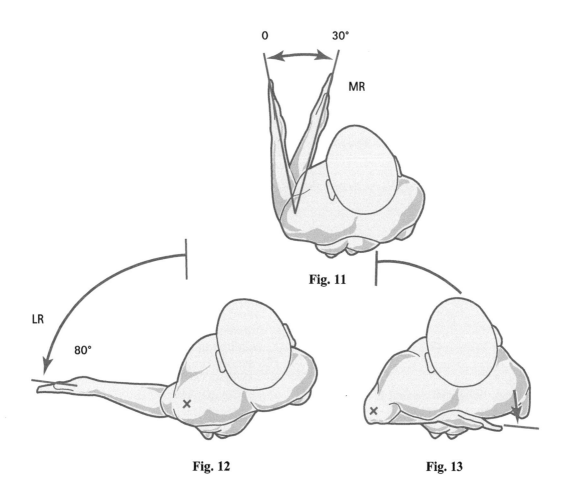

Fig. 11

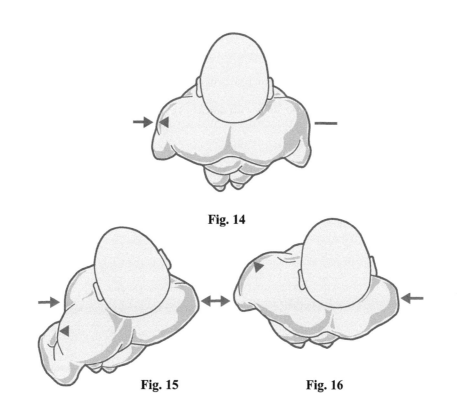

Fig. 12

Fig. 13

Fig. 14

Fig. 15

Fig. 16

Horizontal flexion-extension

These movements of the upper limb take place (Figs 17-19) in the horizontal plane (Plane C, Fig. 20) about a vertical axis or, more accurately, about a series of vertical axes, since they involve both the shoulder joint (Axis 4, Fig. 2, p. 5) and the scapulo-thoracic 'joint'.

Reference position (Fig. 18)
The upper limb is abducted at 90° in the coronal plane, calling into play the following muscles:
- deltoid (essentially acromial fibres III, Fig. 101, p. 63)
- *supraspinatus*
- *trapezius*: superior (acromial and clavicular) and inferior (tubercular) fibres
- *serratus anterior.*

Horizontal flexion (Fig. 17)
Combined with adduction, horizontal flexion has a range of 140° and mobilizes the following muscles:
- deltoid (a variable contribution from antero-medial fibres I, antero-lateral fibres II and lateral fibres III)
- *subscapularis*
- *pectoralis major* and *pectoralis minor*
- *serratus anterior.*

Horizontal extension (Fig. 19)
Combining extension and adduction, horizontal extension has a more limited range of 30-40° and calls into action the following muscles:
- deltoid (a variable contribution from postero-lateral fibres IV and V, postero-medial fibres VI and VII and lateral fibres III)
- *supraspinatus* and *infraspinatus*
- *teres major, teres minor* and the rhomboids
- *trapezius* (all fibres, including the transverse fibres)
- *latissimus dorsi*, acting as an antagonist-synergist with the deltoid, which cancels its strong adductor function.

The **overall range** of this movement of flexion and extension falls short of 180°. Movement from the extreme anterior position to the extreme posterior position successively mobilizes, like a scale played on the piano, the various fibres of the deltoid (p. 63), which is the dominant muscle involved.

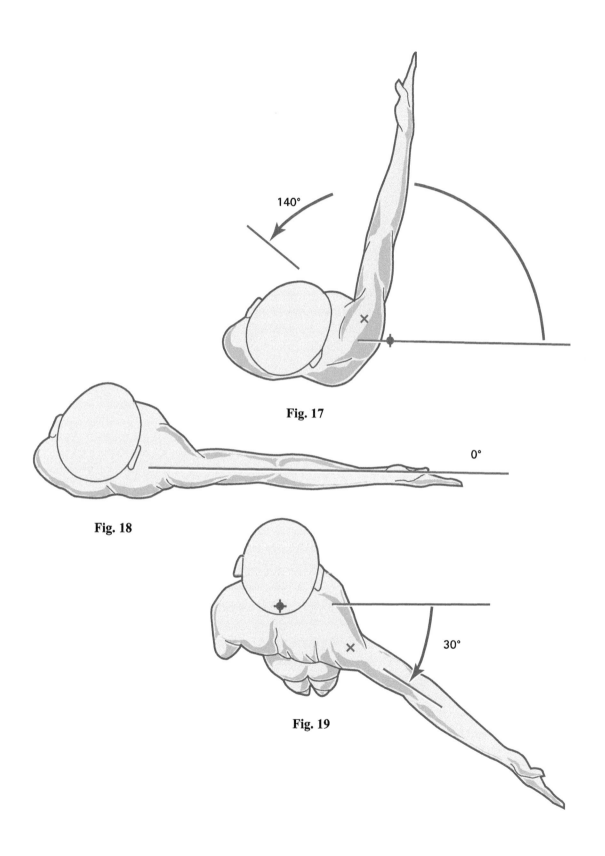

Fig. 17

140°

0°

Fig. 18

Fig. 19

30°

13

The movement of circumduction

Circumduction combines the elementary movements about the three cardinal axes (Fig. 20) up to their maximal ranges. The arm describes a conical surface in space, the **cone of circumduction.** Its apex lies at the theoretical centre of the shoulder and its side is equal to the length of the upper limb, but its base is far from being a regular circle, deformed as it is by the presence of the trunk. This cone demarcates in space a **spherical sector of accessibility**, wherein the hand can grasp objects and bring them to the mouth without displacement of the trunk. Figure 20 shows in red the tracing of the path of the tips of the fingers representing the base of the cone of circumduction distorted by the trunk.

The three orthogonal planes of reference (perpendicular to each other) meet at a point lying at the centre of the shoulder, as follows:

- **Plane A: sagittal**, or rather parasagittal, since the true sagittal plane coincides with the long axis of the body. This is the plane of flexion and extension.
- **Plane B: coronal.** This is parallel to the plane of the back and is the plane of abduction and adduction.
- **Plane C: transverse**, perpendicular to the long axis of the body. This is the plane of horizontal flexion-extension, taking place only in the horizontal plane.

Starting from the reference position with the upper limb hanging vertically alongside the body, the base of the cone successively traverses sectors III-II-VI-V-IV. Inside the cone the upper limb can explore sector I. Sectors VII and VIII (not shown) are nevertheless accessible because of flexion at the elbow. Thus the hand can reach all parts of the body, and this makes grooming more efficient in humans than in animals.

The red arrow that extends the axis of the arm indicates the axis of the cone of circumduction and corresponds more or less to the position of function of the shoulder (Fig. 21) and to the **position of equilibrium** of the periarticular muscles. This explains why this position is favoured as the **position of immobilization** in fractures of the shoulder and of the upper limb. This position of the hand lies in sector IV, appropriately named the **sector of preferential accessibility**, and it satisfies the need to keep working hands under visual control (Fig. 22). This need is also satisfied by the partial overlapping of the two sectors of accessibility of the upper limbs in front of the trunk, allowing the two hands to work together under stereoscopic visual control, which is also the result of the overlapping of the visual fields of the two eyes over a sector of 90°. Thus the visual fields and the sectors of accessibility overlap almost exactly.

This congruence has been achieved during phylogeny by the downward migration of the foramen magnum, which faces posteriorly in the crania of quadrupeds. As a result, the human face can look forwards with respect to a vertical cervical column and the eyes can glance in a direction perpendicular to the long axis of the body, whereas in quadrupeds the direction of the gaze coincides with the axis of the body.

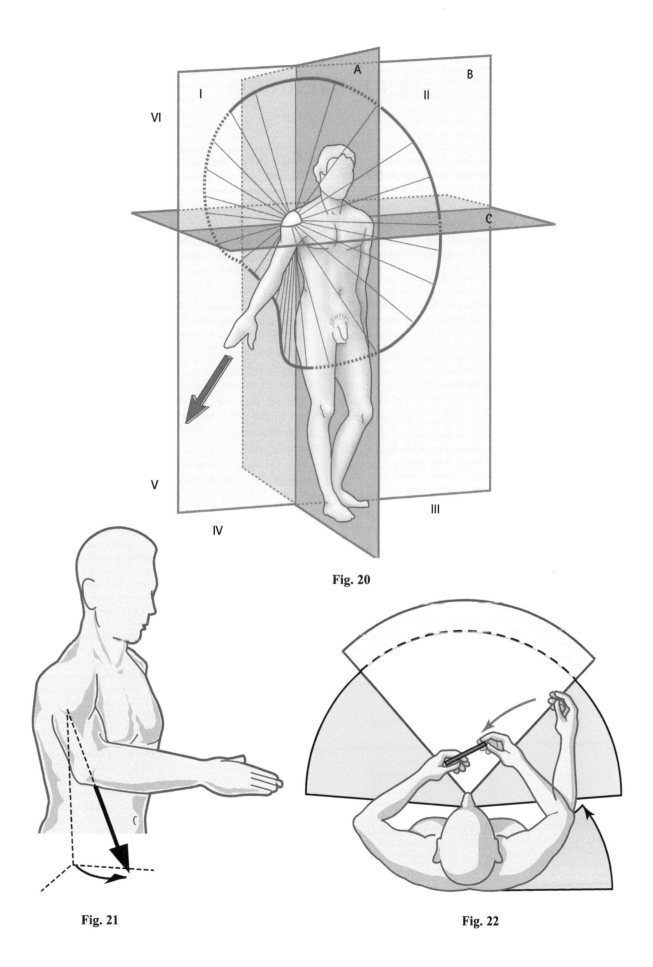

Fig. 20

Fig. 21

Fig. 22

Quantitation of shoulder movements

The quantitation of the movements and positions of joints with three degrees of freedom, particularly the shoulder, is difficult because of certain ambiguities in terminology. For example, if abduction is defined as a movement of the upper limb away from the median plane of the body, the definition is only valid up to 90°, since past that point the upper limb moves towards the body and the term 'adduction' would be more appropriate. In practice, however, abduction is still used in order to stress the continuity of the movement.

Quantitation of axial rotation is even harder. If it is difficult to quantitate a movement in the cardinal planes, it is even more difficult to do so in intermediate planes. At least two coordinates are needed, whether a system of rectangular or polar coordinates is used.

Using the **system of rectangular coordinates** (Fig. 23), one measures the angle of projection of the arm (P) on the three reference planes, i.e. coronal (C), sagittal (S) and transverse (T). The scalar coordinates X, Y and Z precisely define the point P on the sphere whose centre coincides with that of the shoulder. In this system it is impossible to take into account the axial rotation of the arm.

The **system of polar coordinates** (Fig. 24), used by sailors, allows the measurement of the axial rotation of the arm. As on the globe, the position of the point P is defined by two angles:

1) Angle α, corresponding to the **longitude**; this is the **angle of protraction.**

2) Angle β, corresponding to the **latitude**; this is the **angle of flexion.**

Note that only two angles suffice. Instead of β one could use the angle γ, which lies in the coronal plane and also defines the latitude. The advantage of this system lies in the fact that from the angle of elevation ω one can deduce the extent of axial rotation of the arm.

This latter system is therefore more precise and more complete than the former. It is actually the only system that allows the cone of circumduction to be represented as a closed loop on the surface of a sphere, just as the circular course of a boat is traced on the surface of a globe. Nevertheless, it is not used in practice because of its complexity for non-sailors.

There is, however, another method of quantitating the axial rotation of the arm in any position relative to the position of reference, and this consists of **observing the return of the hand to the position of reference via the meridian** (Fig. 25), as, for example, from the position of the hand that allows one to comb one's hair. From here the elbow is moved down vertically towards the position of reference, i.e. the meridian corresponding to the starting point. If care is taken to avoid any voluntary rotation of the arm during this downward movement, the amount of axial rotation can be measured by the usual criteria. In this case, it is close to the maximum, i.e. 30°. This method is one I have personally developed.

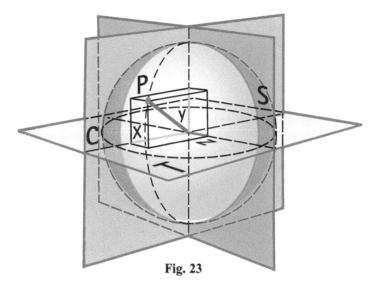

Fig. 23

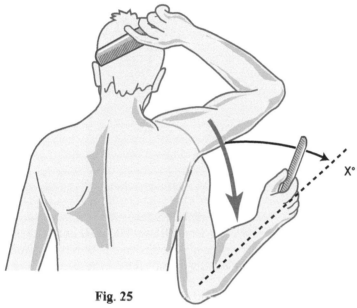

Fig. 25

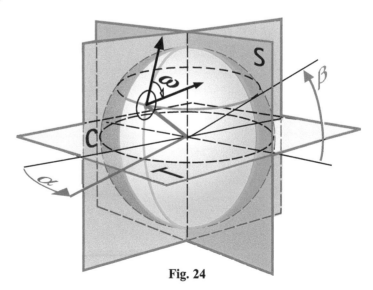

Fig. 24

Codman's 'paradox'

Codman's manœuvre (Figs 26-30) is carried out as follows:
- In the position of reference (Fig. 26, lateral view, and Fig. 27, posterior view), the upper limb hangs down vertically alongside the trunk, with the thumb facing anteriorly (Ant) and the palm of the hand medially.
- The limb is then abducted to +180° (Fig. 28).
- From this vertical position with the palm facing laterally the limb is extended −180° in the sagittal plane (Fig. 29).
- It is now back in its original position (Fig. 30) alongside the body, except that the palm now faces laterally and the thumb posteriorly.
- This was called a 'paradox' by Codman, who could not explain why, after two successive movements of abduction and extension, there followed a 180° change in the orientation of the palm.

In reality, it is due to an **automatic medial rotation** of the limb on its long axis, also called **conjunct rotation** by **MacConaill**, and typically seen in joints with two axes and two degrees of freedom. It can be explained by using **Riemann's curved geometry** as applied to the surface of a sphere. Since **Euclid**, it has been known that on a flat surface the sum of the angles of a triangle is 180° (two right angles). If, on the surface of a sphere (e.g. an orange), one cuts a triangle bounded by the meridians 0° and 90° and by the equator at its base (Fig. 31), one obtains a 'pyramid' with a curved triangular base (Fig. 32). The sum of the angles of this triangle is greater than 180°, since they add up to 270° (three right angles).

Let us now indulge in a purely fanciful **thought experiment**, as enjoyed by Einstein (Fig. 34). You start from the South Pole and proceed north along the 90° meridian. Once you reach the North Pole, go back down towards the South Pole along the 0° meridian, without doing a 90° turn, and walk 'crab-fashion', leading with your side. Admittedly, it would be very uncomfortable to cover 20 000 km like this! When you arrive after all these efforts, you will find yourself back-to-back with your starting position: you will have unwittingly rotated through 180°! In this way you have carried out experimentally the conjunct rotation of MacConaill. In **curved geometry**, the sum of the angles of **two trirectangular triangles** (Fig. 33) is 540° (6 × 90°) and exceeds by 180° the sum of the angles of two triangles (360°) lying in a flat plane. This discrepancy accounts for the half-turn that you have made on yourself. Normally, however, the shoulder does not work like this, since after two complete cycles, it should have 'rotated' through 360°, which is a physiological impossibility. This is why the shoulder, like the hip, is a joint with three axes and three degrees of freedom; it has a **voluntary axial rotation**, called **adjunct rotation** by MacConaill. In conclusion, the shoulder can go through **successive cycles** ad infinitum, as in swimming, and these cycles are called **ergonomic**, because at every moment its adjunct rotation offsets and cancels its conjunct rotation. Codman's 'paradox' is seen only when the shoulder is used as a biaxial joint, where the adjunct rotation does not offset the conjunct rotation.

One can say that Codman's paradox is a false paradox, and it is easy to understand why the joints at the roots of limbs have three degrees of freedom so that their movements are not limited by conjunct rotation during movement of the limb in space.

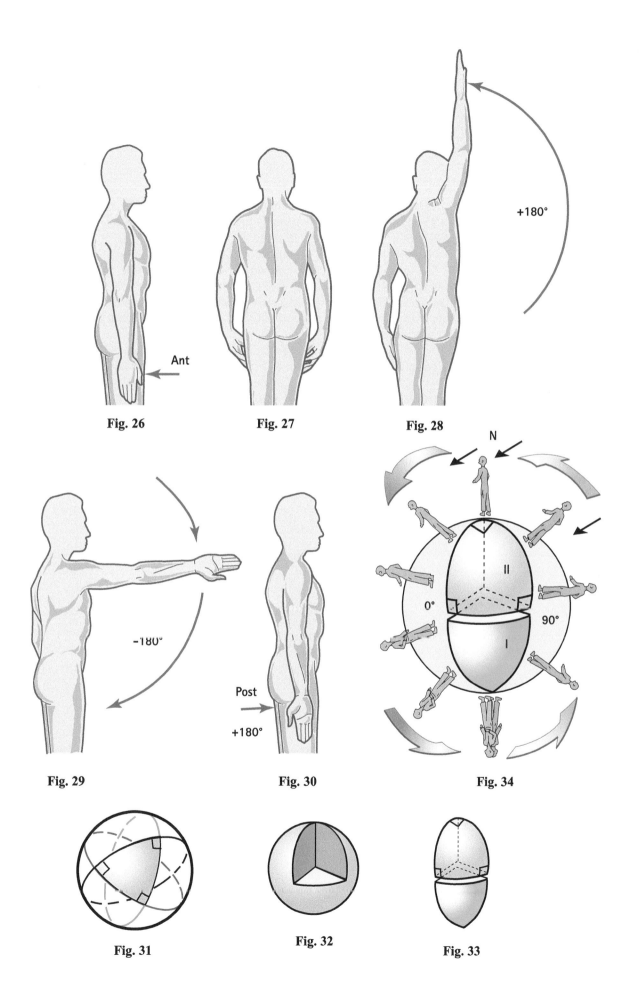

Fig. 26

Ant

Fig. 27

Fig. 28

+180°

Fig. 29

−180°

Fig. 30

Post
+180°

Fig. 34

N

II

0°

90°

I

Fig. 31

Fig. 32

Fig. 33

Movements used for assessing the overall function of the shoulder

In practice some everyday movements permit a good evaluation of shoulder function, such as combing one's hair, slipping on a jacket or an overcoat, and scratching one's back or the back of one's neck. It is possible, however, to use a manœuvre known as the **triple point test**, which relies on the fact that in normal people the hand can reach a **triple point** on the posterior aspect of the contralateral scapula by three different routes. Figure 35 shows the path covered by circumduction in blue dotted lines and the three sets of possible routes to this triple point, as follows:

- in pale blue, the **anterior contralateral route** (C), passing on the other side of the head
- in green, the **anterior ipsilateral route** (I), passing on the same side of the head
- in red, the **posterior route** (P), which goes straight to the back on the same side.

The points reached by the tips of the fingers along each of these routes are mapped in five stages. Stage 5 is shared by all three routes and is the **triple point** (large red dot) located on the contralateral scapula.

The **anterior contralateral route** (Fig. 36, anterior view; Fig. 38, posterior view) starts at the mouth (1) and proceeds to the opposite ear (2), the back of the neck (3), the trapezius (4) and finally the scapula (5). It **evaluates horizontal adduction or flexion.**

The **anterior ipsilateral route** (Fig. 37, posterior view) goes through the same stages but on the same side: the mouth (1), the ear (2), the back of the neck (3), the trapezius (4) and the scapula (5). It **evaluates lateral rotation**, which is maximal at stage 5. In this diagram the ipsilateral and posterior routes are combined.

The **posterior route** (Fig. 35) starts at the buttock (1) and proceeds to the sacral region (2), the lumbar region (3), the tip of the scapula (4) and finally the body of the scapula (5). It **evaluates medial rotation**, which is maximal at the triple point. The first stage (1) is very important, as it is the minimum requirement for ensuring posterior perineal hygiene, which determines the patient's functional autonomy. In this figure the contralateral and posterior routes are combined.

It is clear that the results of this test will depend on the functional integrity of the elbow. This test is therefore also useful for obtaining an overall functional assessment of the upper limb.

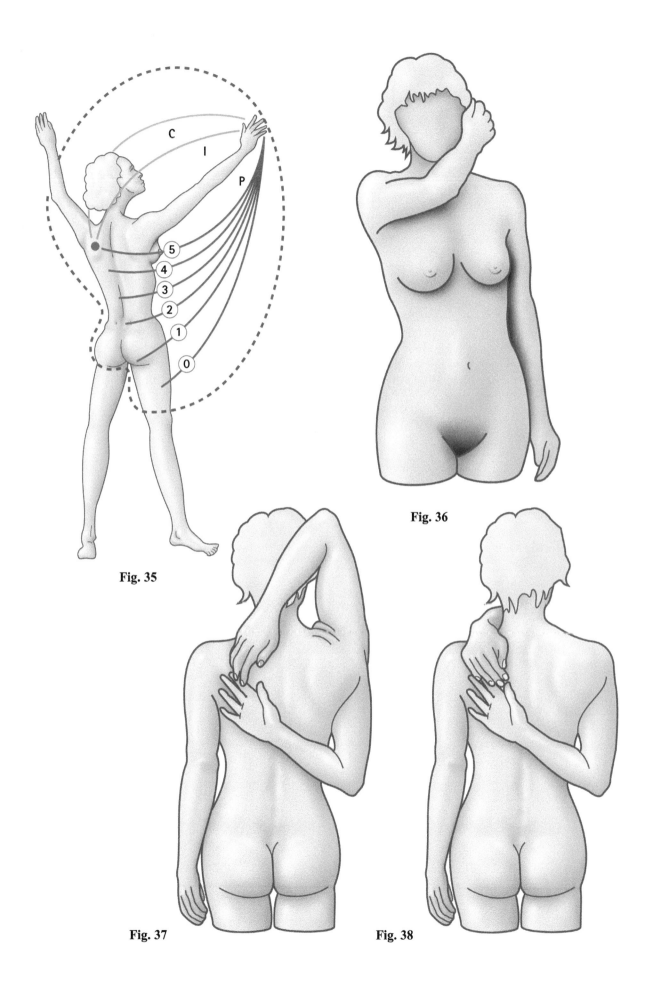

Fig. 35

Fig. 36

Fig. 37

Fig. 38

21

The multiarticular complex of the shoulder

The shoulder comprises not one but five joints that together form **the articular complex of the shoulder** (Fig. 39). We have already described its movements involving the upper limb. The five joints fall into two groups.

First group: two joints
1) The **shoulder (gleno-humeral) joint**, which is a true joint anatomically, with two articular surfaces lined by hyaline cartilage. It is the most important joint of this group.
2) The **subdeltoid 'joint'** or second shoulder joint', which is not an anatomical but a physiological joint, as it consists of two surfaces sliding with respect to each other. The subdeltoid 'joint' is linked mechanically to the shoulder joint because any movement in the latter brings about movement in the former.

Second group: three joints
1) The **scapulo-thoracic 'joint'**, which again is a physiological rather than an anatomical joint. It is the most important joint of this group but cannot function without the other two, which are mechanically linked to it.
2) The **acromio-clavicular joint**, a true joint, located at the lateral end of the clavicle.
3) The **sterno-costo-clavicular joint**, a true joint, located at the medial end of the clavicle.

The articular complex of the shoulder can be schematized as follows:
- **first group**: a true main joint (the shoulder joint) linked to a 'false' joint (the subdeltoid 'joint')
- **second group**: a 'false' main joint (the scapulo-thoracic joint) associated with two true mechanically linked joints (the acromio-clavicular and the sterno-clavicular joints).

In each group the joints are mechanically linked, i.e. they must function in concert. In practice, both groups also work simultaneously with a variable contribution from each set, depending on the type of movement.

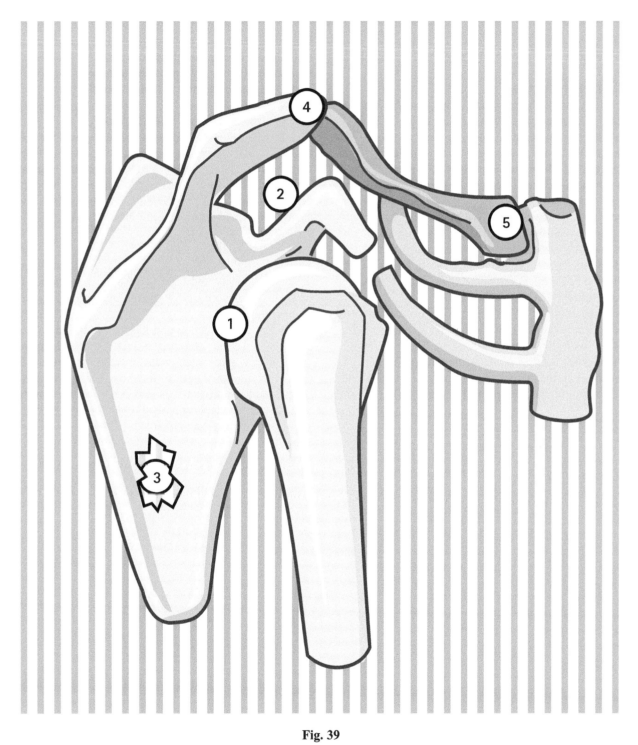

Fig. 39

The articular surfaces of the shoulder joint

These are spherical surfaces typical of the ball-and-socket joint, with three axes and three degrees of freedom (Fig. 18, p. 13).

The head of the humerus

Facing superiorly, medially and posteriorly (Fig. 40), this corresponds to a third of a sphere with a radius of 3 cm. In effect this sphere is far from regular, since its vertical diameter is 3-4 cm greater than its antero-posterior diameter. Furthermore, a coronal cut (Fig. 42) shows that its radius of curvature decreases slightly in a supero-inferior direction and that it contains not one centre of curvature but a series of spirally arranged centres of curvature. Thus, when the superior portion of the humeral head is in contact with the glenoid cavity, the mechanical support is maximal and the joint is most stable, the more so as the middle and inferior fibres of the gleno-humeral ligament become taut. This position of abduction at 90° corresponds to the locked or the **close-packed position** of MacConaill.

Its axis forms an angle of 135° (the angle of inclination) with the axis of the humeral shaft and an angle of 30° (the **retroversion angle**) with the coronal plane.

It is separated from the rest of the proximal epiphysis of the humerus by the anatomical neck, which makes an angle of 45° with the horizontal plane (the angle of declination).

It is flanked by two tuberosities, which receive the insertions of the periarticular muscles:
- the lesser tuberosity, pointing anteriorly
- the greater tuberosity, pointing laterally.

The glenoid cavity of the scapula

This lies (Fig. 41) at the supero-lateral angle of the scapula and points laterally, anteriorly and slightly superiorly. It is biconcave vertically and transversely, but its concavity is irregular and less marked than the convexity of the humeral head. Its margin is slightly raised and is grooved antero-superiorly. The glenoid cavity is much smaller than the humeral head.

The glenoid labrum

This is a ring of fibrocartilage (gl) attached to the margin of the glenoid cavity and filling in the antero-superior groove. It deepens the glenoid cavity so as to make the articular surfaces more congruent.

It is triangular in section and has three surfaces:
- an inner surface attached to the margin of the glenoid
- an outer surface giving attachment to the capsular ligaments
- a central or axial surface lined by cartilage continuous with that of the glenoid cavity and in contact with the humeral head.

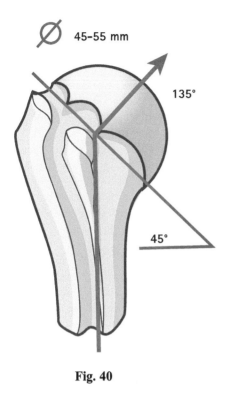

Fig. 40

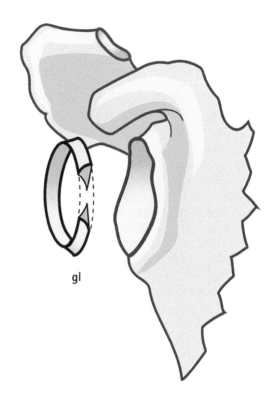

gl

Fig. 41

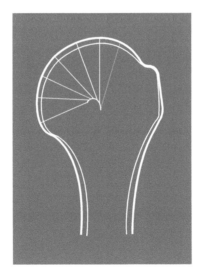

Fig. 42

Instantaneous centres of rotation

The centre of curvature of an articular surface does not necessarily coincide with its centre of rotation, since other factors, i.e. the shape of the articular surface, mechanical factors within the joint and muscular contractions, come into play.

In the past the **humeral head** was likened to a portion of a sphere, and this led to the belief that it had a fixed and unchangeable centre of rotation. The studies of L.R. Fisher et al. have shown that there exists a series of instantaneous centres of rotation (ICRs), corresponding to the centre of a movement occurring between two very close positions. These centres are determined by a computer from a series of radiographs taken in succession.

Thus during **abduction**, when only the component of rotation of the humerus in the coronal plane is considered, there are two sets of ICRs (Fig. 43, humeral head seen from front), which for unknown reasons are separated by a distinct gap (3-4). The first set lies within a circular domain (C_1), located near the infero-medial aspect of the humeral head and having as its centre the barycentre of the ICRs and as its radius the mean of the distances between the barycentre and each ICR. The second set lies within another circular domain (C_2) located in the upper half of the humeral head. These two domains are separated by a gap.

During abduction the shoulder joint can thus be likened to two joints (Fig. 44, anterior view of humeral head):

- During abduction up to 50°, rotation of the humeral head occurs around a point located somewhere within circle C_1.
- At the end of abduction from 50° to 90° the centre of rotation lies within circle C_2.
- At about 50° abduction there is a discontinuity so that the centre of rotation lies superior and medial to the humeral head.

During **flexion** (Fig. 45, lateral view) a similar analysis fails to discover any discontinuity in the path of the ICRs, which lie within a single circular domain located in the inferior part of the humeral head midway between its two borders.

During **axial rotation** (Fig. 46, superior view) the circular domain of the ICRs lies perpendicular to the inner cortical margin of the shaft and is equidistant from the two borders of the head.

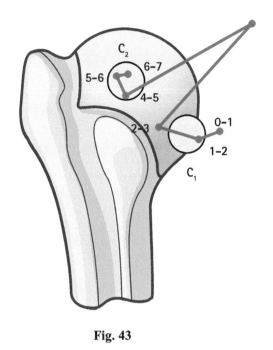

Fig. 43

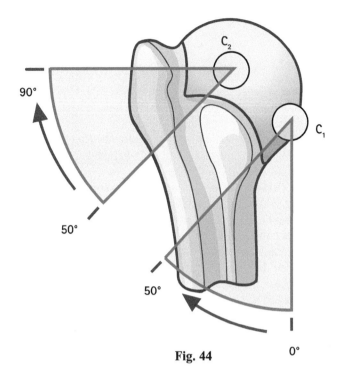

Fig. 44

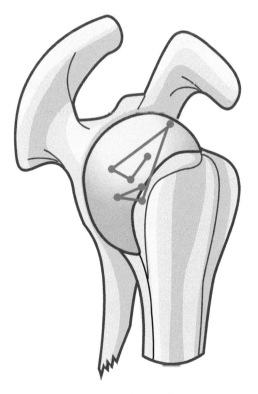

Fig. 45

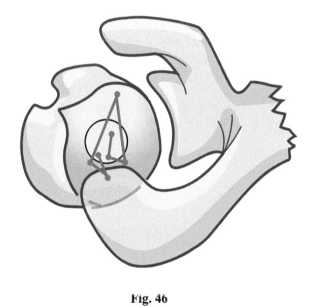

Fig. 46

The capsulo-ligamentous apparatus of the shoulder

This apparatus is loose enough to allow great mobility but is not by itself strong enough to ensure the coaptation of the articular surfaces.

To show the articular surfaces and the capsule (Figs 47-50, according to Rouvière) the joint has been opened and the flaps have been turned back on both sides.

An **intra-articular view of the superior extremity of the humerus** (Fig. 47) reveals the following:

- the **humeral head** (1), surrounded by the capsular cuff
- the **frenula capsulae** (2), i.e. synovial folds on the inferior pole of the capsule
- the **superior band** (4) **of the gleno-humeral ligament**, which thickens the superior part of the capsule
- the **cut tendon of the long head of the biceps** (3)
- the **tendon of the subscapularis** (5), cut near its insertion into the lesser tuberosity.

A lateral view of the scapula (Fig. 48) reveals:

- The **glenoid cavity** (2), surrounded by the glenoid labrum, which bridges over the **groove in the glenoid margin**.
- The **cut tendon of the long head of the biceps** (3), which inserts into the supraglenoid tubercle of the scapula and sends two bands of fibres to contribute to the formation of the glenoid labrum. This tendon is thus intracapsular.
- The **capsule** (8), reinforced by these ligaments:
  - the coraco-humeral ligament (7)
  - the gleno-humeral ligament (Fig. 49), with its three bands: superior (9), middle (10) and inferior (11).
- The **coracoid process**, seen in the background after resection of the scapular spine (15).
- The **infra-glenoid tubercle** (17, Fig. 48), to which is attached the long head of the triceps, which is therefore extracapsular.

An **anterior view of the shoulder** (Fig. 49) clearly shows the anterior ligaments:

- The **coraco-humeral ligament** (3), stretching from the coracoid process (2) to the greater tuberosity, into which is inserted the *supraspinatus* (4).

- The space between the two insertions of the coraco-humeral ligament and the intertubercular groove, which forms the **point of entry of the tendon of the long head of the biceps (6) into the joint cavity** after its course in the intertubercular gutter, transformed into the **bicipital groove** by the **transverse humeral ligament**.
- The **gleno-humeral ligament** with its supraglenoid suprahumeral superior (1), its supraglenoid prehumeral middle (10) and its preglenoid subhumeral inferior (11) bands. This complex forms a **Z** spread over the anterior aspect of the capsule. Between these bands there are **two points of weakness**:
  - the foramen of Weitbrecht (12) and the foramen of Rouvière (13)
  - and the long tendon of the triceps (14).

A **posterior view of the open joint** (Fig. 50) clearly shows the ligaments after removal of the humeral head. The laxity of the capsule in the cadaver allows the articular surfaces to be separated by at least 3 cm, revealing:

- The middle (2) and inferior (3) bands of the gleno-humeral ligament, seen on their deep aspects. On top lies its **superior band**, as well as the **coraco-humeral ligament** (4), to which is attached the **coraco-glenoid ligament** (not shown) and the spinohumeral ligament (16), of no mechanical significance.
- The **intra-articular portion of the tendon of the long head of the biceps** (6) in the upper quadrant.
- The **glenoid cavity** (7), reinforced by the **glenoid labrum** (8), lying medially.
- Outside the cavity the **greater trochanter**, with the insertion of three posterior periarticular muscles:
  - *supraspinatus* (11)
  - *infraspinatus* (12)
  - *teres minor* (13).

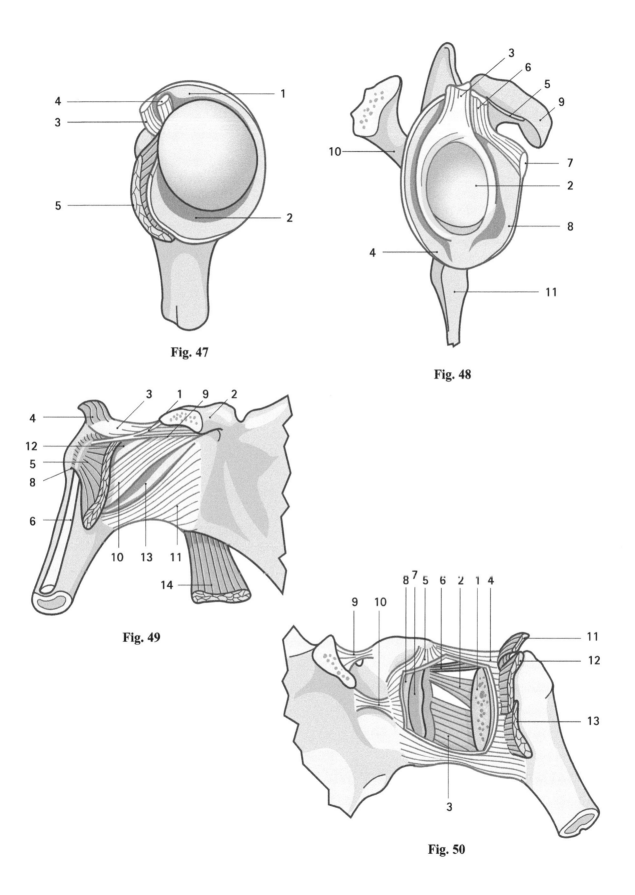

Fig. 47

Fig. 48

Fig. 49

Fig. 50

The intra-articular course of the biceps tendon

A **coronal section of the shoulder** (Fig. 51, inspired by Rouvière) shows the following:

- The irregularities of the bony glenoid cavity are smoothed out by the articular cartilage (1).
- The glenoid labrum (2) deepens the glenoid cavity but the interlocking of the articular surfaces is still poor; hence the frequency of dislocations. The superior margin (3) of the glenoid labrum is not completely tethered to the bone and its sharp central edge lies free in the cavity like a meniscus.
- In the reference position, the superior part of the capsule (4) is taut, while the inferior part (5) is pleated. This 'slack' in the capsule and the unpleating of the frenula capsulae (6) allow abduction to occur.
- The tendon of the long head of the biceps (7) arises from the supraglenoid tubercle of the scapula and the superior margin of the glenoid labrum. As it emerges from the joint cavity in the bicipital groove (8), it slips under the capsule (4).

A **sagittal section of the superior pole of the capsule** (Fig. 52) shows that the tendon of the long head of the biceps is in contact with the synovium in the following three positions:

1) It is pressed against the **deep surface of the capsule** (C) by the synovial lining (S).
2) The synovium forms two tiny recesses between the capsule and the tendon, which is now attached to the capsule by a thin synovial sling called a **mesotendon.**
3) The two synovial recesses have fused and disappeared so that the tendon lies free but surrounded by synovium.

In general, these three positions of the tendon occur successively from the inside to the outside of the joint as the tendon courses away from its origin. **But in every case the tendon, though intra-articular, remains extrasynovial.**

We know now that the tendon of the long head of the biceps plays **an important role in the physiology and pathology of the shoulder.**

When the biceps contract to lift a heavy load, its two heads act together to ensure the coaptation of the articular surfaces of the shoulder. The short head, resting on the coracoid process, lifts the humerus relative to the scapula and, along with the other longitudinal muscles (*triceps, coracobrachialis* and deltoid), prevents the downward dislocation of the humeral head. At the same time the long head of the biceps presses the humeral head against the glenoid cavity, especially during abduction (Fig. 53), since the long head of the biceps is also an abductor. If it is ruptured there is a 20% drop in the strength of abduction. The initial degree of tension of the long head of the biceps depends on the length of its horizontal intra-articular path, which is maximal when the humerus is in the intermediate position (Fig. 56, superior view) and in lateral rotation (Fig. 54). In these positions the efficiency of the long head is at its greatest. In contrast, when the humerus is medially rotated (Fig. 55), the intra-articular path of the biceps and hence its efficiency are minimal.

It is clear also that the biceps, reflected as it is at this level of the bicipital groove without the benefit of a sesamoid bone, is subject to severe mechanical stress that can only be tolerated when the muscle is in excellent condition. If the collagen fibres degenerate with age, the slightest effort can lead to rupture of the intra-articular portion of the tendon as it enters the bicipital groove, giving rise to a clinical picture associated with periarthritis of the shoulder.

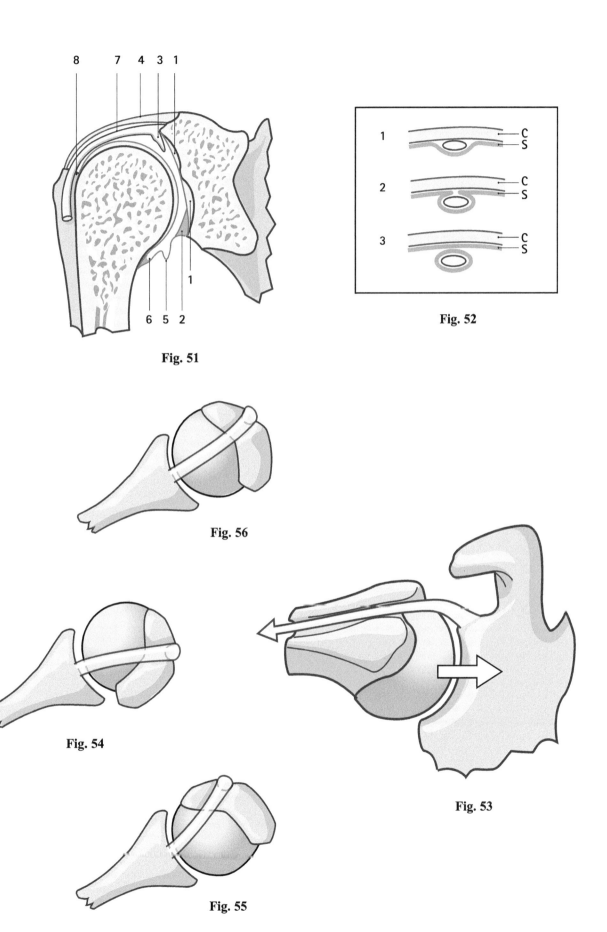

Fig. 51

Fig. 52

Fig. 56

Fig. 54

Fig. 53

Fig. 55

The role of the gleno-humeral ligament

During abduction

- The **reference position** is shown in Figure 57, with the middle (light green) and the inferior (dark green) bands.
- During **abduction** (Fig. 58) the middle and inferior bands of the gleno-humeral ligament become taut, while the superior band and the coraco-humeral ligament (not shown here) relax. Thus in abduction the ligaments are maximally stretched and the articular surfaces achieve maximal contact because the radius of curvature of the humeral head is greater superiorly than inferiorly. Hence abduction corresponds to the locked or **close-packed position** of MacConaill.

Abduction is also checked when the greater tuberosity hits the upper part of the glenoid and the glenoid labrum. This contact is delayed by lateral rotation, which pulls back the greater tuberosity near the end of abduction, draws the bicipital groove under the acromio-coracoid arch and slightly slackens the inferior fibres of the gleno-humeral ligament. As a result abduction reaches 90°.

When abduction is combined with 30° flexion in the plane of the scapula, the tightening of the gleno-humeral ligament is delayed and abduction can reach up to 110° at the shoulder.

During axial rotation

- **Lateral rotation** (Fig. 59) stretches all three bands of the gleno-humeral ligament.
- **Medial rotation** (Fig. 60) relaxes them.

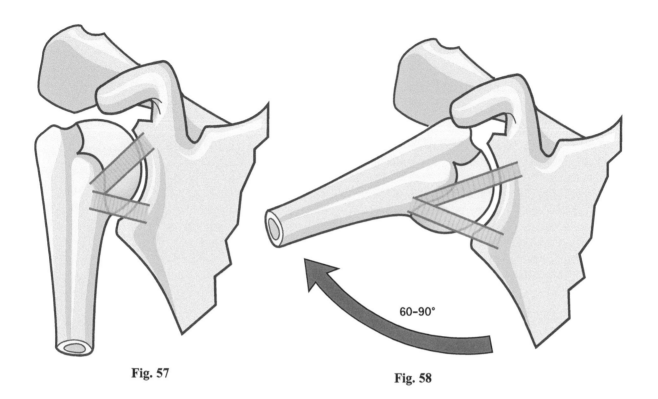

Fig. 57

Fig. 58
60–90°

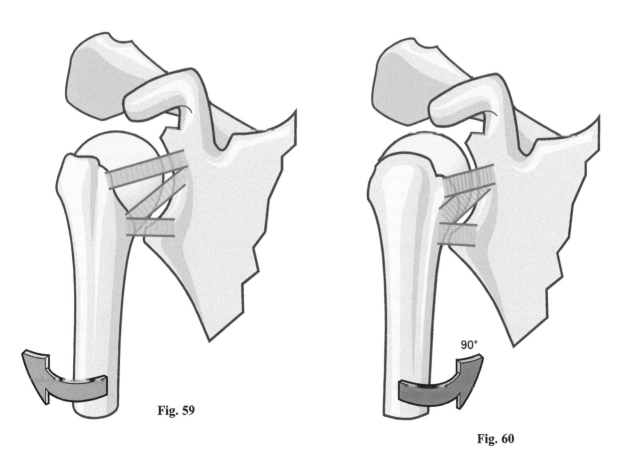

Fig. 59

Fig. 60
90°

The coraco-humeral ligament in flexion and extension

A schematic lateral view of the shoulder joint demonstrates the differential development of tension in the two bands of the coraco-humeral ligament:

- The **reference position** (Fig. 61) shows the coraco-humeral ligament with its two bands, i.e. the posterior (dark green) inserted into the greater tuberosity and the anterior (light green) inserted into the lesser tuberosity. Also visible in the diagram is the point of entry of the long head of biceps into the bicipital groove between the two bands of the coraco-humeral ligament.

- **During extension** (Fig. 62) tension develops mainly in the anterior band.
- **During flexion** (Fig. 63) tension develops mainly in the posterior band.

Medial rotation of the humerus at the end of flexion slackens the coraco- and the gleno-humeral ligaments, thus increasing the range of movement.

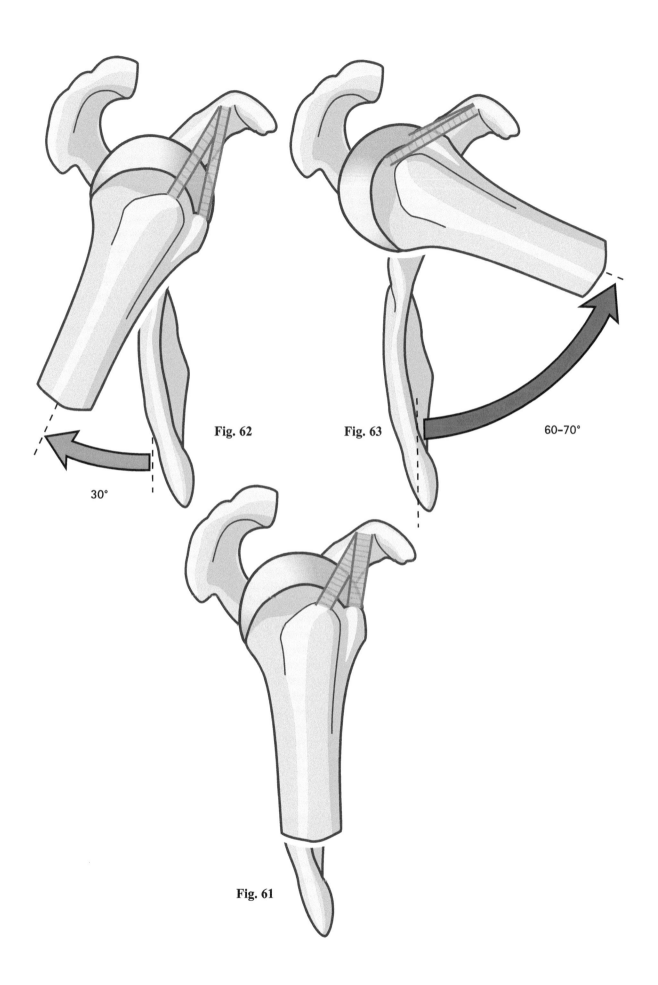

Fig. 62

30°

Fig. 63

60–70°

Fig. 61

Coaptation of the articular surfaces by the periarticular muscles

Because of the great mobility of the shoulder, **coaptation of the articular surfaces cannot be achieved by the ligaments alone**. It requires the help of the **muscles of coaptation**, which fall into two groups:

1) The **transverse muscles**, which press the humeral head against the glenoid cavity because of their orientation (Figs 64-66).

2) The **longitudinal muscles** (Figs 67 and 68), which support the upper limb and prevent downward dislocation when heavy loads are carried in the hand. They 'bring back' the humeral head towards the glenoid. **The syndrome of the 'droopy shoulder'** occurs when these muscles are deficient or paralysed. In contrast, when their action is predominant, upward dislocation is prevented by the 'recentring' action of the transverse muscles of coaptation.

These two groups of muscles therefore act as **antagonists-synergists as their point of dynamic equilibrium is shifted during abduction**.

In Figure 64 (**posterior view**) the **transverse muscles of coaptation** are three in number:

1) *supraspinatus* (1), arising from the supraspinatus fossa of the scapula and inserting into the superior impression on the greater tuberosity

2) *infraspinatus* (3), arising from the infraspinatus fossa and inserting into the postero-superior impression on the greater tuberosity

3) *teres minor* (4), arising from the lower part of the infraspinatus fossa and inserting into the postero-inferior impression on the greater tuberosity.

Figure 65 (**anterior view**) shows:

- *supraspinatus* (1), already seen in Figure 64
- the powerful *subscapularis* (2), arising from the entire floor of the subscapularis fossa of the scapula and inserted into the lesser tuberosity
- the tendon of the long head of the biceps (5), which arises from the supraglenoid tubercle of the scapula and is bent as

it enters the bicipital groove. As a result, it plays a crucial role in ensuring the transverse coaptation of the articular surfaces of the shoulder by '**bringing back the humerus**' while flexing the elbow when a load is lifted by the hand.

Figure 66 (**superior view**) again shows the following two muscles: the *supraspinatus* (1) and the tendon of the long head of the biceps (5), both lying above the joint. Hence, their role as the **superior buttress** of the joint.

Figure 67 (**posterior view**) shows three **longitudinal muscles of coaptation**:

1) The deltoid, with its lateral (8) and posterior (8') bands, 'lifts' the humeral head during abduction.

2) The long head of triceps (7) arises from the infraglenoid tubercle of the scapula and brings back the humeral head towards the glenoid cavity during extension of the elbow.

In Figure 68 (**anterior view**) the **longitudinal muscles of coaptation** are more numerous:

1) The deltoid (8), with its lateral (8) band and its anterior (clavicular) band (not shown).

2) The tendon of the long head of the biceps (5), along with the short head of the biceps (5') arising from the coracoid process close to the *coraco-brachialis* (6). The biceps lifts back the humeral head during flexion of the elbow and shoulder.

3) The clavicular part of the *pectoralis major* (9), which contributes to the action of the anterior band of the deltoid while being mainly a flexor and an adductor of the shoulder.

The predominance of the longitudinal muscles of coaptation can in the long term cause wear and tear on the muscles of the 'cuff', which act as cushions between the humeral head and the acromion and can even cause rupture of some of these muscles, particularly the **supraspinatus**. As a result, the humeral head directly hits the inferior aspect of the acromion and of the acromio-coracoid ligament, causing a painful syndrome classically called periarthritis of the shoulder and now renamed '**syndrome of rotator cuff rupture**'.

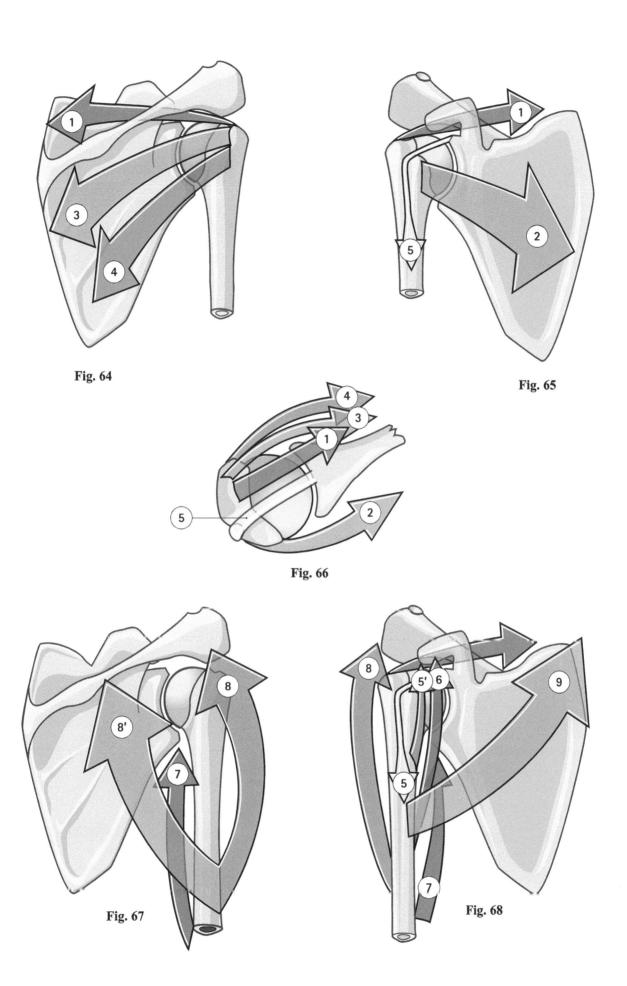

Fig. 64

Fig. 65

Fig. 66

Fig. 67

Fig. 68

The subdeltoid 'joint'

The subdeltoid 'joint' is really a **'false joint'**, since it has no articular cartilages and consists simply of a slit between the deep surface of the deltoid and the 'rotator cuff'. Some authors have described a **serous bursa**, which facilitates the gliding movements in the 'joint'.

A **view of the opened subdeltoid joint** (Fig. 69, inspired by Rouvière), after the deltoid (1) has been cut transversely and pulled back, shows the deep surface of the gliding plane, i.e. the 'rotator cuff' of the shoulder, made up of the upper extremity of the humerus (2) and the attached muscles:

- the *supraspinatus* (3)
- the *infraspinatus* (4)
- the *teres minor* (5), lying behind the *subscapularis* (not shown here)
- the tendon of the long head of the biceps as it runs along the bicipital groove (9) to enter the 'joint'.

Sectioning of the deltoid has opened the serous bursa, whose cut edges are seen (7).

This gliding plane is extended anteriorly by the fused tendons of the *coraco-brachialis* (14) and of the short head of the biceps (13) as they insert into the coracoid process to form the 'ante-rior buttress' of the 'joint'. Also visible in the background are the tendons of the long head of the triceps (6), of the *pectoralis major* (15) and of the *teres major* (16).

The functions of these muscles can be deduced from the two **coronal sections of the shoulder**: one in the reference position with the arm hanging vertically alongside the body (Fig. 70), and the other in abduction with the arm in the horizontal position (Fig. 71).

Figure 70 shows the muscles previously mentioned, a **section of the shoulder joint** (8) with the **glenoid labrum**, and the inferior recess of the capsule. The **subdeltoid serous bursa** (7) lies between the deltoid and the superior extremity of the humerus. Figure 71 shows how abduction due to contraction of the *supraspinatus* (3) and of the deltoid (1) has caused the **serous bursa** (7) to sprawl with its two walls sliding with respect to each other. The section through the shoulder joint (8) illustrates the stretching of the inferior recess of the capsule, whose redundancy is necessary for the full range of abduction at the shoulder. Also seen is the stretched tendon of the long head of the triceps (6), which forms the **inferior buttress of the shoulder joint**.

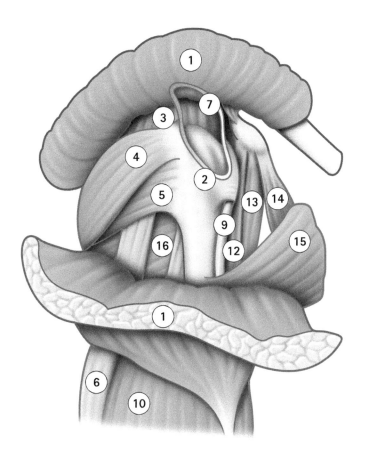

Fig. 69

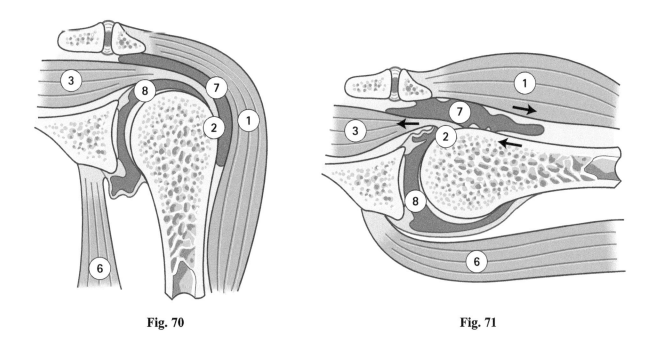

Fig. 70

Fig. 71

The scapulo-thoracic 'joint'

This is also a **'false joint'**, since it contains no articular carti-lages and consists of **two gliding planes** illustrated in the **horizontal section of the thorax** (Fig. 72).

The **left side of the section** shows the contents of the thoracic wall with oblique cuts of the ribs and of the intercostals, as well as the humerus with the insertion of the *pectoralis major* flanked laterally by the deltoid. Because of its twisted shape the scapula (yellow) has a double profile anterior to the *subscapularis* and posterior to the *infraspinatus*, the *teres minor* and the *teres major*. It is the *serratus anterior*, extending as a muscular sheet from the medial border of the scapula to the lateral thoracic wall, which gives rise to **two gliding spaces**:

* **the space between the scapula padded by the subscapularis and the serratus anterior** (1)
* **the space between the thoracic wall and the serratus anterior** (2).

The right side of the section reveals the functional architecture of the shoulder girdle:

* The scapula lies in a plane forming a **30° angle** with the plane of the back, which is parallel to the coronal plane. This angle represents the **physiological plane of abduction at the shoulder**.

* The clavicle, shaped like an italicized S, runs obliquely posteriorly and laterally, forming an **angle of 30°** with the coronal plane. It articulates anteriorly and medially with the sternum at the **sterno-costo-clavicular joint**, and laterally and posteriorly with the scapula at the **acromio-clavicular joint**.

* The angle between the clavicle and the scapula is open medially and is 60° in the reference position but can vary with movements of the shoulder girdle.

In a posterior view of the thoracic skeleton and of the shoulder girdle (Fig. 73) it is customary to show the scapula lying in a coronal plane. In reality it lies in an oblique plane and should appear tilted. In the normal position the scapula extends up and down from the second (2) to the seventh (7) rib. Its supero-medial angle corresponds to the first thoracic spinous process. The medial tip of its spine lies at the level of the third spinous process. Its medial or spinal border lies at a distance of 5-6 cm from the interspinous line. Its inferior angle lies at a distance of 7 cm from the interspinous line.

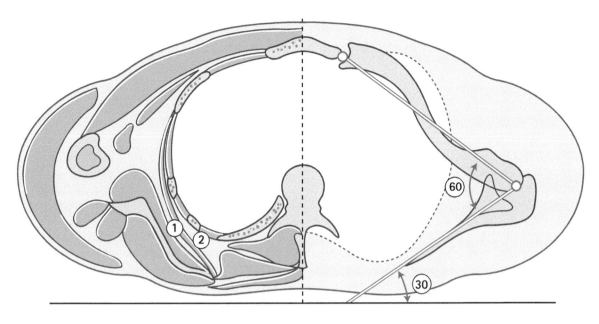

Fig. 72

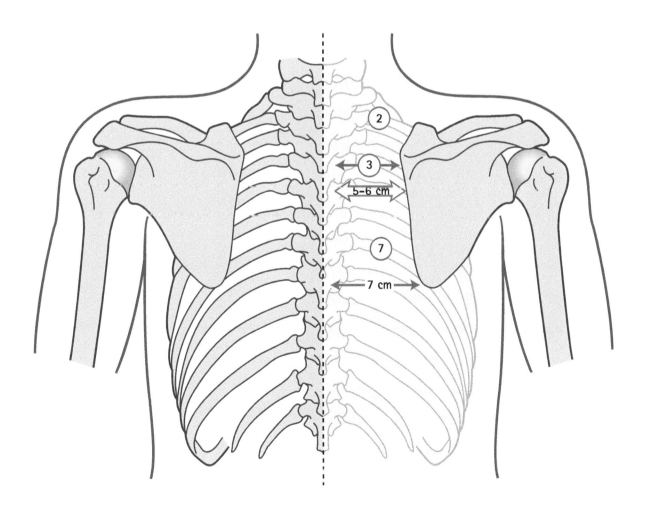

Movements of the shoulder girdle

Analytically three types of movement of the scapula and therefore of the shoulder girdle are recognized: lateral, vertical and rotational. In fact, these three types of movement are always interrelated but to a variable degree.

A **horizontal section** (Fig. 74) shows that the lateral movements of the scapula depend on rotation of the clavicle about the sterno-costo-clavicular joint, thanks to the mobility of the acromio-clavicular joint.

- When the shoulder is pulled back in the movement of **retraction** (right half of the section), the clavicle assumes a more oblique direction posteriorly and the angle between the scapula and the clavicle increases to **70°**.
- When the shoulder is pulled forward in the movement of **protraction** (left half of the section), the clavicle moves closer to the coronal plane (forming an angle of less than 30° with it), the plane of the scapula gets closer to the sagittal plane, the angle between the scapula and the clavicle tends to close down to **below 60°**, and the glenoid cavity faces anteriorly. At this point the transverse diameter of the thorax is maximal.

Between these two extreme positions the plane of the scapula has changed from 30° to 45°.

A **posterior view** (Fig. 75) shows that protraction brings the medial border of the scapula to within 10-12 cm of the interspinous line.

A **posterior view** (Fig. 76) also illustrates the vertical movements of the scapula, which range from 10-12 cm and are of necessity associated with some tilting and raising or lowering of the clavicle.

A **posterior view** (Fig. 77) also demonstrates the tilting movements of the scapula. This rotation occurs around an axis perpendicular to the plane of the scapula and passing through a centre close to its superolateral angle:

- When the scapula rotates 'downwards' (right side), its inferior angle is displaced medially while the glenoid tends to face inferiorly.
- When the scapula rotates 'upwards' (left side), its inferior angle is displaced laterally while the glenoid cavity tends to face superiorly.

The range of that rotation is 45-60°. The displacement of the inferior angle is 10-12 cm, and that of the superolateral angle is 5-6 cm. Most important, however, is the change in the orientation of the glenoid cavity, which plays an essential role in the movements of the shoulder.

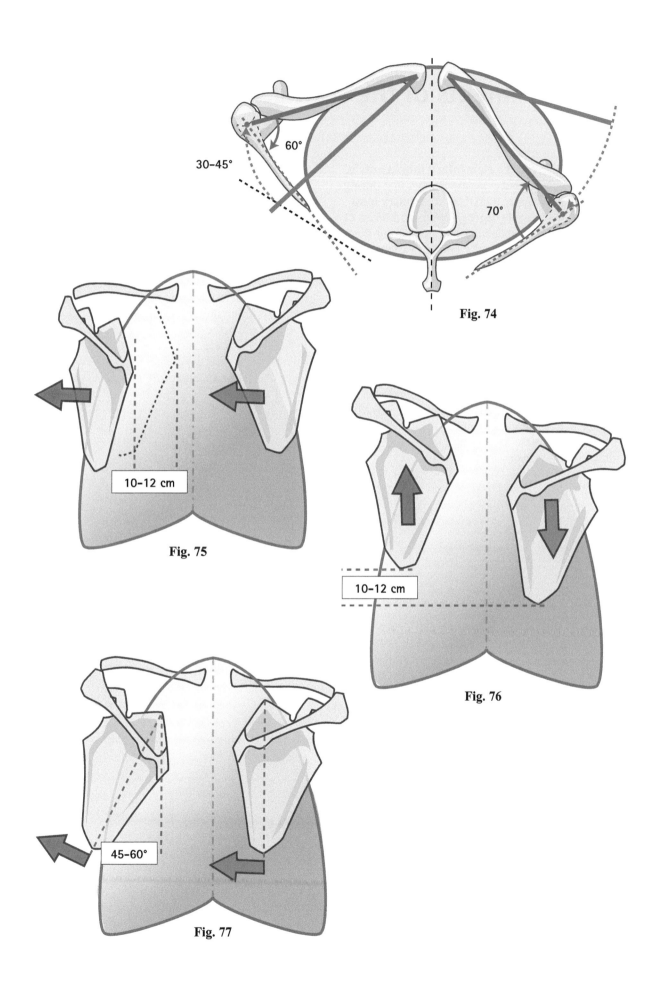

60°

30–45°

70°

Fig. 74

10–12 cm

Fig. 75

10–12 cm

Fig. 76

45–60°

Fig. 77

The real movements of the scapulo-thoracic 'joint'

We have previously described the **elementary movements of the scapulo-thoracic 'joint'** but it is now known that during abduction or flexion of the upper limb these elementary movements are combined to a variable degree. By taking a series of radiographs (Fig. 78) during abduction and comparing them with photographs of a stripped scapular bone in various positions, J.-Y. de la Caffinière has been able to study the components of its real movements. Views taken in perspective of the acromion (above), of the coracoid and of the glenoid cavity (above and to the right) reveal that during active abduction the scapula exhibits four movements:

1) **Elevation** of 8-10 cm without any associated forward displacement, as usually believed.
2) **Angular rotation** of 38°, increasing almost linearly as abduction increases from 0° to 145°. From 120° abduction onwards the degree of angular rotation is the same in the shoulder joint and in the scapulo-thoracic 'joint'.
3) **Tilting** around a transverse axis running obliquely medio-laterally and postero-anteriorly, so that the tip of the scapula moves forwards and upwards, while its upper part moves backwards and downwards. This movement recalls that of a man bending over backwards to look at the top of a skyscraper. The range of tilting is 23° during abduction from 0° to 145°.
4) **Swivelling** around a vertical axis with a biphasic pattern:
   - initially, during abduction from 0° to 90°, the glenoid cavity paradoxically shifts 10° to face posteriorly
   - as abduction exceeds 90°, the glenoid cavity shifts 6° to face anteriorly, and thus just fails to resume its initial position in the antero-posterior plane.

During abduction, the glenoid cavity undergoes a complex series of movements, i.e. elevation, medial displacement and a change in orientation, so that the greater tuberosity of the humerus just 'misses' the acromion anteriorly and slides under the acromio-coracoid ligament.

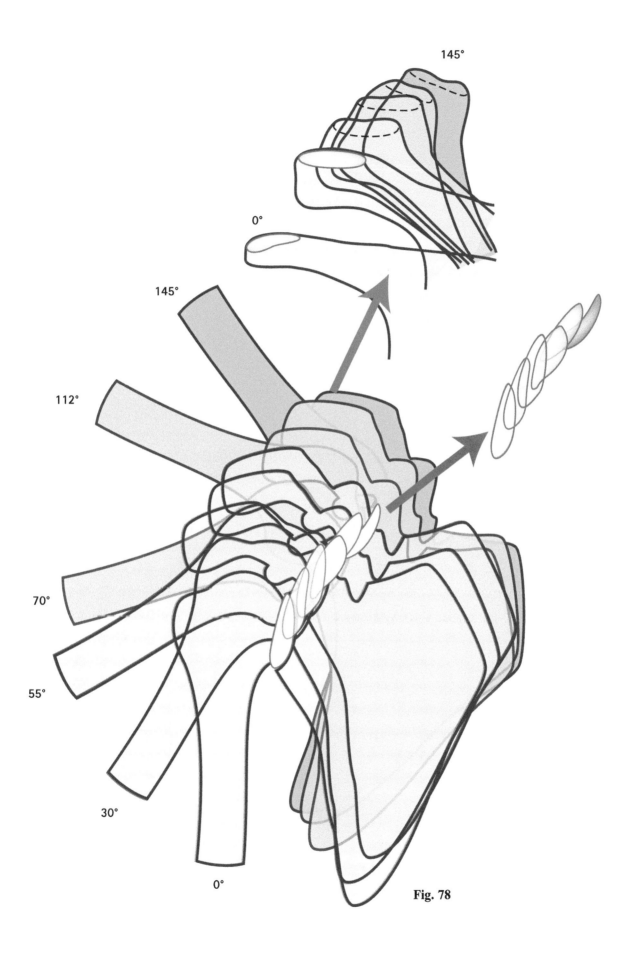

Fig. 78

The sterno-costo-clavicular joint

Like the trapezo-metacarpal joint, this joint belongs to the **toroid** type, since its saddle-shaped articular surfaces correspond to segments cut from the interior surface of a **torus**, which closely resembles the 'inner tube' of a tyre. The two surfaces shown separated in Figure 79 exhibit an **inverse double curvature**: convex in one direction and concave in another, as if 'cut out' of the inner surface of a torus. The concave curvature of one surface fits the convex curvature of the other. The small surface (1) is clavicular and the large surface (2) is sterno-costal. The small surface is in reality longer horizontally than vertically and thus 'overhangs' the sterno-costal surface anteriorly and especially posteriorly.

Such joints have **two perpendicular or orthogonal axes** in space (Fig. 80). Axis 1 corresponds to the concave curvature of the sterno-costal surface and to the convex curvature of the clavicular surface. Axis 2 corresponds to the convex curvature of the sterno-costal surface and to the concave curvature of the clavicular surface. The two axes of these surfaces coincide exactly, just as the curvatures do. These surfaces are termed saddle-shaped or sellar, because the clavicular surface fits easily into the costo-sternal surface, just as a rider sits on the saddle of his horse.

- Axis 1 allows movements of the clavicle in the vertical plane.
- Axis 2 allows movements of the clavicle in the horizontal plane.

This type of joint corresponds to the universal joint. It has **two degrees of freedom**, but by combining these two elementary movements it can also undergo axial rotation, i.e. **conjunct rotation**. The clavicle also undergoes passive movements of axial rotation.

The **right sterno-costo-clavicular joint** (Fig. 81) is shown here opened anteriorly. The posteriorly tilted clavicle (1) displays its articular surface (2) after the superior sterno-clavicular (3), the anterior sterno-clavicular (4) and the costo-clavicular (5) ligaments have been cut. Only the posterior ligament (6) is left uncut. The sterno-costal surface (7) is clearly seen with its two curvatures.

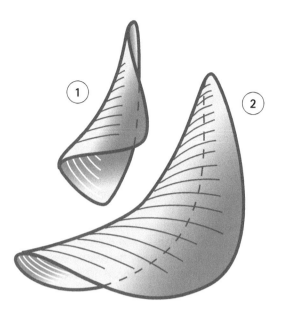

Fig. 79

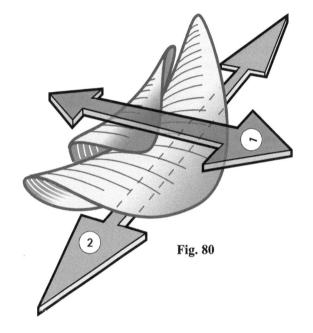

Fig. 80

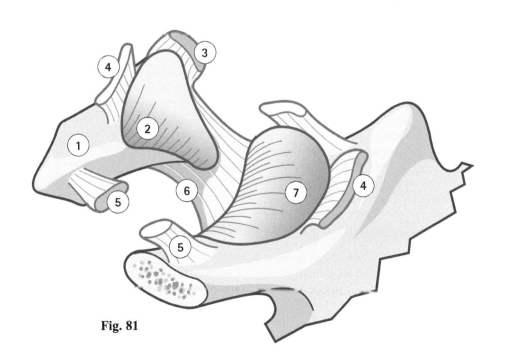

Fig. 81

The movements

Figure 82 (the **sterno-costo-clavicular joint**, inspired by Rouvière) consists of a **coronal section** on the right and an **anterior view of the joint** on the left.

The **coronal section** shows the costo-clavicular ligament (1), attached to the superior aspect of the first rib and running superiorly and laterally towards the inferior surface of the clavicle.

- Very often the **two articular surfaces** do not have the same radii of curvature and congruence is restored by a meniscus (3), just like a saddle between the rider and the horse. This **meniscus** divides the joint into two secondary cavities that may or may not communicate with each other, depending on whether the meniscus is perforated centrally or not.
- The **sterno-clavicular ligament** (4), lining the superior aspect of the joint, is strengthened superiorly by the **interclavicular ligament** (5).

The **anterior view** shows the following:

- The **costo-clavicular ligament** (7) and **the subclavius muscle** (6).
- **Axis X**, horizontal and slightly oblique anteriorly and laterally, which corresponds to the movements of the clavicle in the vertical plane with a range of 10 cm for elevation and 3 cm for depression.
- **Axis Y**, lying in a vertical plane obliquely, inferiorly and slightly laterally, which traverses the mid-portion of the costo-clavicular ligament and corresponds to the movements of the clavicle in the horizontal plane. The range of these movements is as follows: the lateral extremity of the clavicle can move 10 cm anteriorly and 3 cm posteriorly. From a strictly mechanical viewpoint, the real axis (Y′) of this movement is parallel to axis Y but lies medial to the joint.

There is also a third type of movement, i.e. a 30° **axial rotation** of the clavicle. Until now it used to be thought that this rotation was only possible because of the 'slack' in the joint due to the laxity of the ligaments, but, as in all joints with two degrees of freedom, the sterno-clavicular joint also produces a **conjunct rotation** during rotation about its two axes. This idea is confirmed by the fact that in practice this axial rotation of the clavicle is seen only during elevation-retraction or depression-protraction.

Movements of the clavicle in the horizontal plane (Fig. 83, superior view)

- The bold outline shows the position of the clavicle at rest.
- Point Y′ corresponds to the mechanical axis of movement.
- The two red crosses represent the extreme positions of the clavicular insertion of the costo-clavicular ligament.

A section taken at the level of the costo-clavicular ligament (inset) shows the tension developed in the ligament in the extreme positions:

- protraction (A) is checked by the tension developed in the costo-clavicular ligament and the anterior capsular ligament (7).
- retraction (P) is checked by the tension developed in the costo-clavicular ligament and in the posterior capsular ligament (6).

Movements of the clavicle in the coronal plane (Fig. 84, anterior view)

The red cross represents the axis X. When the lateral extremity of the clavicle is raised (shown in bold outline), its medial extremity slides inferiorly and laterally (red arrow). The movement is checked by the tension developed in the costo-clavicular ligament (striped band) and by the tone of the subclavius muscle (6).

When the clavicle is lowered, its medial extremity rises. This movement is limited by the tension developed in the superior capsular ligament (4) and by contact between the clavicle and superior surface of the first rib.

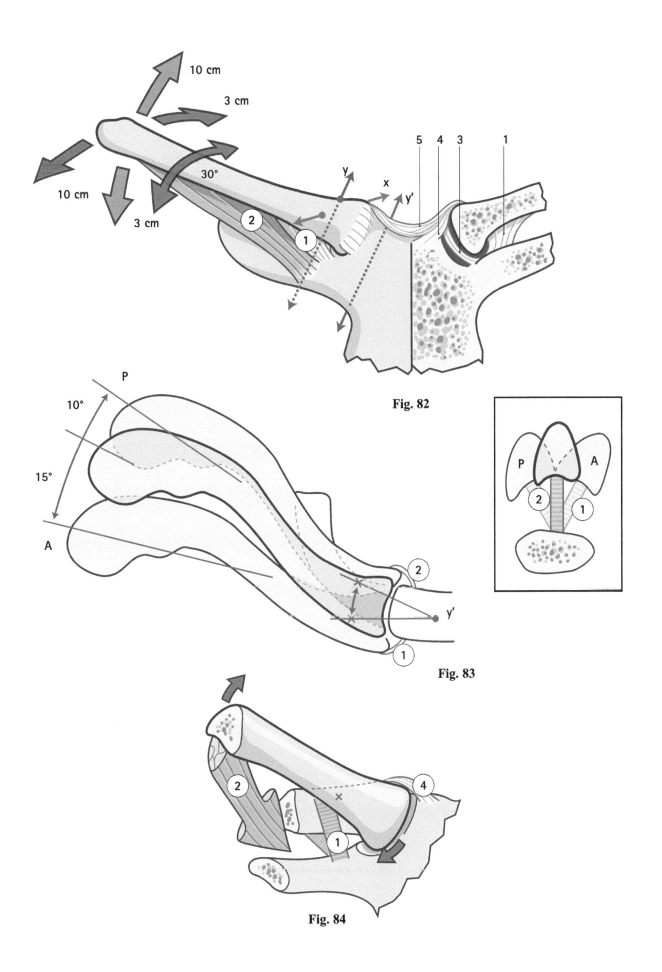

Fig. 82

Fig. 83

Fig. 84

The acromio-clavicular joint

A blown-up posterior view (Fig. 85) illustrates features of this plane joint, characterized by great instability due to absence of interlocking of the articular surfaces and great susceptibility to dislocation due to the weakness of its ligaments.

- The **spine of the scapula** (1), continuous laterally with the **acromion** (2), bears on its antero-medial aspect an oval, flat or slightly convex **articular surface** (3) facing superiorly, anteriorly and medially.
- The lateral extremity of the **clavicle** (4) bears on its inferior aspect an **articular surface** (5), which is similar to the scapular articular surface and faces inferiorly, posteriorly and laterally in such a way that the clavicle appears to be 'poised' over the acromion.
- This joint overhangs the **glenoid cavity of the scapula** (10) and is very exposed. A coronal section (inset) reveals the weakness of the **superior acromio-clavicular ligament** (12).
- The articular surfaces are often convex and not congruent, so that in one-third of cases congruence is restored by an intra-articular fibrocartilaginous **meniscus** (11).

In fact, the stability of this joint depends on **two extra-articular ligaments** that bridge the **coracoid process** (6), which is attached to the superior border of the supraspinatus fossa (9) and the **inferior aspect of the clavicle**. These ligaments are:

- the **conoid ligament** (7), which runs from the 'elbow' of the coracoid process to the conoid tubercle near the posterior border of the inferior aspect of the clavicle
- the **trapezoid ligament** (8), inserted into the coracoid process anterior to the conoid ligament, and running superiorly and laterally to attach itself to a rough triangular area continuous anteriorly and laterally with the conoid tubercle of the clavicle.

An **anterior view of the coracoid process seen in isolation** (Fig. 86) reveals the arrangement of the **conoid** (7) and **trapezoid** (8) ligaments, which together form a solid angle open anteriorly and medially. The conoid ligament lies in the coronal plane and the trapezoid ligament runs obliquely, so that its anterior border faces anteriorly, medially and superiorly.

The acromio-clavicular and the sterno-costo-clavicular joints are called into action during flexion-extension (F) at the shoulder (Fig. 87), because the tilt of the scapula subjects the clavicular buttress to a **torsion R** that is normally dissipated in these two joints. For a range of movement of 180° incorporating extension E and flexion F, a movement of 60° is absorbed by the slack in these joints, and the remaining 30° movement is the result of conjunct rotation at the sterno-costo-clavicular joint. The mobility of the acromio-clavicular joint is very typical and illustrates perfectly the mode of action of arthroidal joints, which depends only on the mechanical play in the joint responsible for its six degrees of freedom. The small surfaces do not stay congruent in harmony with each other; they move away from each other, slide and 'gape' in all directions. Relatively weak ligaments and more powerful muscles only limit their ranges of motion. The scapula, hanging from the distal extremity of the clavicle, can be compared to the **swingle**, which is the movable part of the now obsolete agricultural implement, the **flail**, and was used to beat the wheat. (Fig. 87bis: young boy beating the wheat with a flail) The combine harvester, a large machine that leaves on the field only straw and bags of wheat, has replaced it. Incidentally, these machines also produce unemployment.

The flail (from Latin flagellum: a whip) resembles a whip with a long handle attached by a leather strap to a long flat piece (known as the swingle) used to beat the ears of wheat and cause them to break and release the grain.

The swingle is attached to the handle by soft leather and able to move in all directions (as shown in Figure 87ter, illustrating the mechanical principle of the flail). This degree of mobility is the **maximum attainable** at a synovial joint, which explains why dislocations of the acromio-clavicular joint are the most frequent.

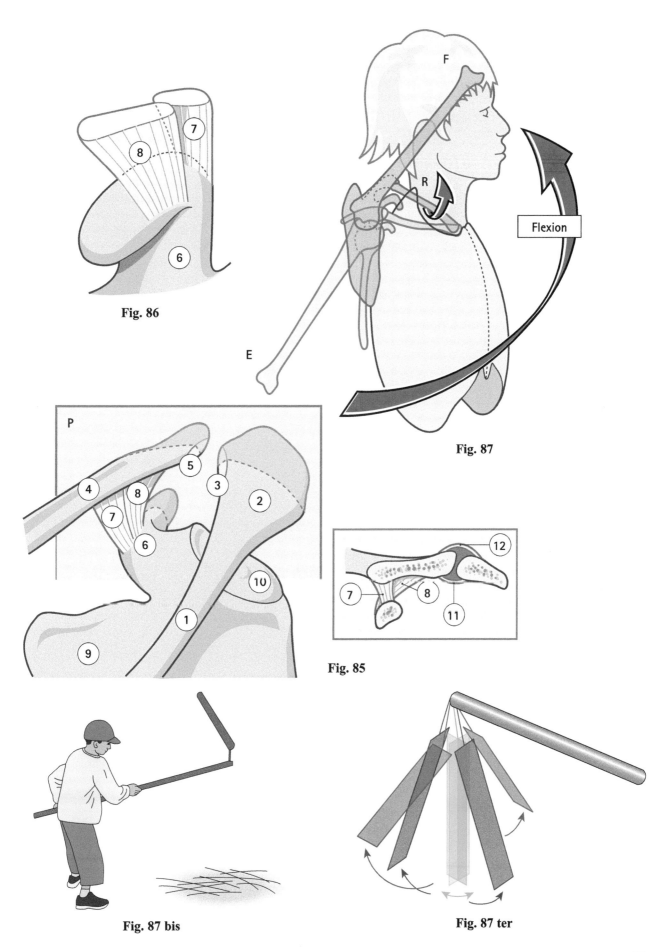

Fig. 86

Fig. 87

Fig. 85

Fig. 87 bis

Fig. 87 ter

In Figure 88 (**supero-lateral view of the right acromio-clavicular joint**, inspired by Rouvière) the following can be seen:

- The superficial portion of the **acromio-clavicular ligament** (11) cut to show its **deep aspect**, which strengthens the capsule (15).
- The **conoid** (7), the **trapezoid** (8) and the **medial coraco-clavicular** (12) **ligaments**.
- The **coraco-acromial ligament** (13), which plays no part in joint control but helps to form the **supraspinatus canal** (Fig. 96, p. 61). The view of the glenoid cavity (10) shows how close the tendons of the rotator cuff are to the coraco-acromial ligament.

- Superficially (not shown in this figure) is attached the **delto-trapezial aponeurosis**, made up of collagen fibres linking the muscle fibres of the deltoid and the trapezius. This recently described structure plays an important role in the coaptation of the articular surfaces as the only one responsible for limiting the degree of dislocation of the acromio-clavicular joint.

The medial end of the clavicle is shown 'running away' (Fig. 89, an infero-medial view, inspired by Rouvière). The structures already described can be seen, as well as the coracoid ligament (14), which bridges the suprascapular notch and plays no mechanical role.

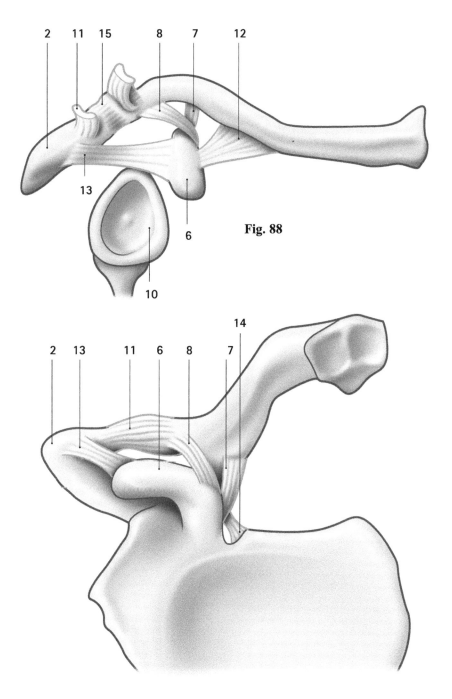

Fig. 88

Fig. 89

The role of the coraco-clavicular ligaments

A diagram of the acromio-clavicular joint (Fig. 90, **superior view**) shows the role of the conoid ligament (7):
- the scapula seen from above with the coracoid process (6) and the acromion (2)
- the contours of the clavicle in its initial position (4, dotted lines) and in its final position (4′, solid line).

The diagram demonstrates how, as the angle between the clavicle and the scapula gets wider (small red arrow), movement is limited by the stretching of the conoid ligament (shown by two green bands representing its two successive positions).

Another similar view (Fig. 91, **superior view**) shows the role of the **trapezoid ligament** (8); with closing of the angle between the clavicle and the scapula (small red arrow) the trapezoid ligament is stretched and limits movement.

Axial rotation in the acromio-clavicular joint can be clearly seen in this antero-medial view (Fig. 92), which also shows the following:
- the cross indicating the centre of rotation of the joint
- the initial position of the scapula (lightly shaded) with its inferior half removed

- the final position of the scapula (darkly shaded) after it has rotated at the tip of the clavicle **like the beater of a flail at the tip of the handle**.

One can see the stretching of the conoid (light green) and of the trapezoid (dark green) ligaments. The 30° range of this rotation is added to a 30° rotation in the sterno-costo-clavicular joint to allow the 60° tilting of the scapula.

With the use of serial photography Fischer et al. have revealed the **full complexity of the movements at the acromio-clavicular joint**, which is a partly interlocked plane joint.

During **abduction**, when the scapula is taken as the fixed base of reference, the following can be seen:
- a 10° elevation of the medial extremity of the clavicle
- a 70° widening of the scapulo-clavicular angle
- a 45° axial rotation of the clavicle posteriorly.

During **flexion** the elementary movements are similar, though the widening of the scapulo-clavicular angle is less marked.

During **extension** the scapulo-humeral angle closes.

During **medial rotation** the only movement is an opening of the scapulo-clavicular angle up to 13°.

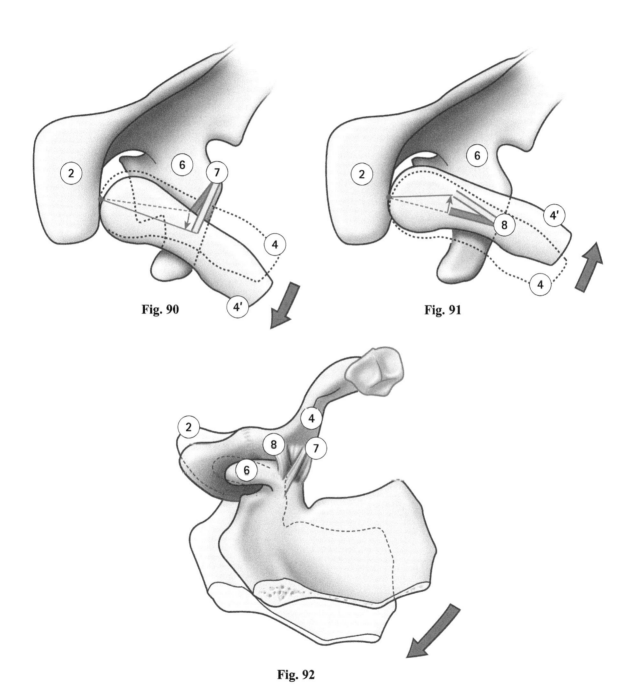

Fig. 90

Fig. 91

Fig. 92

Motor muscles of the shoulder girdle

The right half of the diagram of the thorax (Fig. 93) represents a posterior view and reveals the following.

Trapezius
Trapezius consists of three parts with different actions:
- The **upper acromio-clavicular fibres** (1) raise the shoulder girdle and prevent it from sagging under the weight of a load; they hyperextend the neck and turn the head to the other side when the shoulder is stationary (see Volume 3).
- The **intermediate horizontal fibres** (1'), arising from the vertebral spines, bring the medial edge of the scapula 2-3 cm closer to the midline and press the scapula against the thorax; they move the shoulder girdle posteriorly.
- The **lower fibres** (1''), running obliquely inferiorly and medially, pull the scapula inferiorly and medially.

Simultaneous contraction of these three sets of fibres:
- draws the scapula inferiorly and medially
- rotates the scapula superiorly for 20°, playing a minor part in abduction but a major part in the carrying of heavy loads
- prevents the arm from sagging and the scapula from being pulled off the thorax.

Rhomboid muscles
Running obliquely, superiorly and medially, the rhomboid muscles (2):
- draw the inferior angle of the scapula supero-medially and so elevate the scapula, rotating it inferiorly so that the glenoid cavity faces inferiorly
- fix the inferior angle of the scapula against the ribs; rhomboid paralysis is followed by separation of the scapulae from the thoracic wall.

Levator scapulae
Levator scapulae **(3), sloping obliquely, superiorly and medially, has the same actions as the rhomboids:**
- It draws the supero-medial angle of the scapula superiorly and medially by 2-3 cm (as in shrugging of the shoulders).
- It is active during the carrying of a load, and its paralysis leads to sagging of the shoulder girdle.
- It produces a slight downward rotation of the glenoid cavity.

Serratus anterior (see also Fig. 94, 4')
Figure 93 shows the anterior aspect of its left half with *pectoralis minor* and *subclavius*.

Pectoralis minor
Running obliquely, anteriorly and inferiorly, *pectoralis minor* (5):
- depresses the shoulder girdle so that the glenoid cavity faces inferiorly (e.g. during movements on parallel bars)
- pulls the scapula laterally and anteriorly so that its posterior edge is pulled off the thorax.

Subclavius
Running obliquely, inferiorly and medially, and almost parallel to the clavicle, *subclavius* (6):
- lowers the clavicle and so the shoulder girdle
- presses the medial extremity of the clavicle against the manubrium sterni and thus ensures the coaptation of the articular surfaces of the sterno-costo-clavicular joint.

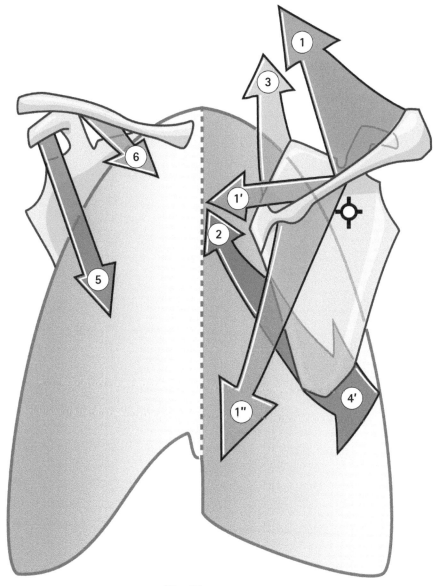

Fig. 93

The **diagrammatic profile of the thorax** (Fig. 94) shows:
- The *trapezius* (1), which elevates the scapular girdle.
- The *levator scapulae* (3).
- The *serratus anterior* (4 and 4′), lying on the deep surface of the scapula and spreading over the postero-lateral wall of the thorax. It is made up of two parts:
  - The **upper part** (4), running horizontally and anteriorly, draws the scapula 12-15 cm anteriorly and laterally and stops it from moving back when a heavy object is being pushed forwards. Its paralysis is easily detected clinically. If a patient leans forward against a wall, the scapula detaches itself from the thorax on the paralysed side.
  - The **lower part** (4′), running obliquely, anteriorly and inferiorly, tilts the scapula superiorly by pulling its inferior angle laterally and causing the glenoid cavity to face superiorly. It is active in flexion and abduction of the arm, and in the carrying of loads (e.g. a bucket of water), only when the arm is already abducted beyond 30°.

The **horizontal section of the thorax** (Fig. 95), highlighting the scapular girdle, allows one to visualize the actions of the muscles:
- **On the right side**: the *serratus anterior* (4) and the *pectoralis minor* (5) pull the scapula laterally and increase the distance between its spinal (medial) border and the vertebral spines. The *pectoralis minor* and *subclavius* (not shown here) depress the scapular girdle.
- **On the left side**: the intermediate fibres of the *trapezius* (not shown here) and the rhomboids (1) bring the spinal border of the scapula closer to the vertebral spines. The rhomboids also elevate the scapula.

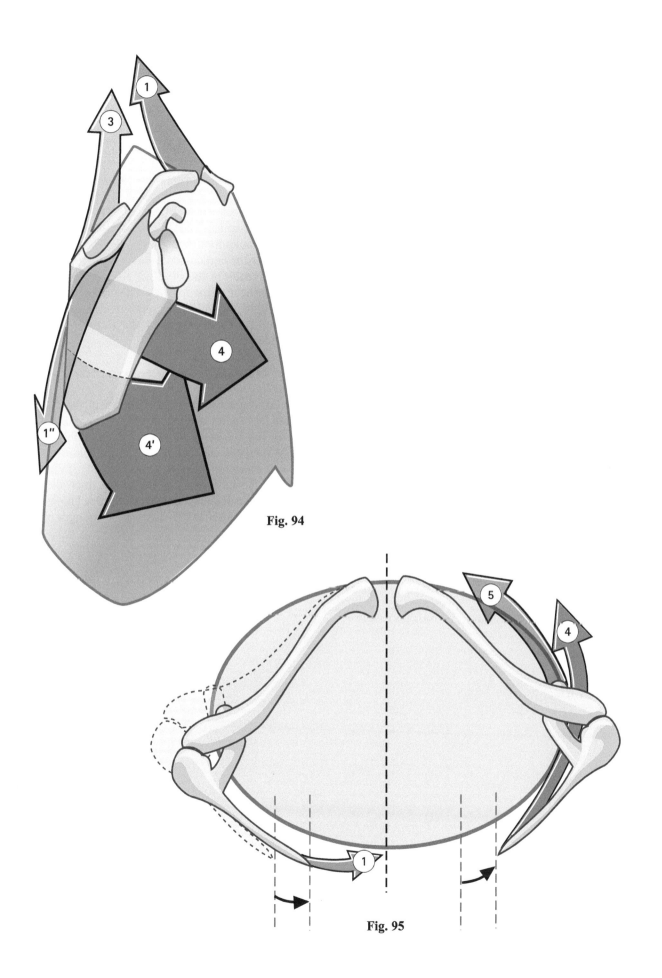

Fig. 94

Fig. 95

59

The supraspinatus and abduction

Figure 96 (**lateral view of the scapula**) clearly shows the **supraspinatus canal** (*), bounded as follows:
- posteriorly by the spine of the scapula and the acromion (a)
- anteriorly by the coracoid process (c)
- superiorly by the coraco-acromial ligament (b), directly continuous with the acromion, thus creating a fibro-osseous arch, called the **coraco-acromial arch**.

The supraspinatus canal forms a **rigid and inextensible ring**, so that:
- If the supraspinatus tendon is thickened by an inflammatory or degenerative process, the muscle has difficulty sliding in the canal.
- If the muscle develops a nodular swelling, it gets stuck in the canal until the nodule is able to glide through eventually. This phenomenon is known as '**jumping shoulder**'.
- If the muscle ruptures as a result of a degenerative process, this leads to '**rotator cuff rupture**', with the following consequences:
  - the **loss of complete active abduction**, which does not go beyond the horizontal plane
  - the **direct application of the humeral head against the coraco-acromial arch**, responsible for the pain associated with the syndrome of 'rotator cuff rupture'.

Surgical repair of the tendon is difficult because of the small size of the canal, and this difficulty justifies the use of **inferior acromioplasty** (the full-thickness resection of the lower half of the acromion) **coupled with resection of the coraco-acromial ligament**.

An **antero-superior view of the shoulder joint** (Fig. 97) shows how the supraspinatus (2), stretching from the supraspinatus fossa of the scapula to the greater tuberosity of the humerus, glides under the coraco-acromial arch (b).

A **posterior view of the shoulder joint** (Fig. 98) demonstrates the arrangement of the four abductor muscles:
- the deltoid (1), which cooperates with the *supraspinatus* (2) to form the **force couple of the abductor muscles** of the shoulder
- the *serratus anterior* (3) and the *trapezius* (4), forming the **force couple of abductor muscles** at the scapulo-thoracic 'joint'.

The following muscles are not shown in the figure, but are none the less useful in abduction: the *subscapularis*, the *infraspinatus* and the *teres minor*, which pull the humeral head inferiorly and medially and form with the deltoid a second force couple of abductor muscles at the shoulder joint. Finally the tendon of the long head of the biceps (not shown) plays a substantial role in abduction, since it is now known that rupture of the tendon causes a 20% loss in the strength of abduction.

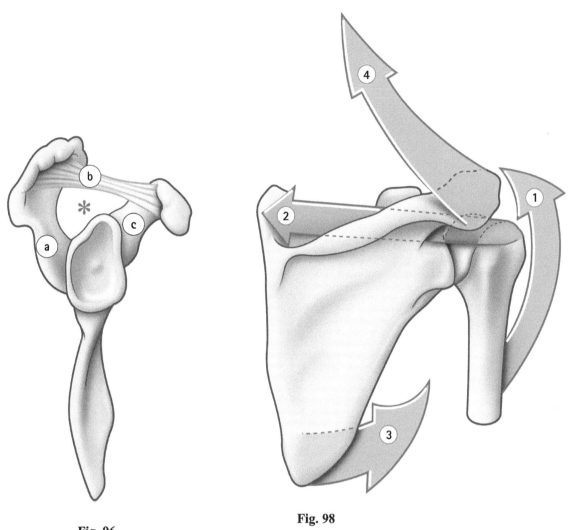

Fig. 96

Fig. 98

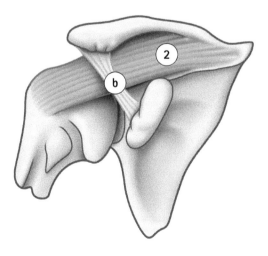

Fig. 97

The physiology of abduction

Though at first sight abduction appears to be a simple process involving two muscles, the deltoid and the *supraspinatus*, there is controversy regarding their respective contributions. Recent electromyographic studies (J.-J. Comtet and J. Auffray, 1970) have shed new light on the problem.

Role of the deltoid

According to Fick (1911), the deltoid (black cross in Figs. 99 and 100) is made up of seven functional components (Fig. 101, horizontal cut through the inferior part of the muscle):

- the anterior (clavicular) band contains two components: I and II
- the middle (acromial) band contains only one component: III
- the posterior (spinal) band contains four components: IV, V, VI and VII.

When the position of each component is considered with regard to the axis of pure abduction AA′ (Fig. 100, anterior view, and Fig. 99, posterior view), it is evident that some components, i.e. the acromial band (III), the most lateral portion of component II of the clavicular band, and component IV of the spinal band, lie lateral to the abduction axis and from the start produce abduction (Fig. 101). The other components (I, V, VI, VII), on the other hand, act as adductors when the upper limb hangs down vertically alongside the body. Thus these latter components antagonize the former, and they start to abduct only when during abduction they are progressively displaced lateral to the abduction axis AA′. Thus for these components there is inversion of function, depending on the starting position of the movement. Note that some components (VI and VII) are always adductors, regardless of the degree of abduction.

Strasser (1917) by and large agrees with this view but notes that when abduction takes place in the plane of the scapula, i.e. with an associated 30° flexion and around an axis BB′ (Fig. 101), perpendicular to the plane of the scapula, nearly the whole of the clavicular band is abductor from the start.

Electromyographic studies have shown that different portions of the muscle are successively recruited during abduction and that the more strongly adductor the fibres are at the start, the later they are recruited, as if they were under the command of a central keyboard as in a musical scale. Thus the abductor components are not opposed by the antagonistic adductor components. This is an example of the reciprocal innervation of Sherrington.

During **pure abduction**, the order of recruitment is as follows:
1) acromial band III
2) components IV and V almost immediately after
3) finally, component II after 20-30° abduction.

During **abduction associated with 30° flexion**:
1) Components III and II contract from the very start.
2) Components IV, V and I are progressively recruited later.

During **lateral rotation of the humerus associated with abduction**:
1) Component II contracts at the start.
2) Components IV and V are not recruited even at the end of abduction.

During **medial rotation of the humerus associated with abduction** the order of recruitment is reversed.

To sum up, the deltoid, active from the very start of abduction, can by itself complete the full range of abduction. It achieves maximal efficiency at about 90° abduction when, according to Inman, it generates a force equivalent to 8.2 times the weight of the upper limb.

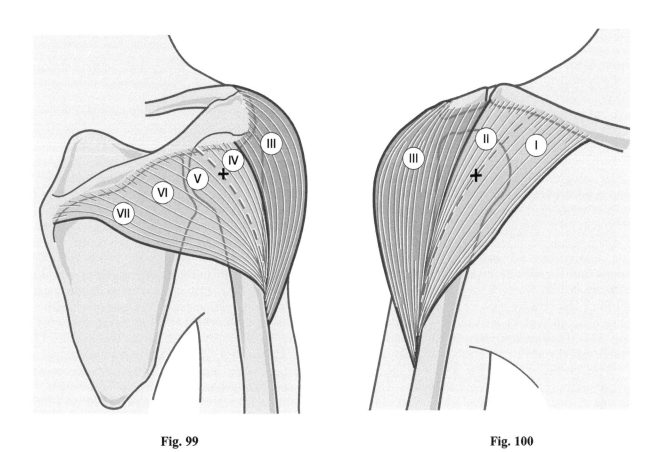

Fig. 99

Fig. 100

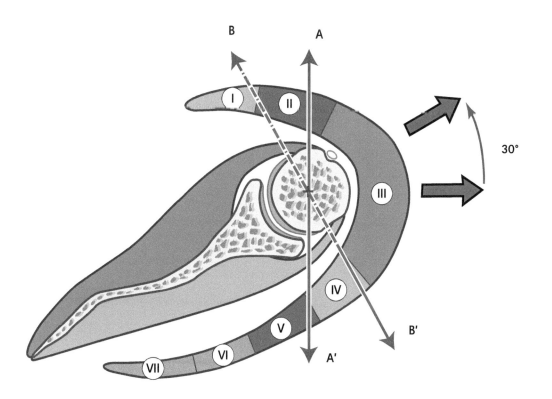

Fig. 101

Role of the rotator muscles

Previously the synergistic deltoid and *supraspinatus* muscles were considered to play an important, if not fundamental, role in abduction, but current thinking is that the other muscles of the rotator cuff are also indispensable for the efficiency of the deltoid (Inman). In fact, during abduction (Fig. 102), the force exerted by the deltoid **D** can be resolved into a longitudinal component **Dr**, which will be applied to the centre of the humeral head as a force **R** after subtraction of the longitudinal component **Pr** of the weight of the upper limb **P** (acting through its centre of gravity). This force **R** can in turn be resolved into a force **Rc**, which presses the humeral head against the glenoid cavity, and a stronger force **RI**, which tends to dislocate the head superiorly and laterally. If the rotator muscles (*infraspinatus*, *subscapularis* and *teres minor*) contract at this point, their overall force **Rm** directly opposes the dislocating force **RI**, preventing dislocation of the humeral head superiorly and laterally (Fig. 104). Thus the force **Rm**, which tends to lower the upper limb, and the elevating component of **Dt** act as a functional couple producing abduction. The force generated by the rotator muscles is maximal at 60° abduction. This has been confirmed electromyographically for the infraspinatus (Inman).

Role of the supraspinatus

The *supraspinatus* has long been viewed as the 'abduction starter'. Studies (B. Van Linge and J.-D. Mulder) producing paralysis of the muscle by anaesthetizing the suprascapular nerve have shown that it is not essential for abduction even at the start. The deltoid by itself is enough to produce complete abduction.

But the *supraspinatus* can by itself produce a range of abduction equal to that produced by the deltoid, as shown by Duchenne de Boulogne's electrical experiments and clinical observations, following isolated paralysis of the deltoid.

Electromyography reveals that the *supraspinatus* contracts during the full duration of abduction and achieves peak activity at 90° abduction, just like the deltoid.

At the start of abduction (Fig. 103; De = deltoid; Pt = tangential component) its tangential component of force **Et** is proportionately greater than that of the deltoid **Dt**, but it has a shorter leverage. Its radial component **Er** presses the humeral head strongly against the glenoid cavity and thus significantly opposes superior dislocation of the head provoked by the radial component of the deltoid **Dr**. It also ensures coaptation of the articular surfaces just as the rotator muscles do. Likewise it tenses the superior fibres of the capsule and opposes inferior subluxation of the humeral head (Dautry and Grosset).

The *supraspinatus* is thus a synergist of the other muscles of the cuff, i.e. the rotators. It is a powerful helper of the deltoid, which on its own tires rapidly.

All in all, its action is important **qualitatively** in helping to keep the articular surfaces together and **quantitatively** in improving the endurance and power of abduction. Though it can no longer enjoy the title of abduction starter, it is clearly useful and effective, particularly at the start of abduction.

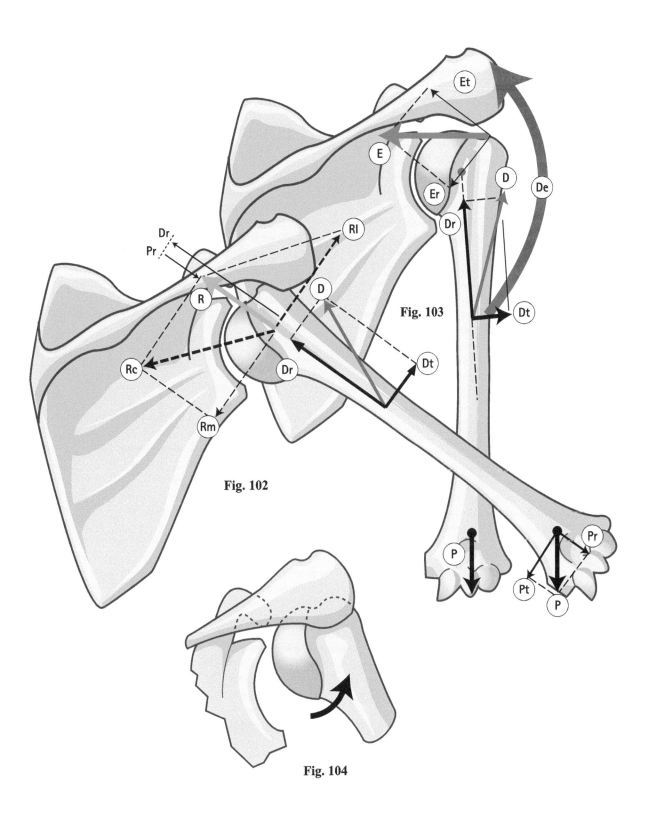

Fig. 102

Fig. 103

Fig. 104

The three phases of abduction

The first phase of abduction (Fig. 105): 0-60°

The muscles involved are essentially the deltoid (1) and the *supraspinatus* (2), which form a functional couple at the level of the shoulder joint. It is in this joint that the movement of abduction starts. This first phase ends near 90°, when the shoulder 'locks' as a result of the greater tuberosity hitting the superior margin of the glenoid cavity. Lateral rotation and a slight flexion of the humerus displace the greater tuberosity posteriorly and delay this mechanical block. Thus abduction combined with 30° flexion and taking place in the plane of the scapula is the true physiological movement of abduction (Steindler).

The second phase of abduction (Fig. 106): 60-120°

When the shoulder reaches its full range of motion, abduction can only proceed with participation of the shoulder girdle.
The movements are these:
*   A 'swing' of the scapula with anticlockwise rotation (for the right scapula), causing the glenoid cavity to face more superiorly. The range of this movement is 60°.
*   Axial rotation mechanically linked at the sterno-costo-clavicular and the acromio-clavicular joints, each joint contributing up to 30°.

The muscles involved in this second phase are these:
*   *trapezius* (2 and 4)
*   *serratus anterior* (5).

These muscles form a functional couple of abduction at the level of the scapulo-thoracic 'joint'. This movement is checked at about 150° (90° + 60° due to rotation of the scapula) by the resistance of the stretched adductors: *latissimus dorsi* and *pectoralis major.*

The third phase of abduction (Fig. 107): 120-180°

To allow the limb to reach the vertical position, movement of the spinal column becomes necessary. If only one arm is abducted, lateral bending of the spinal column produced by the contralateral spinal muscles (6) is adequate. If both arms are abducted, they can come to lie parallel vertically only by being maximally flexed. For the vertical position to be reached, exaggeration of the lumbar lordosis is necessary and this is achieved by the action of the spinal muscles.

This division of abduction into three phases is, of course, artificial; in fact, these various combinations of muscular movements run into one another. Thus it is easy to observe that the scapula begins to 'swing' before the arm has reached 90° abduction; likewise, the spinal column begins to bend before 150° abduction is reached.

At the end of abduction all the muscles are in a state of contraction.

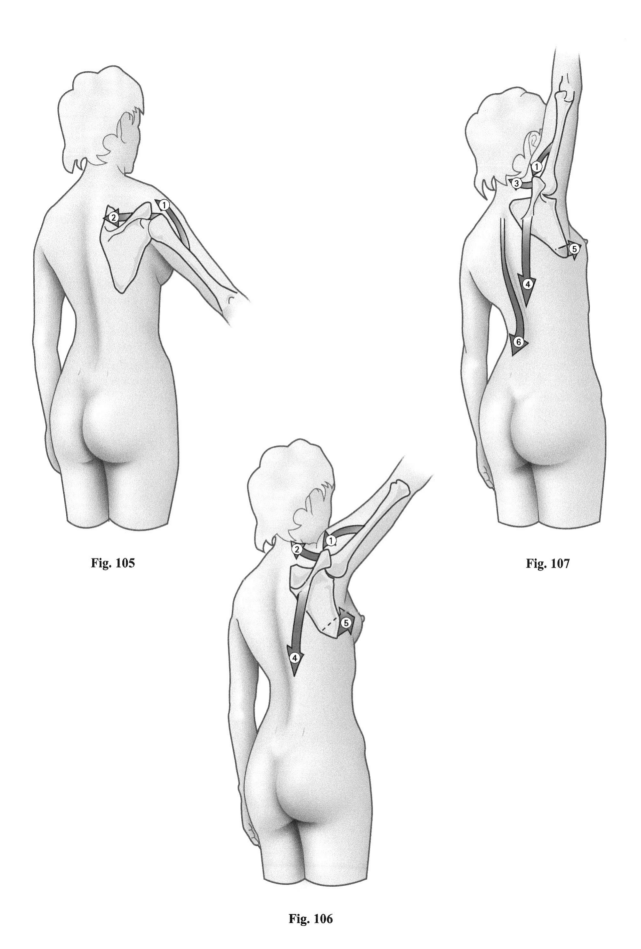

Fig. 105

Fig. 106

Fig. 107

67

The three phases of flexion

The first phase of flexion (Fig. 108): 0-50/60°

The muscles involved are these:
- the anterior clavicular fibres of the deltoid (1)
- the *coraco-brachialis* (2)
- the superior clavicular fibres of the *pectoralis major* (3).

This movement of flexion at the shoulder is limited by two factors:

1) tension developed in the coraco-humeral ligament
2) resistance offered by *teres minor, teres major* and *infraspinatus.*

The second phase of flexion (Fig. 109): 60-120°

The shoulder girdle participates as follows:
- 60° rotation of the scapula so that the glenoid cavity faces superiorly and anteriorly
- axial rotation mechanically linked at the sterno-costo-clavicular and acromio-clavicular joints, each joint contributing 30°.

The muscles involved are the same as in abduction: the *trapezius* (not shown) and the *serratus anterior* (6).

This flexion at the scapulo-thoracic 'joint' is limited by the resistance of the *latissimus dorsi* (not shown) and the inferior fibres of the *pectoralis major* (not shown).

The third phase of flexion (Fig. 110): 120-180°

The raising of the upper limb is continued by the action of the deltoid (1), the *supraspinatus* (4), the inferior fibres of the *trapezius* (5) and the *serratus anterior* (6).

When flexion is checked at the shoulder and in the scapulo-thoracic joints, movement of the spinal column becomes necessary.

If one arm is flexed, it is possible to complete the movement by shifting into the position of maximal abduction and then bending the spinal column laterally. If both arms are flexed, the terminal phase of the movement is identical to that of abduction, i.e. exaggeration of the lumbar lordosis by the lumbar muscles (not shown).

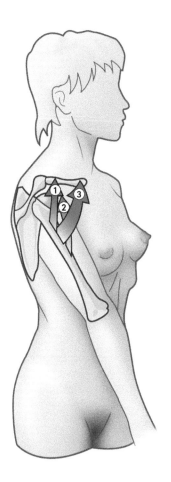

Fig. 108

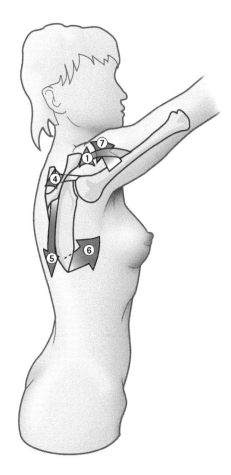

Fig. 109

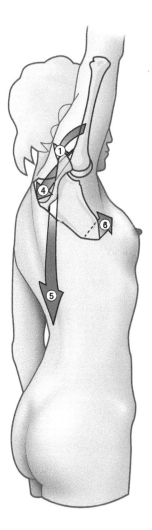

Fig. 110

69

The rotator muscles

A **superior view of the shoulder joint** (Fig. 111) shows the rotator muscles:

Medial rotators (see also Fig. 112):
1) *latissimus dorsi* (1)
2) *teres major* (2)
3) *subscapularis* (3)
4) *pectoralis major* (4).

Lateral rotators (see also Fig. 113):
5) *infraspinatus* (5)
6) *teres minor* (7).

Against the numerous and powerful medial rotators, the lateral rotators are weak. They are none the less indispensable for the proper function of the upper limb, because by themselves they can act on the hand as it lies in front of the trunk and move it anteriorly and laterally. This medio-lateral movement of the right hand is essential for writing.

It should be noted that, though these muscles have a separate nerve supply (the supra-scapular nerve for the infraspinatus and the circumflex nerve for the teres minor), these two nerves come from the same root (C5) of the brachial plexus. So both muscles can be paralysed simultaneously as a result of traction injuries of the brachial plexus caused by a fall forward on the shoulder (a motorcycle accident).

But rotation at the shoulder does not account for the whole range of rotation of the upper limb. There are in addition changes in the direction of the scapula (and so of the glenoid cavity) as it moves laterally on the chest wall (Fig. 75, p. 43); this 40-45° change in direction of the scapula produces a corresponding increase in the range of the movement of rotation. The muscles involved are these:
- for lateral rotation (adduction of the scapula): rhomboids and *trapezius*
- for medial rotation (abduction of the scapula): *serratus anterior* and *pectoralis minor*.

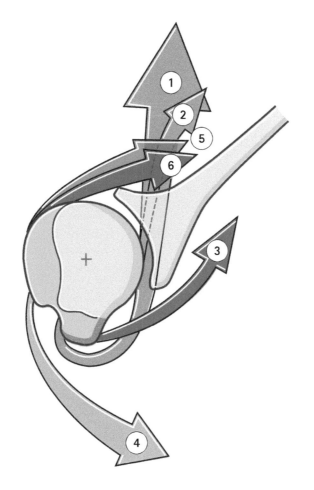

Fig. 111

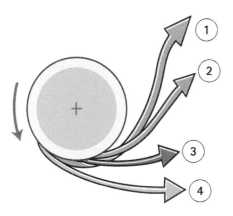

Fig. 112

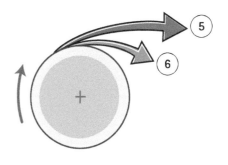

Fig. 113

Adduction and extension

The **adductor muscles** (Fig. 114, anterior aspect, and Fig. 115, postero-lateral aspect, with the same legends) are: *teres major* (1), *latissimus dorsi* (2), *pectoralis major* (3) and rhomboids (4).

Figure 117 is an inset showing two diagrams explaining the actions of the two muscular couples producing adduction:

- Figure 117a: The synergistic action of the rhomboids (1)-*teres major* (2) couple is indispensable for adduction. If the *teres major* alone contracts and the upper limb resists adduction, there follows upward rotation of the scapula on its axis (marked with a cross). Contraction of the rhomboids prevents this scapular rotation and allows the *teres major* to adduct the arm.
- Figure 117b: Contraction of the very powerful adductor, *latissimus dorsi* (3), tends to displace the humeral head inferiorly (black arrows). The long head of the triceps (4), which is a weak abductor, opposes this inferior displacement by contracting simultaneously and lifting the humeral head (small white arrows). This is another example of antagonism-synergism.

The **extensor muscles** (Fig. 116, postero-lateral aspect) produce extension at two levels:

1) **Extension at the shoulder joint**:
   - *teres major* (1)
   - *teres minor* (5)
   - posterior spinal fibres of the deltoid (6)
   - *latissimus dorsi* (2).

2) **Extension at the scapulo-thoracic 'joint'** by adduction of the scapula:
   - rhomboids (4)
   - middle transverse fibres of the *trapezius* (7)
   - *latissimus dorsi* (2).

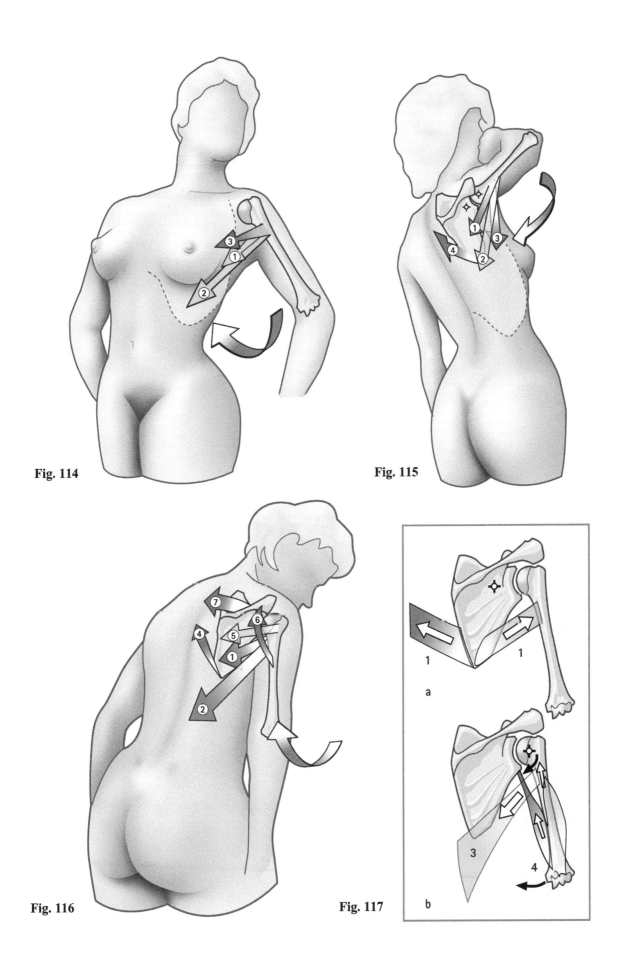

Fig. 114

Fig. 115

Fig. 116

Fig. 117

'Hippocratic' measurement of flexion and abduction

Current examination methods, such as radiology, computed tomography (CT) and magnetic resonance imaging (MRI), have not always been available to doctors. These advanced methods are very useful and often indispensable for refining a diagnosis or establishing the location and significance of a lesion, but during the initial clinical examination doctors must be able to diagnose and evaluate the patient using only their five senses, as did Hippocrates, the founder of medicine.

It is quite possible to evaluate the function of a joint without the use of any measuring instrument, not even a gonlometer or a protractor, **if one considers the human body as its own system of** reference. This system can be used even where no technical device is available; **one must go back to Hippocrates**. This is perfectly applicable to the examination of the shoulder.

For **flexion** (Figs 119 and 120) and **extension** (Fig. 118), one must remember that:

* When the fingers touch the mouth (Fig. 119), flexion at the shoulder equals **45°**. This movement allows food to be brought to the mouth.

* When the hand rests on top of the head (Fig. 120), flexion at the shoulder equals **120°**. This movement allows personal haircare, e.g. combing. As already shown on page 21 the 'triple point test' also provides an excellent tool in the clinical overall assessment of the shoulder joint.

For **extension** (Fig. 118), when the hand rests on the iliac crest, extension at the shoulder is up to **40-45°**.

For **abduction** (Figs 121 and 122):

* When the hand rests on the iliac crest, abduction at the shoulder is up to **45°**.

* When the fingers touch the top of the head (Fig. 122), abduction at the shoulder is up to **120°**. This movement allows personal haircare, e.g. combing.

This method can be applied to almost any joint, as we shall see later.

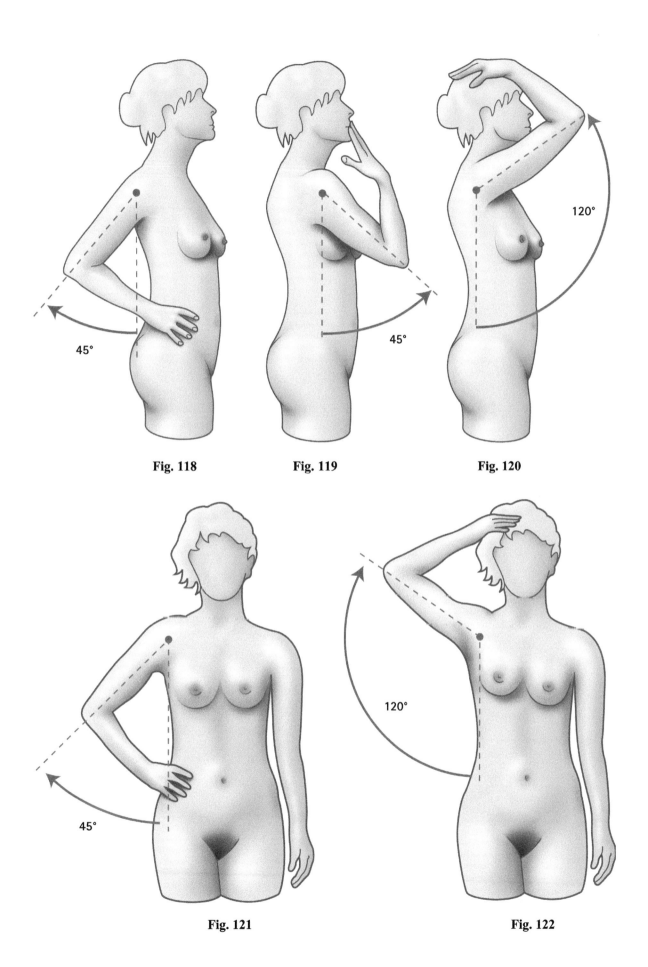

Fig. 118 **Fig. 119** **Fig. 120**

Fig. 121 **Fig. 122**

75

Chapter 2

THE ELBOW

Anatomically, the elbow consists of a single joint with a single joint cavity.

Physiologically, however, it has **two distinct functions**:

- **flexion-extension**, involving two joints: the humero-ulnar and the humero-radial joints

- **pronation-supination**, involving the superior radio-ulnar joint.

In this chapter only flexion and extension will be discussed.

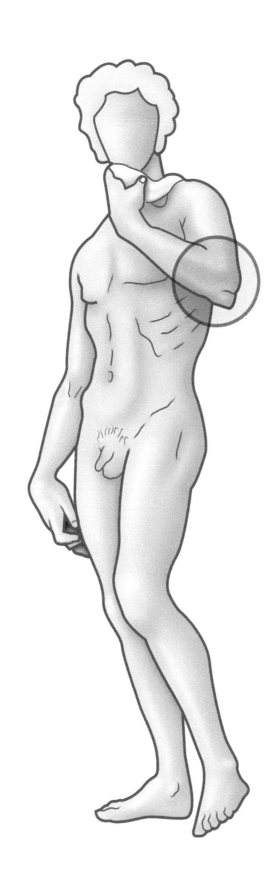

Movement of the hand towards or away from the body

The elbow is the **intermediate joint** of the upper limb, forming the mechanical link between the first segment (the **upper arm**) and the second segment (the **forearm**). It allows the forearm, which can assume any position in space thanks to movements at the shoulder, to move its functional extremity (the hand) to any distance from the body.

Flexion at the elbow underlies the ability to carry food to the mouth. Thus the extended and pronated forearm (Fig. 1) takes hold of the food and carries it to the mouth as a result of combined flexion and supination. In this respect the biceps, which performs these two movements, can be called **the feeding muscle**. It is therefore clear that flexion at the elbow is **essential for feeding**. If both elbows were locked in full extension or in semi-extension, an individual would be unable to feed himself.

The elbow, the upper arm and the forearm form a **pair of compasses** (Fig. 2), which allows the wrist W_1 to come very close to the shoulder (S) in position W_2, while the elbow undergoes flexion from E_1 to E_2. Thus the hand can easily reach the deltoid and the mouth.

In the **telescopic model** (Fig. 3), which presents another theoretical and imaginable mechanical version, the hand cannot reach the mouth, since the shortest distance possible between the hand and the mouth is the sum of the length of the segment L and the length of its casing (C), which is needed to maintain the rigidity of the system.

Thus, for the elbow the **'compasses' solution** is more logical and better than the **'telescopic' solution**, assuming that the latter is biologically possible.

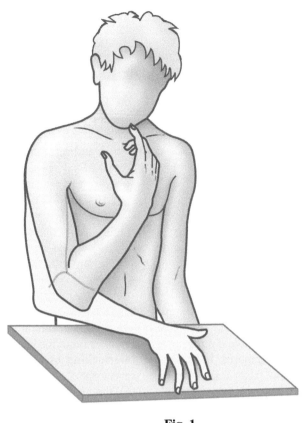

Fig. 1

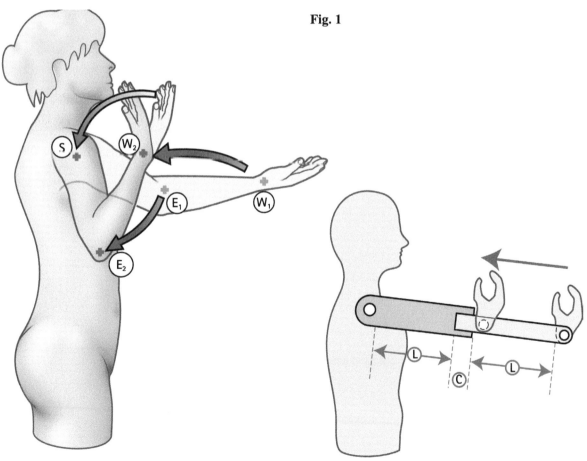

Fig. 2

Fig. 3

The articular surfaces

The **distal end of the humerus** has two articular surfaces (Fig. 4A, inspired by Rouvière):

1) the **trochlea** (2), pulley-shaped (Fig. 4A) with a central groove (1) lying in a sagittal plane and bounded by two convex lips (2)

2) the **capitulum**, a spherical surface (3), lying lateral to the trochlea and facing anteriorly.

The complex formed by the trochlea and the capitulum (Fig. 5) can be compared to a ball and spool threaded on to the same axis T, which constitutes, to a first approximation, the **axis of flexion-extension of the elbow**.

The following two points need to be made:

1) **The capitulum is not a complete sphere but a hemisphere corresponding to the anterior half of a sphere**. Therefore the capitulum, unlike the trochlea, does not extend posteriorly and stops short at the lower end of the humerus. Its surface allows not only flexion-extension, but also axial rotation about axis L (blue arrow, Fig. 5).

2) The **capitulo-trochlear groove** (Figs. 4A and 5) is a zone of transition (4) and has the shape of a segment of a cone, whose wider base rests at the lateral lip of the trochlea. The usefulness of this capitulo-trochlear groove will emerge later.

Figure 5 demonstrates why the medial portion of the joint has only one degree of freedom for flexion-extension, whereas the lateral part has two degrees of freedom for **flexion-extension and axial rotation**.

The **proximal ends of the two bones of the forearm** have two surfaces corresponding to those of the humerus:

1) The **trochlear notch of the ulna** (Fig. 4B), which articulates with the humeral trochlea and has the corresponding shape.

It consists of a longitudinal rounded ridge (10), starting from the olecranon process (11) superiorly and extending anteriorly and inferiorly to the coronoid process (12). On either side of the ridge, which corresponds to the trochlear groove, is a concave surface corresponding to the lips of the trochlea (13). The articular surface is shaped like a single strip of corrugated iron sheet (Fig. 5, double red arrow), with a ridge (10) and two gutters (11).

2) The **cupped proximal surface of the head of the radius** (Fig. 4), with a concavity (14) corresponding to the convexity of the capitulum humeri (3). It is bounded by a rim (15), which articulates with the capitulo-trochlear groove (4).

These two surfaces in effect form a single articular surface as a result of the annular ligament (16), which keeps them together. Figure 6 (anterior view) and Figure 7 (posterior view) show the **interlocking of the articular surfaces**. Figure 6 (right side) reveals the olecranon fossa (5) above the trochlea, the radial fossa (6), the medial epicondyle (7) and the lateral epicondyle (8). Figure 7 (posterior view, left side) also shows the olecranon fossa (21), which receives the beakshaped olecranon process (11).

The **coronal section taken through the joint** (Fig. 8, inspired by Testut) shows that the capsule (17) invests a single anatomical joint cavity with two functional joints (Fig. 9, diagrammatic frontal view):

1) the **joint of flexion-extension**, consisting of the humero-ulnar joint (Fig. 8, 18) and the humero-radial joint (Fig. 8, 19)

2) the **superior radio-ulnar joint** (20), surrounded by the annular ligament (16), is essential for pronation-supination. The olecranon process (8, 11) is also seen, lying inside the olecranon fossa during extension.

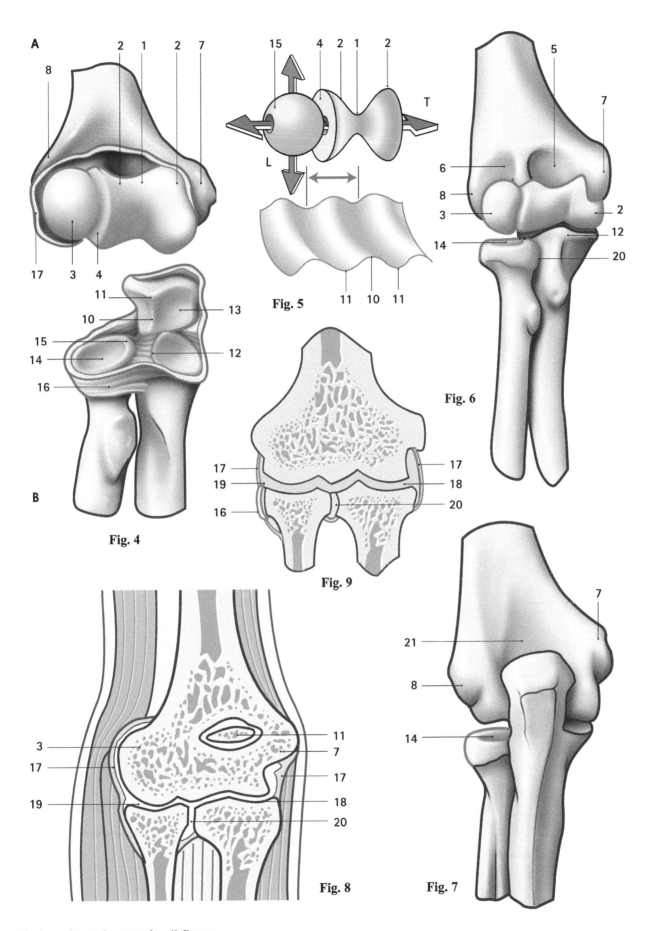

A

Fig. 5

Fig. 4

Fig. 6

Fig. 9

B

Fig. 8

Fig. 7

The legends are the same for all figures.

The distal end of the humerus

This has the shape of an **artist's palette** (Fig. 13, posterior view, and Fig. 14, anterior view) and is flattened antero-posteriorly. On its distal aspect it bears two articular surfaces, the **trochlea** and the **capitulum**. It is important to know the structure and shape of this segment of the humerus to understand the physiology of the elbow.

The humeral palette resembles the **fork of a bicycle** (Fig. 15), with the axis of the articular surfaces running through the distal ends of its two prongs. In fact, its middle portion contains two fossae:

- anteriorly, the **coronoid fossa**, which receives the coronoid process of the ulna during flexion (Figs 12 and 14)
- posteriorly, the **olecranon fossa**, which receives the olecranon during extension (Figs 10 and 13).

These fossae play a vital role in increasing the range of flexion and extension at the elbow by delaying the movement of impact of the coronoid and olecranon processes on the shaft of the humerus. Without them, the trochlear notch of the ulna, which corresponds to a semi-circle, would be able to slide over the trochlea for only a short distance on either side of the intermediate position (Fig. 23).

These two fossae are occasionally so deep that the intervening plate of bone is perforated, and they communicate with each other (as in the fork of a bicycle).

The compact portions of the distal end of the humerus lie on either side of these fossae, forming two divergent pillars (Figs 13-15), the one ending on the medial epicondyle and the other on the lateral epicondyle. This fork-like structure is the reason that it is so difficult to reduce certain fractures of the distal end of the humerus.

The humeral palette as a whole **bulges anteriorly** (Fig. 16, lateral view, red dotted lines) at an angle of 45° with the ulnar shaft, so that the trochlea lies entirely in front of the axis of the shaft. This realignment must be achieved after the reduction of fractures of the distal end of the humerus.

The side view of the humeral palette and of the proximal end of the ulna, first pulled apart (Fig. 17) and then reassembled in extension (Fig. 18) and in 90° flexion (Fig. 19), shows that the anterior bulge of the humeral palette (Fig. 20) promotes flexion only partially because of the obstruction provided by the ulnar coronoid process (red arrow). It is the coronoid fossa that allows flexion (Fig. 21) to be completed by delaying this impact. The two bones are almost parallel (Fig. 21) but are separated (double arrow) by a space that lodges the muscles.

In the absence of these two mechanical factors (Fig. 22) it is obvious that:

- flexion would be limited to 90° by the obstructing coronoid process (Fig. 23)
- during flexion there would be no space left to accommodate the muscles even if a sizeable hole in the distal end of the humerus allowed the two bones to come into direct contact (Fig. 24).

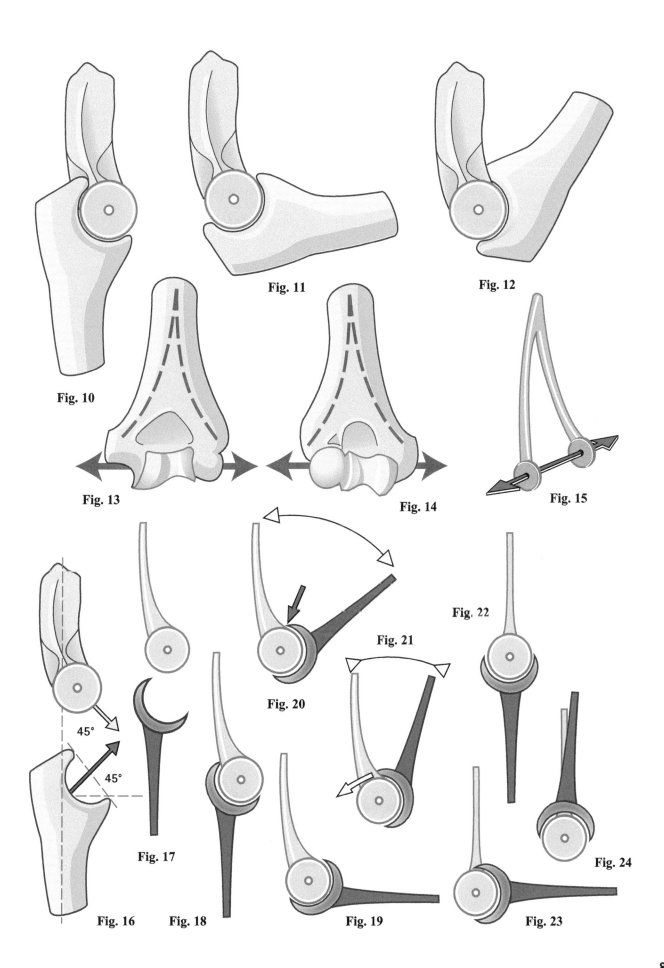

Fig. 10

Fig. 11

Fig. 12

Fig. 13

Fig. 14

Fig. 15

Fig. 16

45°

45°

Fig. 17

Fig. 18

Fig. 19

Fig. 20

Fig. 21

Fig. 22

Fig. 23

Fig. 24

The ligaments of the elbow

The function of these ligaments is to keep the articular surfaces in apposition and to direct movements at the joint. They act like two stays on either side of the joint: the **medial collateral ligament** (Fig. 25, inspired by Rouvière) and the **lateral collateral ligament** (Fig. 26, inspired by Rouvière).

By and large these ligaments are fan-shaped, with their apices attached proximally to the epicondyles of the humerus roughly at the level of the transverse axis XX′ for flexion-extension (Fig. 27, inspired by Rouvière) and their free margins attached distally around the edge of the trochlear notch of the ulna.

A **mechanical model of the elbow** can be constructed as follows (Fig. 28):

- Above, the fork of the distal end of the humerus supports the articular pulley.
- Below, a half-ring (the trochlear notch of the ulna) is continuous with the arm of the lever (the ulnar shaft) and fits into the pulley.
- The ligaments are represented by two stays continuous with the ulnar shaft and inserted at both ends of the axis XX′ of the pulley.

It is easy to see that these lateral 'straps' have two functions (Fig. 29):

- to keep the half-ring encased in the pulley (coaptation of the articular surfaces)
- to prevent any lateral movement.

If one of the ligaments snaps (Fig. 30), e.g. the medial ligament (green arrow), a contralateral movement follows (red arrow), with loss of contact of the articular surfaces. This is the mechanism commonly encountered in lateral dislocation of the elbow, which is, in its first stages, a severe sprain of the elbow due to rupture of the medial ligament.

In greater detail

The **medial collateral ligament** (Fig. 25) consists of three sets of fibres:

1) the **anterior set** (1), with its most anterior fibres (Fig. 27) strengthening the annular ligament (2)
2) the **intermediate set** (3), being the strongest
3) the **posterior set**, the ligament of Bardinet (4), reinforced by the transverse fibres of Cooper's ligament (5).

This diagram also shows the medial epicondyle (6), from which arises the fan-shaped medial collateral ligament, the olecranon (7), the oblique cord (8) and the biceps tendon (9), which is inserted into the radial tuberosity.

The **lateral collateral ligament** (Fig. 26) also consists of three sets of fibres arising from the lateral epicondyle (13):

- the **anterior set** (Fig. 27, 10), which strengthens the annular ligament anteriorly
- the **intermediate set** (11), which strengthens the annular ligament posteriorly
- the **posterior set** (12).

The **capsule** is reinforced anteriorly by the anterior ligament (14) and the oblique anterior ligament (15) and posteriorly by the fibres of the posterior ligament, which run transversely across the humerus and obliquely from humerus to olecranon.

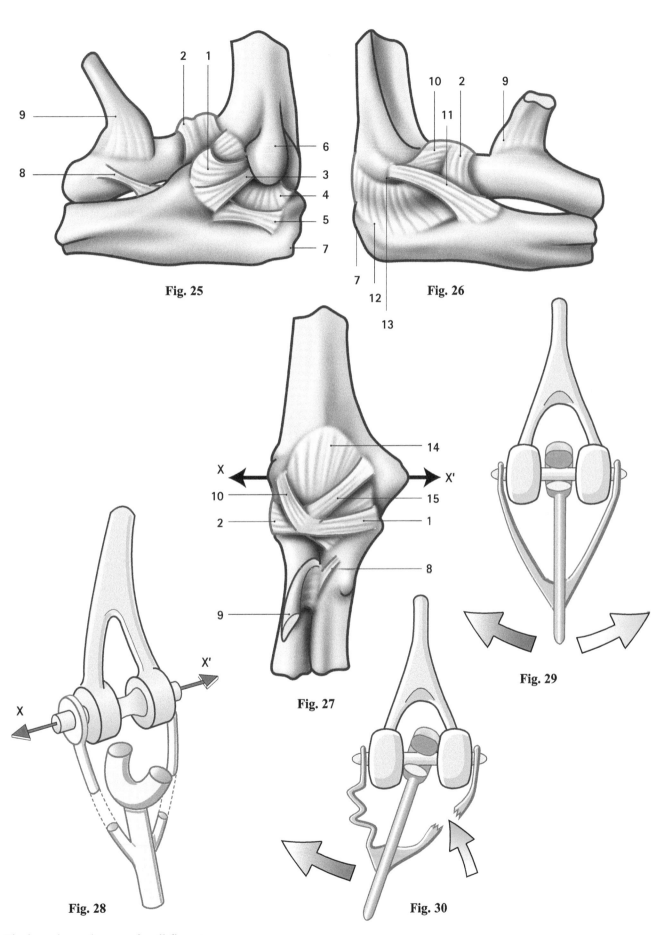

Fig. 25

Fig. 26

Fig. 27

Fig. 28

Fig. 29

Fig. 30

The legends are the same for all figures.

The head of the radius

The shape of the radial head (the proximal radial epiphysis) is entirely determined by its articular function. The purpose of this page is to make the reader understand the shape of the radial head.

- For **axial rotation** (see Chapter 3: Pronation-supination) it is more or less cylindrical.
- For **flexion-extension of the elbow about the intercondylar axis XX′**:
  - The radial head (Fig. 31) must first correspond to the spheroidal capitulum humeri (A). Hence its upper surface is concave and cup-shaped (B). It is as if a half-sphere (C) with a radius of curvature equal to that of the capitulum had been removed from the bone. During pronation-supination the radial head can rotate on the humeral condyle regardless of the degree of flexion or extension of the elbow.
  - But the capitulum (Fig. 32) has a medial border in the shape of a truncated cone, i.e. the **condylo-trochlear groove** (A), so that for congruence during flexion-extension a wedge needs to be removed (C) from the medial aspect of the radial head. This could be achieved by shaving this wedge from the radial head along a plane tangential (B) to that of the trunk of the cone.
  - Finally, the radial head not only glides on the capitulum and the capitulo-trochlear groove while turning on its axis XX′, but it can also simultaneously rotate about its vertical axis (Fig. 33) during pronation-supination (B). Thus the smooth crescent cut along the edge of the radial head (C) extends for some distance along its circumference, as if a shaving had been removed by a razor during rotation of the head (B).

The **articular relationships of the radial head in extreme positions**:

- **In full extension** (Fig. 34) only the anterior half of the articular surface of the radial head is in contact with the capitulum; in fact, the articular cartilage of the capitulum stretches as far as the inferior end of the humerus without extending posteriorly.
- **In full flexion** (Fig. 35) the rim of the radial head reaches beyond the capitulum and enters the radial fossa (Fig. 6, p. 81), which is much less deep than the coronoid fossa.

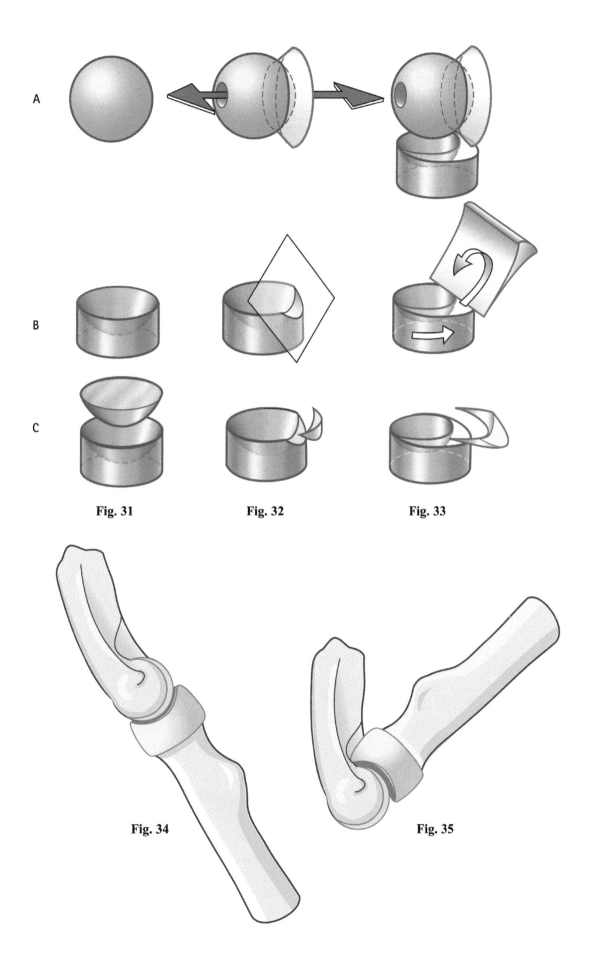

A

B

C

Fig. 31   **Fig. 32**   **Fig. 33**

Fig. 34   **Fig. 35**

The trochlea humeri

When the elbow is fully extended, the axis of the forearm forms with that of the arm an obtuse angle open laterally, and is not collinear with that of the arm. This angle is obviously more marked in women (Fig. 36) and is known as the **carrying angle of the arm** or **cubitus valgus**. It depends on the slope of the trochlear groove, which does not lie in the sagittal plane, as mentioned before (p. 86). In fact, the trochlear groove is not vertical but oblique, with individual variations. The set of diagrams (Figs 39-43) summarizes these different variations and their physiological consequences.

Type I: most frequent type (top row – A)
- **From the front** (Fig. 39, anterior view of the trochlea) the groove is vertical (black arrow); **posteriorly** (Fig. 40, posterior view) it runs obliquely distally and laterally.
- **When viewed in its entirety** (Fig. 41) the trochlear groove spirals around its own axis, whose variations are shown in Figure 37.

The functional consequences are the following:
- **During extension** (Fig. 42, inspired by Roud) the posterior aspect of the groove makes contact with the trochlear notch of the ulna, and its obliquity produces a similar obliquity in the axis of the forearm. Hence, the forearm is slightly oblique inferiorly and laterally, and its axis falls out of line with that of the arm and forms an obtuse angle with that of the latter, i.e. the **carrying angle of the arm** (**cubitus valgus**) (Figs 36 and 37).
- **During flexion** the anterior part of the groove is responsible for the direction of the forearm and, as it lies in the vertical plane, the forearm during flexion (Fig. 43) comes to rest exactly in front of the arm.

Type II: less common type (middle row – B)
- **Anteriorly** (Fig. 39) the trochlear groove runs obliquely proximally and laterally; **posteriorly** the groove (Fig. 40) runs obliquely distally and laterally.

- **When viewed in its entirety** (Fig. 41), the groove traces a true spiral around its axis.
- **During extension** (Fig. 42), the forearm runs obliquely distally and laterally, with a carrying angle similar to the one in type I.
- **During flexion** (Fig. 43) the outward obliquity of the anterior aspect of the groove influences the obliquity of the forearm so that it comes to rest slightly lateral to the arm.

Type III: rare type (bottom row – C)
- **Anteriorly** (Fig. 39) the trochlear groove runs obliquely distally and medially; **posteriorly** (Fig. 40) it runs obliquely distally and laterally.
- **When viewed in its entirety** (Fig. 41), the trochlear groove traces in space either a circle that lies in a plane running obliquely distally and laterally or a very tight spiral that is tilted medially.

The functional effects are the following:
- **During extension** (Fig. 42): the carrying angle of the arm is normal.
- **During flexion** (Fig. 43): the forearm comes to rest medial to the arm.

Another consequence of this spiral configuration of the trochlear groove is that the trochlea has not one axis but a series of instantaneous axes between the two extreme positions (Fig. 37):
- an **axis during flexion** (f), which is perpendicular to that of the flexed forearm F (The most frequent type is illustrated here.)
- an **axis during extension** (e), which is perpendicular to that of the extended forearm (E).

The direction of the axis of flexion-extension changes progressively between the two extreme positions; in other words, it consists of a series of **instantaneous axes** between the two extreme positions (Fig. 38, e and f).

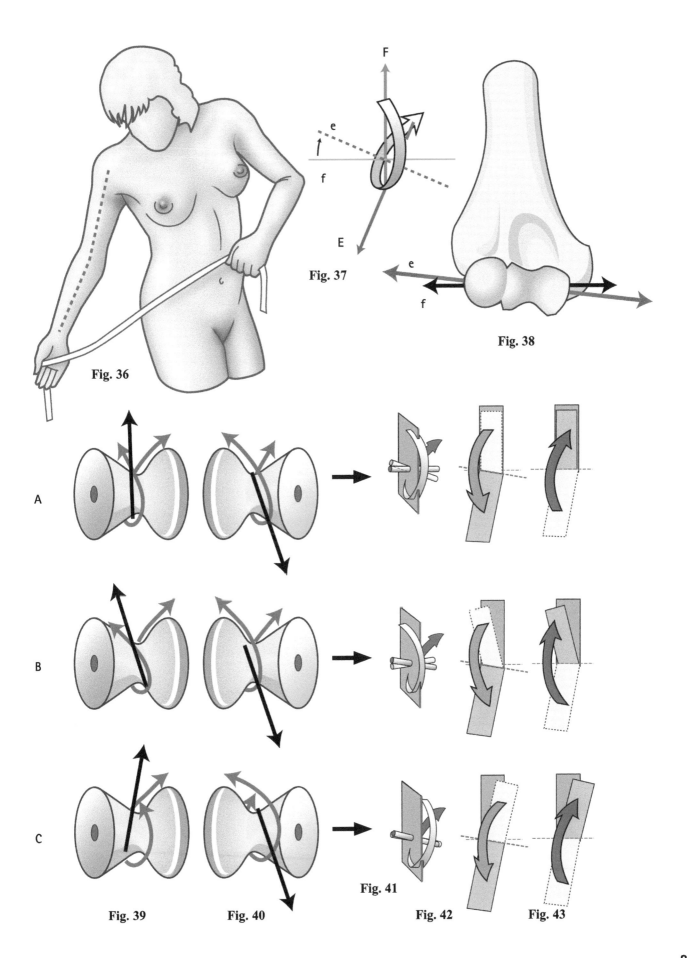

Fig. 36

Fig. 37

Fig. 38

A

B

C

Fig. 39

Fig. 40

Fig. 41

Fig. 42

Fig. 43

The limitations of flexion and extension

Extension is limited (Fig. 44) by three factors:
1) the **impact of the olecranon process** on the deep aspect of the olecranon fossa
2) the **tension developed in the anterior ligament of the joint**
3) the **resistance offered by the flexor muscles** (biceps, brachialis and brachioradialis).

If extension proceeds any further, rupture of one of these limiting structures must occur, as follows:
- The **olecranon is fractured** (Fig. 45, 1) and the capsule is torn (2).
- The olecranon (1) is not fractured (Fig. 46) but the capsule (2) and the ligaments are torn, with posterior dislocation of the elbow (3). The muscles are usually unaffected but the anterior circumflex humeral artery can be torn or at least bruised.

Limitation of flexion depends on whether flexion is active or passive.

If flexion is active (Fig. 47):
- The first limiting factor is the apposition of the anterior muscles of the arm and those of the forearm (white arrows), which harden as they contract. This mechanism explains why active flexion cannot exceed 145°, and the more muscular the subject, the more limited it is.
- The other factors, i.e. impact of the corresponding bony surfaces and tension developed in the capsular ligament, are insignificant.

If flexion is passive (Fig. 48), secondary to an external force (red arrow) that 'closes' the joint, the following occur:
- The relaxed muscles can be flattened against each other and flexion exceeds 145°.
- At this stage the other limiting factors come into play:
  - impact of the radial head against the radial fossa and of the coronoid process against the coronoid fossa
  - tension in the posterior part of the capsule
  - tension developed passively in the triceps.
- Flexion can then reach 160°, since it is augmented by an angle a (Fig. 47).

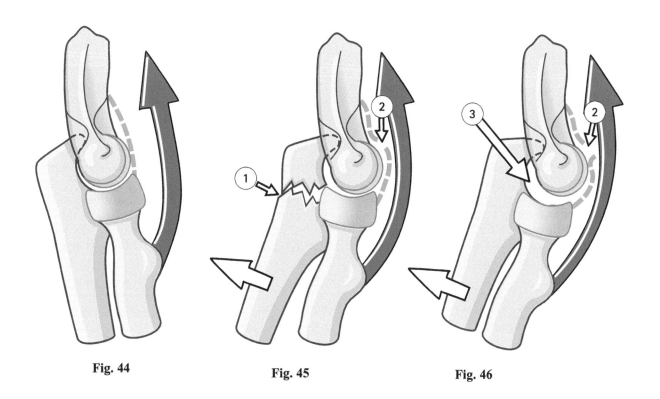

Fig. 44   Fig. 45   Fig. 46

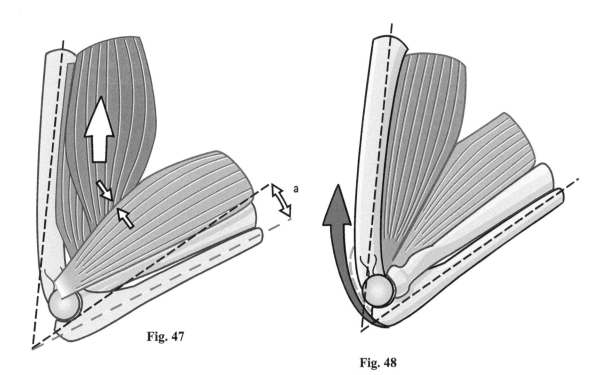

Fig. 47

Fig. 48

The flexor muscles of the elbow

There are **three** flexor muscles:
1) **Brachialis** (1) arises from the anterior aspect of the humerus and is inserted into the tuberosity of the ulna (Fig. 49). Since it spans one joint, it is exclusively a flexor of the elbow and is one of the rare muscles of the body with a single function.
2) **Brachioradialis** (2) arises from the lateral supra-condylar ridge of the humerus and is inserted into the styloid process of the radius (Fig. 49), acting essentially as a flexor of the elbow and becoming a supinator only in extreme pronation and even a pronator in extreme supination.
3) **Biceps brachii** is the main flexor of the elbow (Fig. 50, 3). It is inserted mostly into the radial tuberosity, and as a biarticular muscle it arises not from the humerus but from the scapula by **two heads**:
   – The long head (4) arises from the supraglenoid tubercle and passes through the upper part of the shoulder joint (see Chapter 1: The Shoulder).
   – The short head (5) arises from the coracoid process in conjunction with the coracobrachialis.

By virtue of its two origins the biceps produces articular coaptation of the shoulder, while its long head is an abductor. Its main action is flexion of the elbow. It also plays an important, though secondary, role in supination (see Chapter 3: Pronation-Supination) with maximal efficiency when the elbow is flexed at 90°. It can cause dislocation of the radius (p. 96) when the elbow is flexed.

The flexor muscles work to their best advantage when the elbow is flexed at 90°.

In fact, when the elbow is extended (Fig. 51), the direction of the force exerted by the muscles is nearly parallel (pink arrow) to that of the arm of the lever. The centripetal component C, acting in the direction of the centre of the joint, is the more powerful but mechanically ineffective as a flexor, while the tangential or transverse component T is the only effective force but is relatively weak or almost nil in full extension.

On the other hand, in mid-flexion (Fig. 52), the direction of the force exerted by the muscle is nearly parallel to that of the arm of the lever (pink arrow = biceps; green arrow = brachioradialis) so that the centripetal component is zero and the tangential component coincides with that of the muscular pull, which is then fully utilized for flexion.

The angle of maximum efficiency lies between 80° and 90° for the biceps.

For the *brachioradialis* at 90° flexion, the muscular pull does not yet coincide with the tangential component, and this coincidence occurs only at 100-110°, i.e. at an angle of flexion greater than that for the biceps.

The action of the flexor muscles follows the physical laws governing levers of the third type and so favours range and speed of movement at the expense of power.

There are also three accessory flexor muscles:
* *extensor carpi radialis longus*, lying deep to the brachioradialis (not shown)
* *anconeus* (Fig. 49, 6), mostly an active lateral stabilizer of the elbow
* *pronator teres* (not shown), which, in the syndrome of Volkmann's contracture, becomes a shortened fibrotic cord that prevents full extension of the elbow.

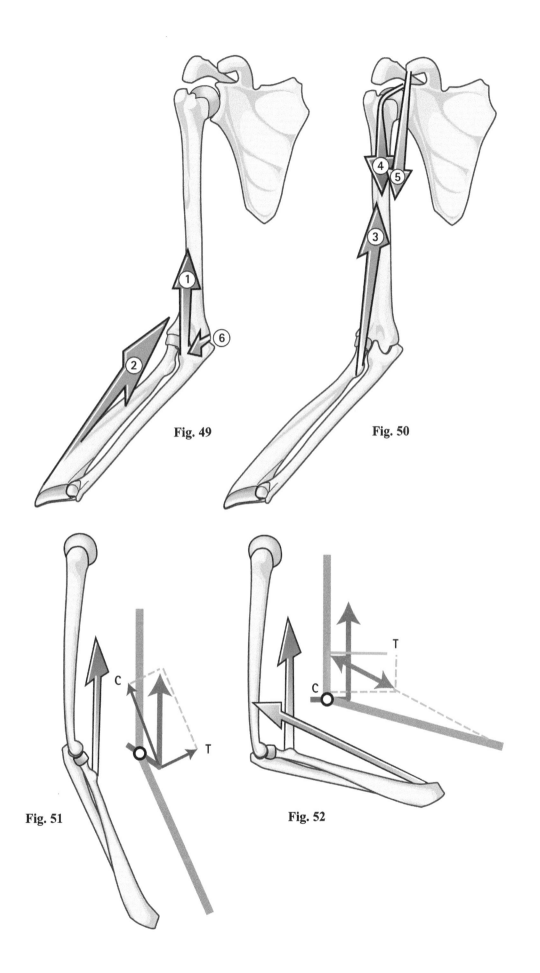

Fig. 49

Fig. 50

Fig. 51

Fig. 52

The extensor muscles of the elbow

Extension of the elbow depends practically on one muscle, i.e. the **triceps brachii** (Figs 53 and 54), as the action of the **anconeus**, although noteworthy for Duchenne de Boulogne, is negligible because of its weakness. According to other authors it has an active external stabilizing function at the elbow.

The **triceps** (Fig. 53, posterior view, and Fig. 54, lateral view) consists of **three fleshy heads**, which converge on a common tendon inserted in the olecranon process but have different sites of origin:

- The **medial head** (1) arises from the posterior surface of the humerus below the spinal groove for the radial nerve.
- The **lateral head** (2) arises from the lateral border of the humeral shaft above the spinal groove.

These two heads are therefore **monoarticular**.

- The **long head** (3) arises not from the humerus but from the scapula at its infraglenoid tubercle and is therefore **biarticular**.

The **efficiency of the triceps** varies according to the degree of flexion of the elbow:

- **In full extension** (Fig. 55), its muscular force can be resolved into two components, i.e. the weak centrifugal component (C), which tends to dislocate the ulna posteriorly, and the more powerful transverse component (T), which is only active in extension.
- **During partial flexion** between 20° and 30° (Fig. 56) the centripetal radial component is eliminated and the only effective tangential component (T) coincides with the muscular pull. Hence in this position the efficiency of the triceps is maximal.
- Subsequently, as the elbow is flexed further (Fig. 57), the effective tangential component (T) decreases as the centripetal component (C) increases.
- **In full flexion** (Fig. 58) the triceps tendon is reflected on to the superior surface of the olecranon as on a pulley, and this arrangement is similar to a displacement of its site of insertion and helps to offset its loss of efficiency. Moreover, its maximally stretched fibres increase its strength of contraction and further compensate for this loss of efficiency.

The **efficiency of the long head of the triceps**, and so of the whole muscle, also depends on the position of the shoulder because it is a biarticular muscle (Fig. 59). It is easy to observe that the distance between its origin and its insertion is greater when the shoulder is flexed at 90° than when the arm hangs down vertically while the elbow stays in the same position. In fact, the centres of the two circles described by the humerus (1) and by the long head of the triceps (2) do not coincide. If the length of the long head of the triceps did not change, its insertion could reach O_1, but, as the olecranon is now at O_2, it follows that the muscle must be passively stretched from O_1 to O_2.

Therefore the triceps are **more powerful** when the shoulder is in flexion or in protraction (wrongly so called), since the long head of the triceps redirects some of the force generated by the flexor muscles of the shoulder (the clavicular fibres of the *pectoralis major* and the deltoid) to enhance the power of the extensors at the shoulder. This exemplifies one of the functions of biarticular muscles. The triceps are at their most powerful when the elbow and the shoulder are flexed at the same time (starting from the position of 90° flexion), e.g. as when a woodcutter strikes with an axe.

For the same reason, the triceps are more powerful when the shoulder is flexed, since its fibres are already pretensioned. The movement of striking a blow forwards is rendered more efficient by the transfer of some of the strength of the shoulder flexors to the elbow.

The triceps (long head) and the latissimus dorsi form a functional adductor couple at the shoulder (Fig. 117, p. 73).

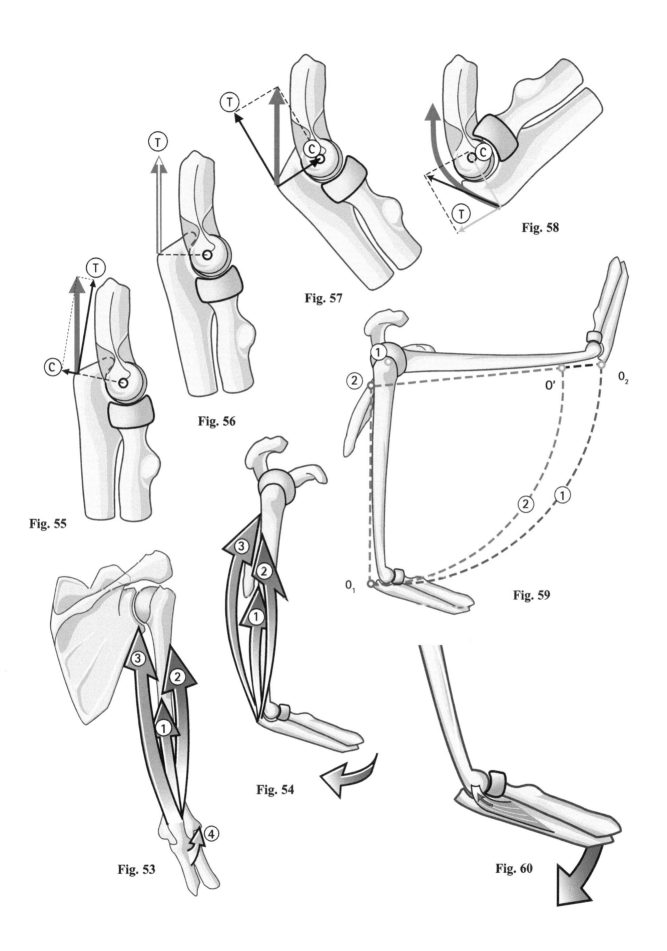

Fig. 58

Fig. 57

Fig. 56

Fig. 55

Fig. 59

Fig. 54

Fig. 53

Fig. 60

Factors ensuring coaptation of the articular surfaces

Coaptation of the articular surfaces in the long axis of the joint precludes dislocation in extension, as when a force is applied downwards (Figs 53 and 60), e.g. when one carries a bucket of water, or when a force is exerted upwards, e.g. when one falls forwards on one's hands with the elbows fully extended.

Resistance to longitudinal traction (Figs 61 and 62)

Since the trochlear notch of the ulna covers an arc of a circle with an apex angle of less than 180°, the soft tissues are responsible for articular coaptation. Thus the apposition of the articular surfaces is achieved by the following:

- the **ligaments**: the medial (1) and the lateral collateral ligaments (2)
- the **muscles**: those of the arm, i.e. **triceps** (3), **biceps** (4) and **coraco-brachialis** (5), and also those of the forearm, i.e. **brachioradialis** (6) and the **muscles attached to the lateral** (7) **and medial** (8) **epicondyles**.

In full extension (Fig. 62) the beak-shaped olecranon hooks over the trochlea in the olecranon fossa, thus imparting some mechanical resistance to elongation of the humero-ulnar joint along its long axis.

On the other hand (Fig. 61), it must be noted that the humero-radial joint is structurally unsuited to withstand excessive traction, as nothing prevents the radial head from being dislocated distally with respect to the annular ligament. This mechanism is thought to operate in the condition of painful pronation in the child (i.e. the so-called 'pulled elbow'). The only structure preventing distal dislocation of the radius relative to the ulna is the **interosseous membrane** (Fig. 32, p. 113).

Resistance to longitudinal compression

This is provided by the bones involved:

- In the radius, pressure is transmitted to the **head** which is liable to fracture (Fig. 65), i.e. fracture by impaction of the neck into the head.
- In the ulna (Fig. 66), it is the **coronoid process** (aptly called the 'console process' by Henle) that transmits the pressure and is liable to fracture, leading to an irreducible posterior dislocation of the elbow, associated with instability of the joint.

Coaptation during flexion

In the position of flexion at 90°, the ulna is perfectly stable (Fig. 63) because the trochlear notch is surrounded by the two powerful musculo-tendinous insertions of the **triceps** (3) and the **coraco-brachialis** (5), which secure close apposition of the articular surfaces. The **anconeus** (not shown) also plays a role in the process. On the other hand, the radius (Fig. 64) is liable to be dislocated proximally as the **biceps contracts** (4). This dislocation is prevented solely by the annular ligament. When the ligament is torn, the simultaneous proximal and anterior dislocation of the radius becomes irreducible and can be produced by the slightest degree of flexion of the arm following contraction of the biceps.

The Essex-Lopresti syndrome

The state of the superior radio-ulnar joint inevitably influences the function of the lower radio-ulnar joint. When the radial head is broken or impacted (Fig. 67) or has been resected (Fig. 68), the shortening of the radius (a) leads to **dislocation of the inferior radio-ulnar joint**, with clinical complications.

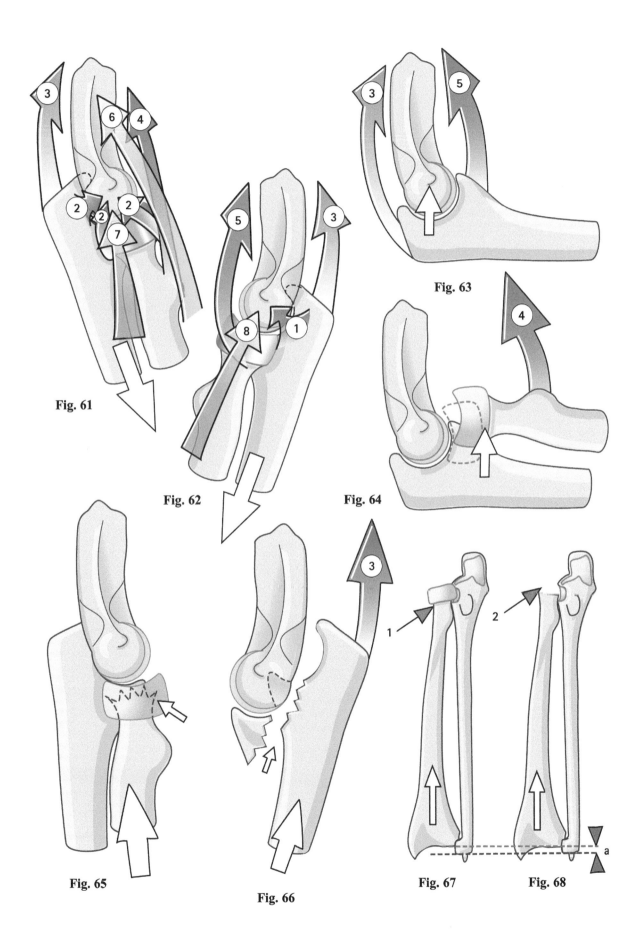

Fig. 61

Fig. 62

Fig. 63

Fig. 64

Fig. 65

Fig. 66

Fig. 67

Fig. 68

The range of movements of the elbow

The **reference position** (Fig. 69), used for measuring the range of movements, is defined as the position achieved when the axes of the arm and of the forearm are collinear.

Extension is the movement of the forearm posteriorly. Since the reference position corresponds to full extension (Fig. 69), the range of extension of the elbow is zero by definition, except in people, e.g. women and children, in whom great laxity of the ligaments (Fig. 70) allows hyperextension (hE) of 5-10° (z). In contrast, relative extension is always possible from any position of flexion. When extension is still incomplete it is quantitated negatively. Thus an extension of –40° corresponds to an extension that falls short of the reference point by 40°, i.e. the elbow is still flexed at 40° when the elbow is being fully extended. In the diagram (Fig. 70) the shortfall in extension is –y when flexion is +x. The angle Dr represents the shortfall in flexion and the useful range of flexion-extension is x-y.

Flexion is the movement of the arm anteriorly so that the anterior surface of the forearm moves towards the anterior surface of the arm. Active flexion has a range of 140-145° (Fig. 71). It is easy to measure without a goniometer using the **closed-fist test**. The distance between the shoulder and the wrist is normally equal to the width of the fist, because the wrist does not touch the shoulder. Passive flexion has a range of 160° when the examiner pushes the wrist towards the shoulder.

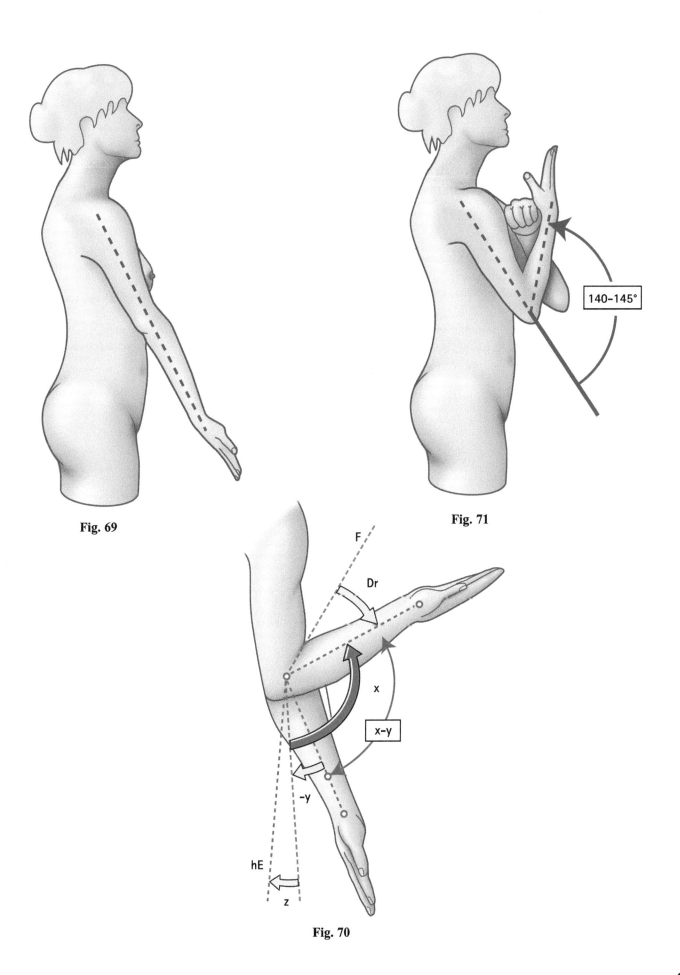

Fig. 69

140–145°

Fig. 71

F

Dr

x

x-y

-y

hE

z

Fig. 70

Surface markings of the elbow

The three visible and palpable markings are these:

1) the **olecranon** (2), **a prominent midline projection (the 'bump' of the elbow)**
2) the **medial epicondyle** (1), medially
3) the **lateral epicondyle** (3), laterally.

In **extension** (Figs 72 and 75) these three landmarks lie in a horizontal plane. Between the olecranon (2) and the medial epicondyle (1) lies the **groove** that contains the **ulnar nerve**, so that any violent blow to the nerve in this position causes an electric shock felt in the territory of supply of the nerve (the medial border of the hand). Laterally, below the epicondyle (3),

can be felt the head of the radius as it rotates during pronation-supination.

In **flexion** (Figs 73 and 76) these three landmarks now form an equilateral triangle lying in the coronal plane tangential to the posterior aspect of the arm (Fig. 74). Figures 75 and 76 show the location of these landmarks on the bone.

When the elbow is dislocated the relationships among these landmarks are disturbed:

- In extension the olecranon reaches above the interepicondylar line (posterior dislocation).
- In flexion the olecranon extends posteriorly beyond the coronal plane of the arm (posterior dislocation).

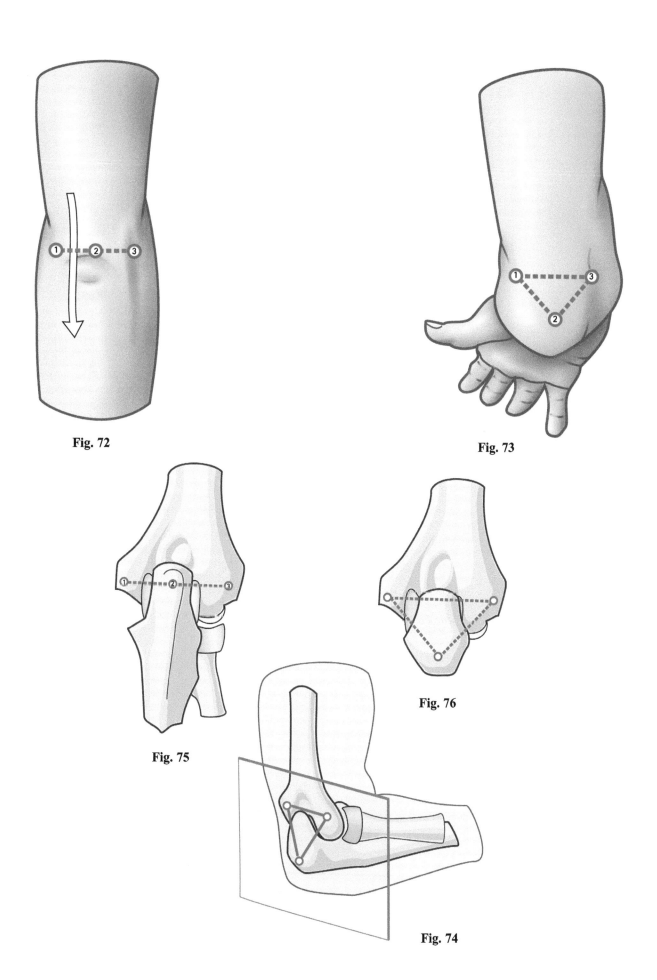

Fig. 72

Fig. 73

Fig. 75

Fig. 76

Fig. 74

101

The efficiency of the flexor and extensor muscles

The positions of function and of immobilization

The **positions of function and of immobilization of the elbow** are defined thus (Fig. 77):

- The elbow is flexed at 90°.
- There is no pronation or supination. (The hand lies in the vertical plane with the thumb upright.)

The relative strength of the muscles

As a whole, the flexors are slightly stronger than the extensors, so that when the arm is relaxed the elbow is slightly flexed; the **more muscular** the subject, the more this is so. The strength of the flexors varies with rotation of the forearm and is greater when the forearm is pronated than when it is supinated, since the biceps are more stretched and thus more efficient and can dislocate the head of the radius. Their flexor efficiency ratio for pronation:supination is 5:3.

Finally, the strength of the muscle varies with the position of the shoulder (S), as shown diagrammatically and comprehensively in Figure 78:

- **The arm lies vertically above the shoulder** (A):
  - The force exerted during extension (e.g. lifting dumbbells) equals 43 kg (arrow 1).

- The force exerted during flexion (e.g. while pulling oneself up) equals 83 kg (arrow 2).
- **The arm is flexed at 90°** (F):
  - The force produced during extension (e.g. while pushing a heavy load forwards) equals 37 kg (arrow 3).
  - The force produced during flexion (e.g. while rowing) equals 66 kg (arrow 4).
- **The arm hangs down vertically alongside the body** (B):
  - The force exerted during flexion (e.g. while lifting a heavy load) equals 52 kg (arrow 5).
  - The force exerted during extension (e.g. while lifting oneself up on parallel bars) equals 51 kg (arrow 6).

Therefore there are preferential positions where the muscle groups achieve maximal efficiency; the arm is below the shoulder for extension (arrow 6) and above the shoulder for flexion (arrow 2).

Thus the muscles of the upper limb are adapted for **climbing** (Fig. 79).

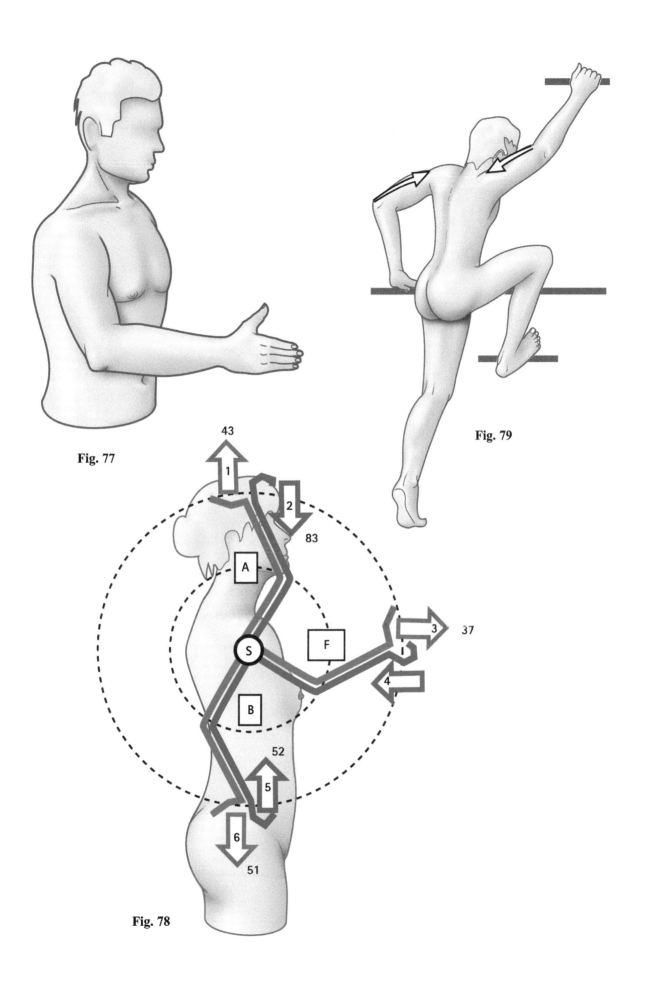

Fig. 77

43

1

2

83

A

F

S

37

3

4

B

52

5

6

51

Fig. 78

Fig. 79

103

Chapter 3

PRONATION-SUPINATION

Pronation-supination is the movement of the forearm around its long axis, and it involves two mechanically linked joints:

- the **superior radio-ulnar joint**, which anatomically belongs to the elbow joint
- the **inferior radio-ulnar joint**, which is anatomically separate from the wrist joint.

This axial rotation of the forearm introduces a **third degree of freedom** into the articular complex of the wrist.

Thus, the hand, the **effector extremity of the upper limb**, can be placed in any position to grasp or support an object. This anatomical arrangement favourably replaces the need to have a triaxial ball-and-socket joint at the shoulder joint, which, as we shall see later, would have given rise to serious mechanical complications.

Axial rotation of the radius is therefore **the only logical and elegant solution**, even if it necessitates the presence of a second bone, the radius, which by itself not only supports the hand but also rotates around the ulna, thanks to the two radio-ulnar joints. This architectural design of the second segment of the anterior and posterior limbs appeared, from the start, 400 million years ago when certain species of fish left the sea to colonize the land and transform into **tetrapod amphibians**, thanks to changes in their fins. Thus our remote marine ancestor, the crossopterygian, already had this bony arrangement.

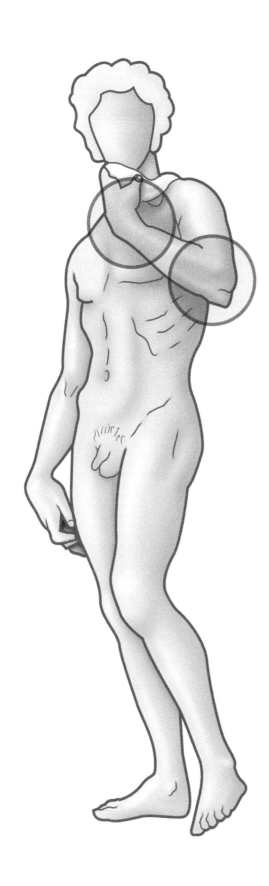

Requirements for measuring pronation-supination

Pronation-supination can only be studied when the elbow is flexed at 90° and resting against the body. In fact, if the elbow is extended, the forearm is collinear with the arm and axial rotation of the former is compounded with that of the latter because of axial rotation at the shoulder.

With the elbow flexed at 90°:

- The **position of reference** or the **intermediate position** or the **position of null rotation** (Fig. 1) is defined as the position attained when the thumb points superiorly. The palm faces medially and there is no pronation or supination of the arm. It is from this position that the ranges of the movements of pronation and supination are measured.

- The **position of supination** is achieved (Fig. 2) with the palm facing superiorly and the thumb pointing laterally.

- The **position of pronation** is achieved (Fig. 3) with the palm facing inferiorly and the thumb pointing medially. In fact, when one views the forearm and the hand head-on, i.e. along their collinear long axes:

  - The hand **in the intermediate position** (Fig. 4) lies in a vertical plane parallel to the sagittal plane of symmetry of the body.

  - The hand **in the position of supination** (Fig. 5) lies in a horizontal plane and so the range of the movement of supination is 90°.

  - The hand **in the position of pronation** (Fig. 6) fails to reach the horizontal plane, and so the range of the movement of **pronation** is 85°. (We shall see later why it falls short of 90°.)

Thus the total amplitude of pronation-supination, i.e. without associated rotation of the forearm, is close to 180°.

When the movements of the rotation of the shoulder are also included, i.e. with the elbow completely extended, the total range of pronation-supination is as follows:

- 360° when the upper limb hangs down vertically alongside the body (the position of reference)
- 270° when the upper limb is abducted to 90°
- 270° when the upper limb is flexed at 90°
- just over 180° when the upper limb lies vertically in full abduction, confirming the fact that, when the arm is abducted at 180°, axial rotation of the shoulder is virtually nil.

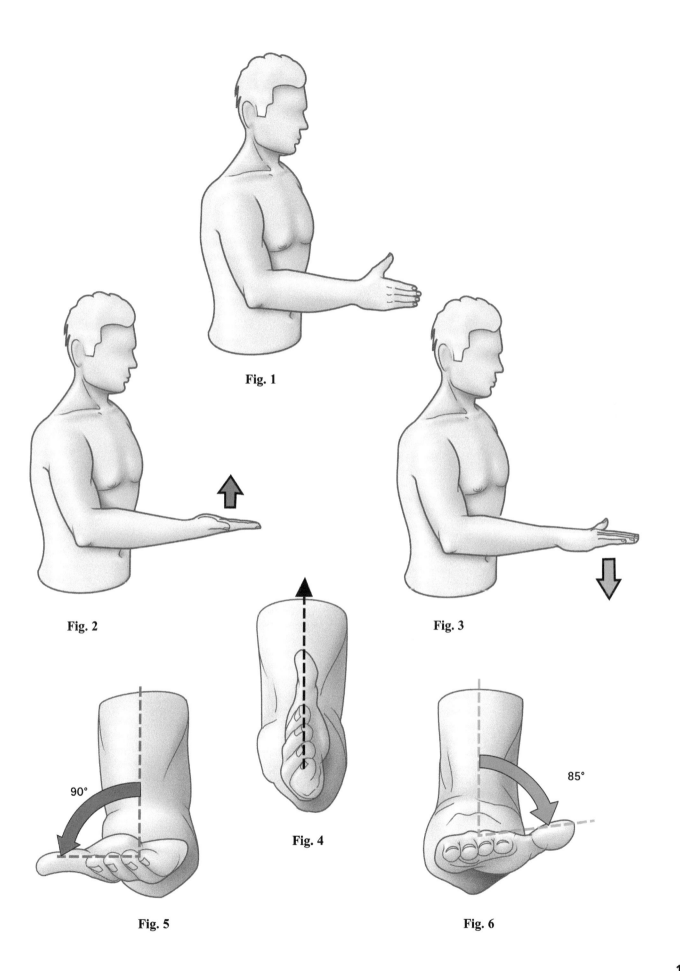

Fig. 1

Fig. 2

Fig. 3

Fig. 4

Fig. 5

Fig. 6

The usefulness of pronation-supination

Of the seven degrees of freedom inherent in the articular chain of the upper limb from shoulder to hand, pronation-supination is one of the most important, since it is indispensable for the control of the orientation of the hand and allows the hand to assume the best position for grasping an object lying within a spherical sector of space centred on the shoulder and for carrying that object to the mouth. Thus pronation-supination is indispensable for **self-feeding**. It also allows the hand to reach any point on the body for protection or **grooming**. In addition it plays an essential role in all actions of the hand, especially in **doing work**.

Thanks to pronation-supination, the hand (Fig. 7) can support a tray, compress an object downwards or lean on a stable object. It also allows one to spin or rotate an object grasped with the middle of the palm and the fingers, as when using a screwdriver (Fig. 8), when the axis of the tool coincides with that of pronation-supination. Since a handle is grasped obliquely by the entire palm (Fig. 9), pronation-supination alters the orientation of the tool as a result of conical rotation. The asymmetry of the hand allows the handle of the tool to lie anywhere in space along the segment of a cone centred on the axis of pronation-supination. Hence the hammer can hit the nail at any controllable angle.

This observation exemplifies one aspect of the **functional coupling of pronation-supination and the wrist joint**, another aspect being the dependence of abduction-adduction of the wrist on pronation-supination. In pronation or in the intermediate position the hand is usually ulnarly deviated in an attempt to bring the dynamic tripod of prehension into line with the axis of pronation-supination. In the position of supination the hand is radially deviated, favouring a supportive grip, e.g. carrying a tray.

This functional coupling makes it imperative to integrate the function of the inferior radio-ulnar joint with that of the wrist, though mechanically the former is linked to the superior radio-ulnar joint.

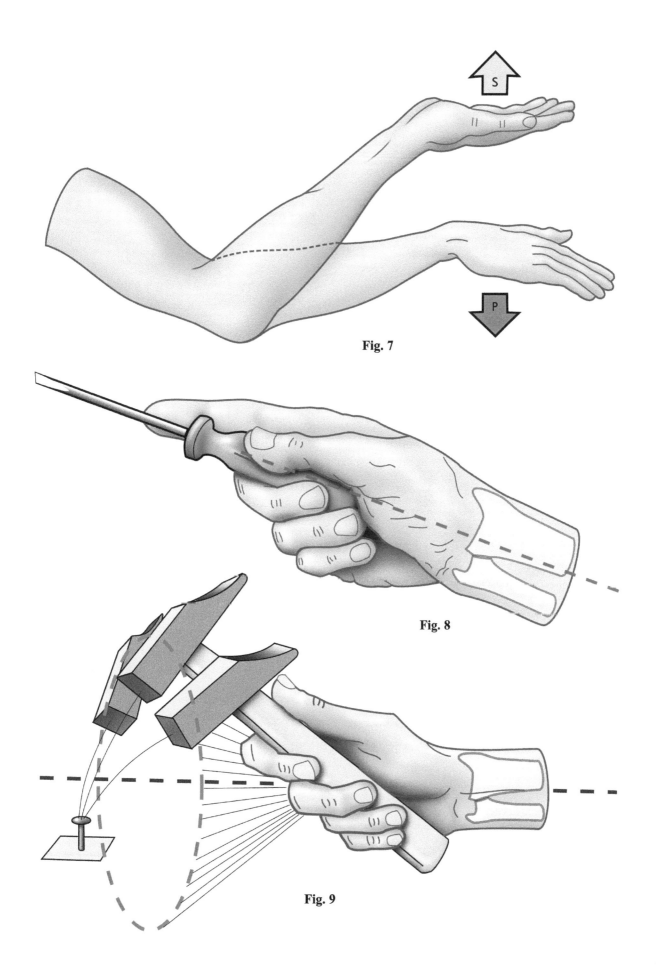

Fig. 7

Fig. 8

Fig. 9

The radio-ulnar complex

The arrangement of the bones

The two bones of the forearm (Fig. 10) are now considered to form a **rectangular radio-ulnar complex** (Fig. 11) split by a diagonal running obliquely and medially (Fig. 12) and demarcating two parts: a medial part corresponding to the ulna and a lateral part corresponding to the radius. This diagonal is effectively the **hinge** (Fig. 13) that allows the lateral (radial) part to rotate anteriorly for 180° and to swing in front of the medial (ulnar) part (Fig. 14).

Such an arrangement would not account for the **cubitus valgus** (Fig. 36, p. 89). Thus, the angles are adjusted at the levels of the oblique interspace of the elbow joint (Fig. 15) so that the hinge is shifted into a vertical position (Fig. 16) and the *cubitus valgus* (red arrow) is restored in extension-supination.

In the anatomical position, corresponding to the position of complete supination, the two bones (Fig. 17, anterior view) are arranged side by side in the same plane and parallel to each other. The diagram (Fig. 18) brings out their overall curvatures in a slightly exaggerated form. A posterior view (Fig. 19) shows the same arrangement but inverted and with similarly inverted curvatures, as illustrated by the diagram in Figure 20. The two bones are joined by the **interosseous membrane** (green and oblique fibres), which forms a flexible hinge.

When the radius is **pronated** (Fig. 21) it crosses the ulna anteriorly (Fig. 22). A posterior view (Fig. 23) shows the opposite, with the ulna partially masking the radius, which is visible only at both ends (Fig. 24).

It is important to point out that the two bones of the forearm in the position of supination are **concave anteriorly** (Fig. 25), as is well demonstrated in the side-view diagram of the two bones (Fig. 26). The importance of this arrangement lies in the fact that during pronation (Fig. 27) the radius crosses over the ulna (Fig. 28), and thus its distal head can extend farther posteriorly with respect to the ulna because the concavities of the two bones face each other.

This biconcave arrangement increases the range of pronation and explains why it is so important to restore it (especially the radial concavity) when one corrects displacements of the bones caused by double fractures of the forearm. To allow the radial shaft to remain buckled anteriorly is to accept beforehand some limitation of pronation.

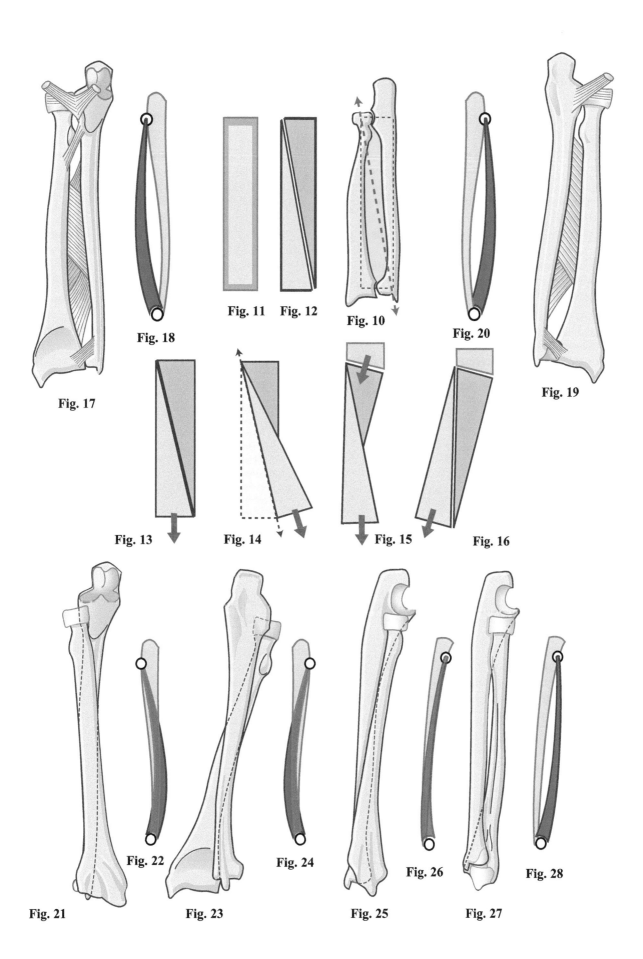

Fig. 17

Fig. 18

Fig. 11   Fig. 12

Fig. 10

Fig. 20

Fig. 19

Fig. 13

Fig. 14

Fig. 15

Fig. 16

Fig. 21

Fig. 22

Fig. 23

Fig. 24

Fig. 25

Fig. 26

Fig. 27

Fig. 28

The interosseous membrane

The interosseous membrane plays an **essential role** in keeping together the two bones of the forearm during pronation-supination (Fig. 29, anterior view; Fig. 30, posterior view) but is not the only structure with this function. The other structures involved include these:

- the **quadrate ligament** (8), joining the superior ends of the two bones
- the **annular ligament** of the superior radio-ulnar joint (9), which is reinforced by the **anterior fibres of the lateral collateral ligament of the elbow** (10), by the **anterior fibres of the medial collateral ligament of the elbow** (11) from farther away, and posteriorly by the **posterior fibres of the medial collateral ligament of the shoulder** (12)
- the **anterior** (13) **and the posterior** (14) **ligaments of the inferior radio-ulnar joint**, as well as the articular disc (not shown), which unite the distal ends of the two bones.

The **interosseous membrane** runs from the medial border of the radius to the lateral border of the ulna. It is made up of two bands of **obliquely criss-crossing fibres**. The description of these fibres is based on the recent work of L. Poitevin (2001), among others.

- The **anterior band** consists of fibres running obliquely inferiorly and medially from the radius with the lowest fibres running the most obliquely. In this continuous band there are three distinct reinforcing bundles:
  - the **proximal bundle** (1), almost horizontal
  - the **middle descending bundle** (2), the central bundle of Hotchkiss
  - the **distal descending bundle** (3), the most oblique.
- The direction of this sheet of fibres (black and red arrows) prevents the radius from being displaced superiorly (white arrow).
- The **posterior band**, much less cohesive, is made up of fibres running obliquely in the opposite direction, i.e. superiorly and medially from the radius. **Two well-defined bundles** can be identified:

- the **proximal ascending bundle** (4), always present and strong
- the **distal ascending bundle** (5), separated from the former by a translucent space (6), which allows the anterior bundle to be seen.
- The direction of these fibres (black and red arrows) prevents the distal displacement of the radius (white arrow).

The two proximal bundles are attached to the medial border of the radius at the level of the clearly visible interosseous tubercle of the radius (7), located 8.4 cm below the interspace of the elbow joint.

This **flexible hinge** (Fig. 31) provides most of the mechanical link between the two bones both transversely and longitudinally:

- After the ligaments of the radio-ulnar joints have been cut, and even after the ulnar and radial heads have been resected, it is by itself able to maintain the contact between the two bones and to prevent displacement of the radius along its long axis.
- Its posterior fibres prevent distal displacement of the radius (Fig. 32), which is not checked by any bony contact.

Proximal displacement of the radius (Fig. 33) stretches its anterior fibres. When the elbow is extended, the radius transmits 60% of the restraining force generated by the membrane while absorbing 82% of the restraining force generated at the wrist joint. In this direction, displacement of the radius is finally checked by the **impact of the radial head on the humeral condyle**. A severe trauma can cause **fracture of the radial head**.

Tears in the interosseous membrane (Figs 34 and 35) are rare and most often go unrecognized. The anterior fibres tear only when the superior radio-ulnar joint is dislocated or when the radial head is broken, since proximal displacement of the radius is normally checked by its impact on the humeral condyle (Fig. 34). When the posterior fibres are torn distal displacement is checked only by direct contact with the carpal bones.

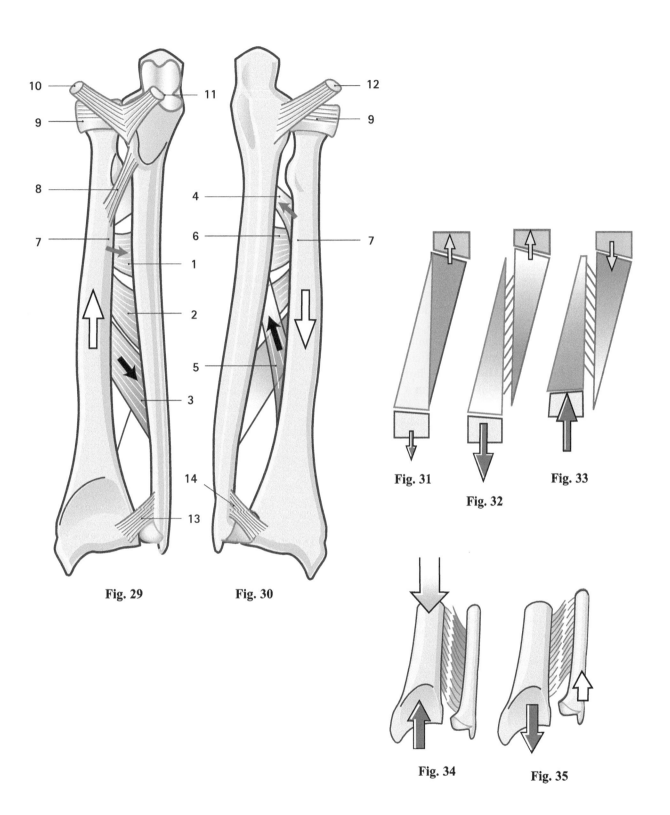

Fig. 29

Fig. 30

Fig. 31

Fig. 32

Fig. 33

Fig. 34

Fig. 35

Downward longitudinal displacement of the radius beyond the ulna is opposed not only by the interosseous membrane but also by the **long muscles** of the hand and of the fingers (Fig. 36), i.e. the flexors (*flexor digitorum superficialis, palmaris longus* and *flexor carpi radialis*) arising from the medial epicondyle, and the extensors (*extensor digitorum communis, extensor carpi radialis longus, extensor carpi radialis brevis, extensor carpi ulnaris*) arising from the lateral epicondyle. Three muscles of the elbow joint (the supinator, the *pronator teres* and the *brachioradialis*) also contribute to this effect (Fig. 37).

When heavy loads are carried or when the arm is stretched lengthwise by the weight of the body, these muscles help to maintain the stability of the radius along its long axis and to keep the articular surfaces of the elbow in close contact.

One can explain **the mechanical role of the fibres of the interosseous membrane** by looking at the movement of one of its elementary fibres (Fig. 38) as follows. Starting from its initial position (1), its lateral edge can move only along a circle with centre (O) anchored in the ulna. Whether this movement (S) occurs superiorly (2) or inferiorly (3), it inevitably brings closer the interosseous margins of the radius and the ulna by a distance **n**. The arrangement of the fibres running obliquely relative to the direction of pull increases its efficiency. One can therefore state that **the combination of two layers of fibres criss-crossing obliquely is more efficient than a single layer of transverse fibres**.

Another mechanism that ensures the approximation of these bones is provided by the attachment of some of the forearm muscles, in particular the flexors, to the anterior and posterior surfaces of the interosseous membrane (Fig. 39). At rest (a), the gap between the two bones is maximal. In contrast, the pull of the flexors (b) stretches the membrane, reduces the gap between the two bones and increases the coaptation of the articular surfaces of both radio-ulnar joints when there is the greatest need.

Finally, the forces acting during rotation are considerable; in men the couple producing pronation generates a force equal to 70 kg/cm and that producing supination 85 kg/cm; in women these values are reduced by 50%. The interosseous membrane acts as a **soft stop** checking pronation, thanks to the muscles of the anterior compartment of the forearm. During supination (Fig. 40) the flexors attached to it (Fig. 41) become more and more compressed (Fig. 42) and stretch the membrane farther, thus bringing the radius and the ulna closer together. The intervening muscles initially prevent the direct contact of the radius and the ulna, which can lead to fractures. In the reference position (the zero position) the fibres of the membrane are maximally stretched, and it is therefore the preferred position of immobilization.

Until now, the interosseous membrane has been the **great unknown in the forearm,** for it certainly plays an essential role. It is possible that selective studies using MRI will further our knowledge of its functional anatomy.

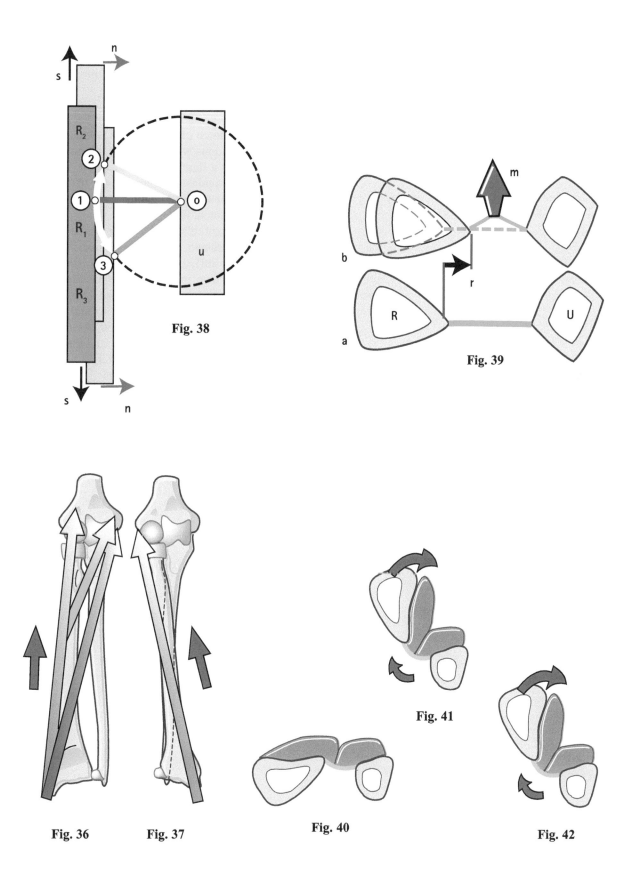

Fig. 38

Fig. 39

Fig. 36   Fig. 37

Fig. 40

Fig. 41

Fig. 42

The functional anatomy of the superior radio-ulnar joint

The **superior radio-ulnar joint** is a **trochoid (pivot) joint** with cylindrical surfaces and **one degree of freedom**, i.e. rotation about the long axis of the two interlocked cylinders. It can therefore be compared mechanically to a system of ball-bearings (Fig. 44). It consists of two nearly cylindrical surfaces.

The **radial head** (Fig. 45) has a cartilage-coated rim (1), which is wider anteriorly and medially and corresponds to the central component (1) of the ball-bearing system. Its superior facet has a **concave surface**, which corresponds to the segment of a sphere (2) and articulates (Fig. 49, sagittal section) with the **capitulum humeri** (9). Since the latter does not extend posteriorly, only the anterior half of the radial head is in contact with it during extension. Its rim is **bevelled** (3), and we have seen the significance of this observation (p. 87).

A fibro-osseous ring (Fig. 43, inspired by Testut), clearly visible after removal of the radial head, corresponds to the outer compartment of the ball-bearing system (Fig. 44, 5 and 6). It consists of the following:

* The **radial notch of the ulna** (6) is coated by cartilage, concave antero-posteriorly and separated by a **blunt ridge** (7) from the **trochlear notch** (Figs 46-48, 8).
* The **annular ligament** (5, shown intact in Figs 43 and 50 and cut in Figs 46 and 47) is made up of a strong fibrous band

attached by its ends to the anterior and posterior margins of the radial notch of the ulna and is lined internally by cartilage continuous with that lining the radial notch. Therefore it serves as a **ligament** by surrounding the radial head and pressing it against the radial notch of the ulna, and also as **an articular surface** in contact with the radial head. Unlike the radial notch, it is flexible.

Another ligament related to the joint is the **quadrate ligament** (4), which is shown cut with the radial head tilted (Fig. 47, inspired by Testut). In Figure 48 (superior view, inspired by Testut) it is shown intact with the olecranon and the annular ligament sectioned. It is a fibrous band inserted into the inferior border of the radial notch of the ulna and into the base of the inner rim of the radial head (Fig. 50, coronal section). Its two borders are strengthened by the radiating fibres of the inferior border of the annular ligament. Inferior to the radial insertion of the ligament lies the radial tuberosity, into which is inserted the biceps (11).

The ligament reinforces the distal aspect of the capsule. The rest of the capsule (10) encloses within a single anatomical cavity the two joints at the elbow: the ulno-humeral and the radio-humeral joints.

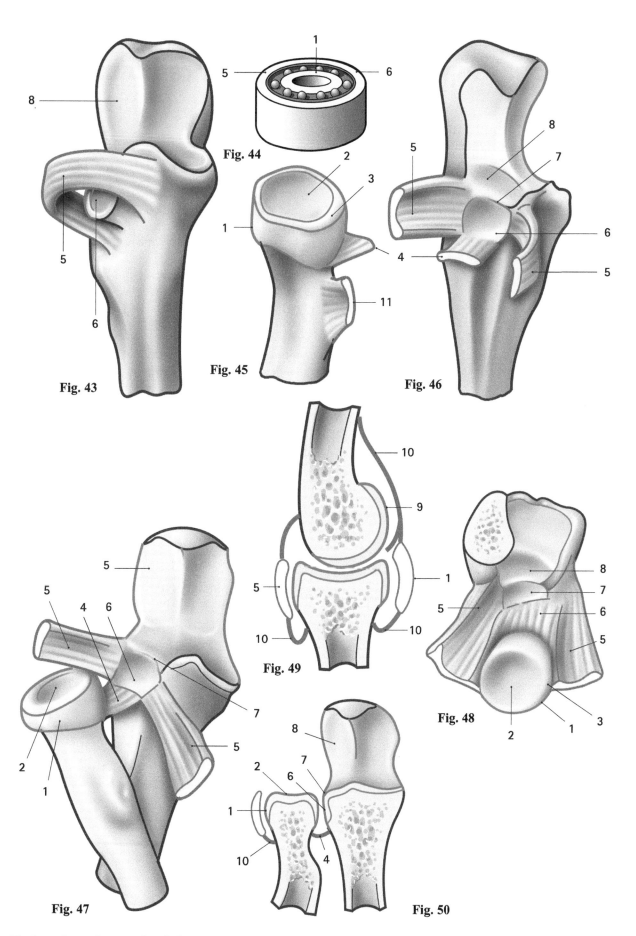

Fig. 43

Fig. 44

Fig. 45

Fig. 46

Fig. 47

Fig. 48

Fig. 49

Fig. 50

The legends are the same for all figures.

The functional anatomy of the inferior radio-ulnar joint

Architecture and mechanical features of the distal end of the ulna

Like its homologue, the superior radio-ulnar joint, the inferior radio-ulnar joint is a **trochoid** (pivot) joint with roughly cylindrical surfaces and only one degree of freedom, i.e. rotation about the axes of the two interlocked cylindrical surfaces. The first of these cylindrical surfaces belongs to the ulnar head. It is possible to view the distal end of the ulna (Fig. 51) as the result of the telescoping of a diaphyseal cylinder (1) into an epiphyseal cone (2), in such a way that the axis of the cone is displaced laterally and falls out of line with that of the cylinder. From this composite structure (Fig. 52) a horizontal plane (3) removes a conical segment (Fig. 53, 4), leaving a distal cup-shaped surface corresponding to the distal end of the ulnar head (7). Next (Fig. 54) a cutting cylinder (5) shaves off a solid crescent (6) and thus shapes (Fig. 55) the outline of the ulnar head (7). Note that the cutting cylinder (5) is concentric neither with the diaphyseal cylinder (1) nor with the epiphyseal cone (2), as it is displaced laterally. Hence the shape of the articular surface, which resembles a crescent 'wrapped' over a cylinder with its anterior and posterior horns 'encasing' the styloid process (8) displaced to the postero-medial aspect of the epiphysis. In reality this surface is not quite cylindrical, but rather conical (Fig. 56). The inferior apex of the cone has an axis (x) parallel to that of the ulnar shaft (y) and the cone has the shape of a cask (Fig. 57), as it has been fashioned by a surface convex outwards (h). All things considered, the distal surface of the ulnar head is not really cylindrical but resembles a conical cask, which, when viewed head-on and to the side, is at its highest (h) anteriorly and slightly laterally.

The inferior surface of the ulnar head (Fig. 58, seen from below) is relatively flat and semi-lunar, with its point of maximal width corresponding to the highest point (h) on its periphery. Thus the following are aligned along the plane of symmetry (arrow): the insertion of the medial fibres of the extensor retinaculum (green square) on the styloid process; the main insertion of the apex of the triangular articular disc (red star) on the styloid process; the centre of curvature of the distal surface of the ulna (black cross); and the highest point on its periphery (h).

On the medial aspect of the distal end of the radius (Fig. 59) lies the **ulnar notch** corresponding to the peripheral surface of the ulnar head. The curvature of this notch is the inverse of that of the ulnar head, i.e. it is concave in both directions and lies along the surface of a cone with an inferiorly pointing apex and a vertical axis (x). In its middle portion its height is equal to that of the outer surface of the ulnar head (h).

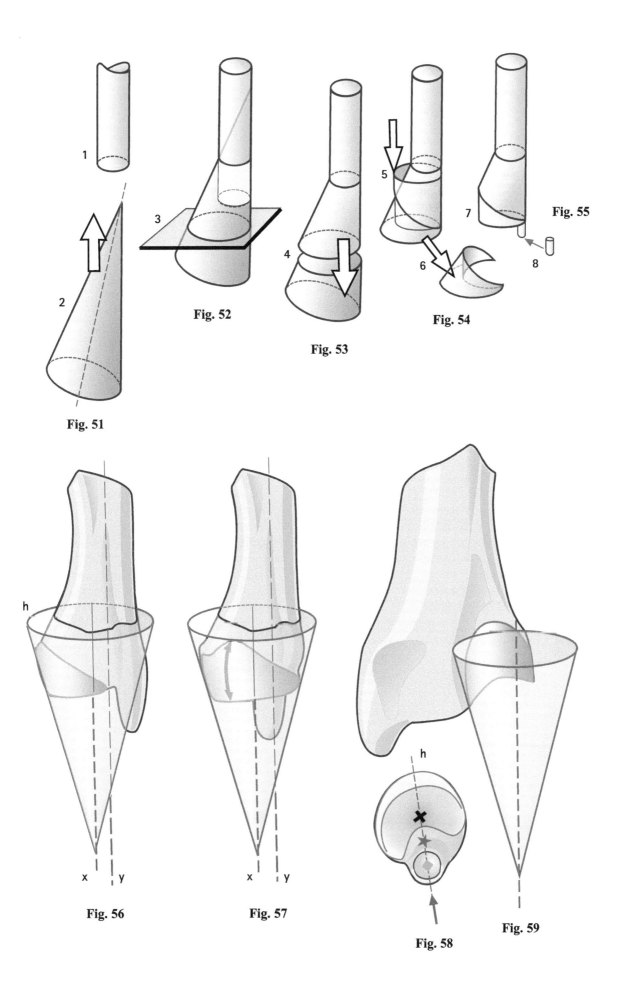

Fig. 51

Fig. 52

Fig. 53

Fig. 54

Fig. 55

Fig. 56

Fig. 57

Fig. 58

Fig. 59

119

Structure of the inferior radio-ulnar joint

The distal end of the radius has **two articular surfaces** (Figs 60 and 61):

- The **first** is its concave inferior (carpal) surface with a lateral area (8) articulating with the scaphoid bone and a medial area (16) articulating with the lunate bone. It is the larger of the articular surfaces and is bounded laterally by the styloid process (1). It will be described in greater detail with the wrist joint.
- The **second**, the **ulnar notch** (3), lies inside the fork formed by the two edges of its interosseous border (2). It faces medially (Fig. 61), and is concave antero-posteriorly and proximo-distally. As shown previously, it can be inscribed on the surface of an inverted cone. It is at its highest in its mid-position and articulates with the head of the ulna (4).

At its distal edge is inserted the **articular disc** (5), which lies in a horizontal plane (Fig. 62, coronal section) and even when normal often has a cleft (6) in the mid-portion of its radial insertion. Its apex is inserted medially into the following:

- the fossa between the styloid process of the ulna (9) and the inferior surface of the ulnar head
- the lateral aspect of the styloid process of the ulna
- the deep aspect of the medial collateral ligament of the wrist.

The articular disc thus fills the gap between the ulnar head and the hamate and acts as an elastic cushion, which is compressed during adduction of the wrist. Its anterior (10) and posterior margins are thickened into genuine ligaments so that it appears biconcave on section (Fig. 61). Its cartilage-coated superior surface articulates with the inferior surface (7) of the ulnar head (Fig. 60). Its cartilage-coated inferior surface is flush medially with the carpal surface of the radius and articulates with the carpal bones. Thus the **articular disc**:

- **binds together** the radius and the ulna
- **provides a dual articular surface** proximally for the ulnar head and distally for the carpal bones.

The ulnar head is not in direct contact with the carpal bones, since the articular disc forms a **partition** between the inferior radio-ulnar and the wrist joints (Fig. 63), which are also anatomically distinct joints unless the markedly biconcave disc is perforated in the middle. Note that such a perforation can also be of traumatic origin. The insertion of its base is incomplete and contains a cleft (6), an age-related change of degenerative origin, according to some authors. Acting as a 'suspended meniscus' the articular disc forms with the ulnar notch of the radius a somewhat flexible articular surface for the ulnar head (Fig. 65). It is also subjected to a variety of stresses: **traction** (blue horizontal arrow), **compression** (red vertical arrows) and **shearing** (green horizontal arrows). These stresses often act in concert, and this explains why the articular disc is often damaged in injuries to the wrist.

The articular disc is the main but not the only structure that binds the inferior radio-ulnar joint (Fig. 66), and it is helped by the anterior (14) and posterior (not shown here) ligaments of the joint and also by other structures whose role has recently been identified:

- the **palmar expansion of the dorsal radio-carpal ligament** (13), which goes round the medial border of the wrist
- the **tendon of the extensor carpi ulnaris** (15), which is surrounded by a **strong fibrous sheath** and runs in a groove lying medial to the styloid process of the ulna on the posterior surface of the ulnar head.

All these structures form what can be called the crossroads of the **medial ligamentous complex of the wrist**.

The direction of the interspace of the radio-ulnar joint varies with individuals. In the vast majority of cases (Fig. 62, coronal section) it is oblique inferiorly and slightly medially (red arrow); more rarely (Fig. 63) it is vertical; and exceptionally (Fig. 64) it is oblique inferiorly and slightly laterally.

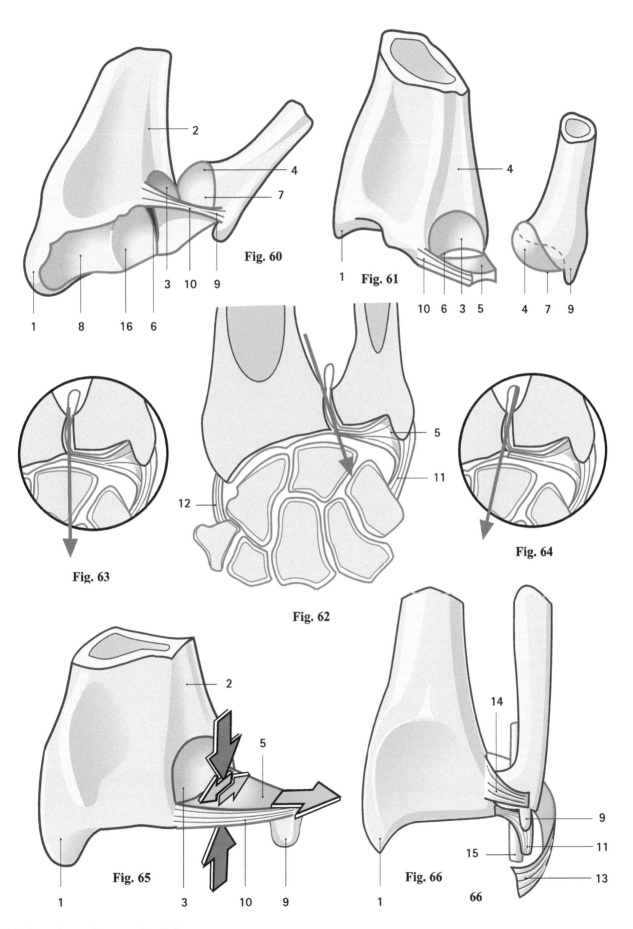

Fig. 60

Fig. 61

Fig. 63

Fig. 62

Fig. 64

Fig. 65

Fig. 66

66

The legends are the same for all figures.

Dynamic features of the superior radio-ulnar joint and ulnar variance

The **main movement** (Fig. 67) is **rotation of the radial head** (1) about its axis within the fibro-osseous ring (2), formed by the **annular ligament and the radial notch of the ulna.** This movement is limited (Fig. 68) by the tension developed in the quadrate ligament (3), which therefore acts as a brake in supination (A) and pronation (B).

On the other hand, the radial head is not quite cylindrical but slightly oval (Fig. 69); its great diameter, lying obliquely antero-laterally, measures 28 mm and its short diameter 24 mm. This explains why the annular cuff of the radial head cannot be bony and rigid. The annular ligament, which makes up about three-quarters of the cuff, is flexible and allows some distortion, while holding the radial head in perfect fit in supination (A) and pronation (B).

There are four **accessory movements**:

1) The cup-shaped surface of the radial head (1) rotates with respect to the capitulum humeri (Fig. 71).

2) The bevelled ridge of the radial head (4) (cf. p.87) glides in contact with the capitulo-trochlear groove of the humerus.

3) The axis of the radial head is translated laterally during pronation (Fig. 70) because of the oval shape of the head. During pronation (B), the great axis of the radial head comes to lie transversely with a lateral shift (e) equal to half the difference between the two axes of the radial head, i.e. 2 mm in position X'.

This lateral displacement is of capital importance; it allows the radius to move out of the way of the ulna just in time for the radial tuberosity to move into the supinator fossa of the ulna, where the supinator is inserted. The white arrow (Fig. 67) indicates this 'creeping' movement of the radial tuberosity 'between' the radius and the ulna.

4) Moreover, we have already seen that during pronation (Fig. 72) the radius, which lies lateral to the ulna (a), overlaps it anteriorly (b) with the following results:

- On the one hand, the axis of the forearm, which was slightly oblique laterally because of the *cubitus valgus,* becomes collinear with the axis of the arm (b) and secondarily with that of the hand.

- On the other hand, the axis of the radius becomes oblique inferiorly and medially so that the plane of the proximal surface of the radial head is tilted distally and laterally during pronation (Fig. 73, b) at an angle (y) equal to that of the lateral inclination of the radius. This accounts for the change in direction of the articular surface of the radial head.

The change in the direction of the axis of the radial shaft takes place around an axis of rotation lying at the centre of the capitulum humeri (Fig. 74), and it comes to lie anterior (red line) to the diagonal of the radio-ulnar complex. As this diagonal is longer than the long side of the rectangle, **during pronation the radius becomes shorter with respect to the ulna** by a distance r, with the following **important** effects on the inferior radio-ulnar joint (Fig. 75):

- In **supination** (a) the distal surface of the ulnar head is overshot by the radius by 1.5-2 mm, the **so-called ulnar variance**, which is clearly seen in anterior radiographs of the wrist in supination and is due to the thickness of the articular disc. This negative ulnar variance can become abnormal as its normal value passes from –2 to 0 or even to +2 during impaction of the radius, which is followed by severe functional disturbances at the wrist joint.

- In **pronation** (b) the relative shortening of the radius (r), which forms an angle (i) with the ulna, allows the ulnar head to overshoot for a distance of 2 mm without any adverse effects on a normal wrist. But if the wrist is abnormal, the already positive ulnar variance with the relative overshoot of the ulnar head can make things worse and increase the pain.

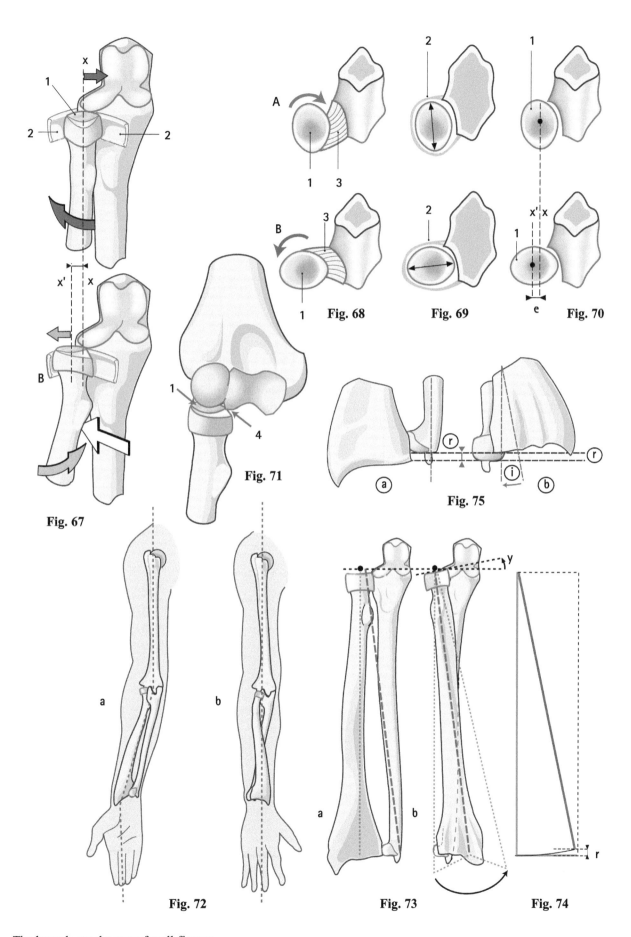

Fig. 67

Fig. 68

Fig. 69

Fig. 70

Fig. 71

Fig. 72

Fig. 73

Fig. 74

Fig. 75

The legends are the same for all figures.

Dynamic features of the inferior radio-ulnar joint

Let us assume at first that the **ulna remains stationary** and **only the radius moves.** In this case (Fig. 76) the axis of pronation-supination extends into the hand along the medial edge of the ulna and the fifth finger (the axis has a red cross). This is the case when the forearm is axially rotated while maintaining contact with the table it is resting on. The dorsal surface of the thumb will touch the table in supination (S), and its palmar surface in pronation (P).

The **main movement** (Fig. 77) is a **rotation** of the distal end of the radius about the ulna. This inferior view reveals the articular surfaces of the radius and ulna after removal of the wrist bones and of the articular disc. The radial epiphysis revolves around the ulnar head, which is taken to be circular and fixed, since the styloid process of the ulna (in yellow) is stationary.

- Supination (S) has a range of 90°.
- Pronation (P) has a slightly smaller range of 85°.

This movement of rotational spin is well demonstrated by comparing the radius to a crank. Starting with **supination** (Fig. 78), the upper branch of the crank (with the handle corresponding to the radial head) rotates around its long axis (dashed red line), while during pronation (Fig. 76) the lower branch of the crank undergoes a **circumferential spin**, i.e. **a rotation combined with a displacement along a circular path** (pink arrow).

The lower branch of the crank turns along the surface of a cylinder, which corresponds to the ulnar head, and its rotation on itself is demonstrated by the change of direction of the red arrow (Fig. 78) towards the blue arrow (Fig. 79). The radial styloid process faces laterally during supination and medially during pronation. This circumferential spin is similar to that of the moon, which rotates around the Earth while maintaining the same face towards it; only recently has the hidden face of our satellite been seen. When the radius revolves around the ulna from supination to pronation, the geometric congruence of the articular surfaces varies (Fig. 80), for these reasons:

- On the one hand, the articular surfaces are not geometrically perfect and have variable radii of curvature, which tend to be shortest at their centres.
- On the other hand, the radius of curvature of the ulnar notch of the radius (blue circle with centre r) is slightly greater than that of the ulnar head (red circle with centre u). It is in the intermediate position, also called 'zero position', that the congruence of the articular surfaces is maximal.

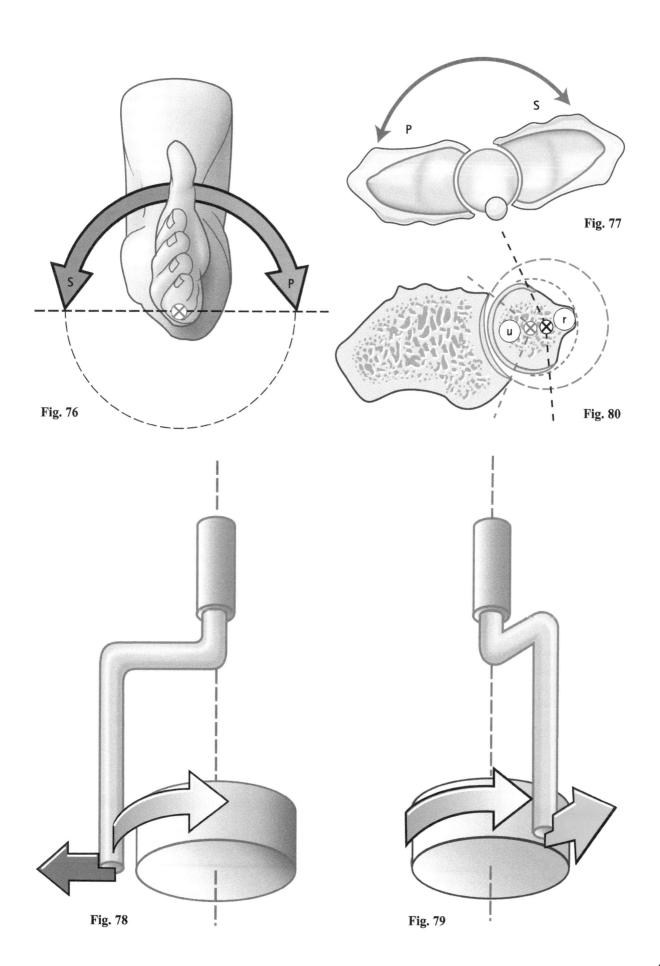

Fig. 76

Fig. 77

Fig. 80

Fig. 78

Fig. 79

It is only in **the intermediate position** (Fig. 81) that articular congruence is maximal. Thus supination (Fig. 82) and pronation (Fig. 83) are associated with a relative loss of congruence, since only a small part of the ulnar head comes into contact with the ulnar notch of the radius. At the same time their radii of curvature are different, adversely affecting articular congruence.

In **full pronation**, there is a true posterior subluxation of the ulnar head (Fig. 88), which tends to 'escape' posteriorly (black arrow), as it is poorly retained by the posterior ligament of the radio-ulnar joint (in green). It is kept in place essentially by the **tendon of the extensor carpi ulnaris** (e.c.u.), which is held in its groove by a **strong fibrous sheath** and 'brings back' the ulnar head towards the ulnar notch of the radius (white arrow); the **pronator quadratus** (p.q.) has a similar function. In the position of maximal congruence, the highest point on the peripheral surface of the ulnar head corresponds to the highest point of the ulnar notch, when the radii of curvature coincide and maximize contact between the articular surfaces.

During movements of pronation-supination (Figs 85-87), the articular disc literally sweeps the inferior surface of the ulnar head like a windscreen wiper. On this inferior surface (Fig. 84), **three points** are aligned along its greater diameter: the centre of the styloid process of the ulna (green square), the site of insertion of the apex of the articular disc (red star) in the groove lying between the styloid process and the articular surface, and the centre of curvature of the periphery of the ulnar head (black cross). Since the ulnar insertion of the articular disc is off-centre, **tension developed in the ligament varies** significantly with its position, being minimal in full supination (Fig. 87) and in full pronation (Fig. 86), owing to its relative shortening (e). The shortening is explained by the fact that, when a radius of the large circle (e.g. one fibre of the articular disc) 'sweeps' the surface of the small circle, it behaves like a secant of the small circle whose length varies with its position. This accounts for the variations in the tension developed by the fibres of the articular disc.

Consequently, the **tension is maximal in the position of maximal articular congruence**, i.e. the position corresponding to the highest point on the periphery of the ulnar head, since the length of the ligament between its insertion and the periphery of the head coincides with the longest diameter. The articular disc, however, is reinforced by two **bands** (one anterior and one posterior), which are moderately stretched in the intermediate position (Fig. 85). **In supination** the anterior band (Fig. 87) is stretched maximally and the posterior is maximally relaxed, while **in pronation** (Fig. 86) the opposite occurs; this is the result of the different excursions of the articular disc. These diagrams also show that, because of the differential distribution of tension in the disc, the small cleft at the base of its insertion becomes distorted. Likewise, the central cleft, if of traumatic origin and not a normal variation, will tend to enlarge during pronation-supination. Thus there is a position of maximal stability for the radio-ulnar joint that corresponds roughly to the intermediate position. It is the **'close-packed' position of Mac-Connaill** with maximal congruence of the articular surfaces combined with maximal stretching of the ligaments, but, since it is an intermediate position, it cannot be viewed as a truly locked position. The differential actions of the articular disc and interosseous membrane are as follows:

- **In full pronation and in full supination**, the articular disc is partially relaxed, while the interosseous membrane is stretched. Note that the anterior and posterior ligaments of the inferior radio-ulnar joint, which are weak condensations of the capsule, play no role in keeping the articular surfaces together or in limiting joint movements.

- **In the position of maximal stability**, i.e. in the intermediate position, the articular disc is stretched, while the interosseous membrane is relaxed, except insofar as it is retightened by the muscles attached to it.

- On the whole, the articular surfaces of the joint are kept together by two anatomical structures: the **interosseous membrane**, whose essential role is underestimated, and the **articular disc**.

Pronation is checked by the presence of the muscles of the anterior compartment of the forearm and the impact of the radius on the ulna. Hence the importance of the slight anterior concavity of the radial shaft, which delays the impact.

Supination is checked by the impact of the posterior end of the ulnar notch of the radius on the ulnar styloid process cushioned by the intervening tendon of the extensor carpi ulnaris. It is not restricted by any ligament or direct bony impact, but it is checked by the tonus of the pronators.

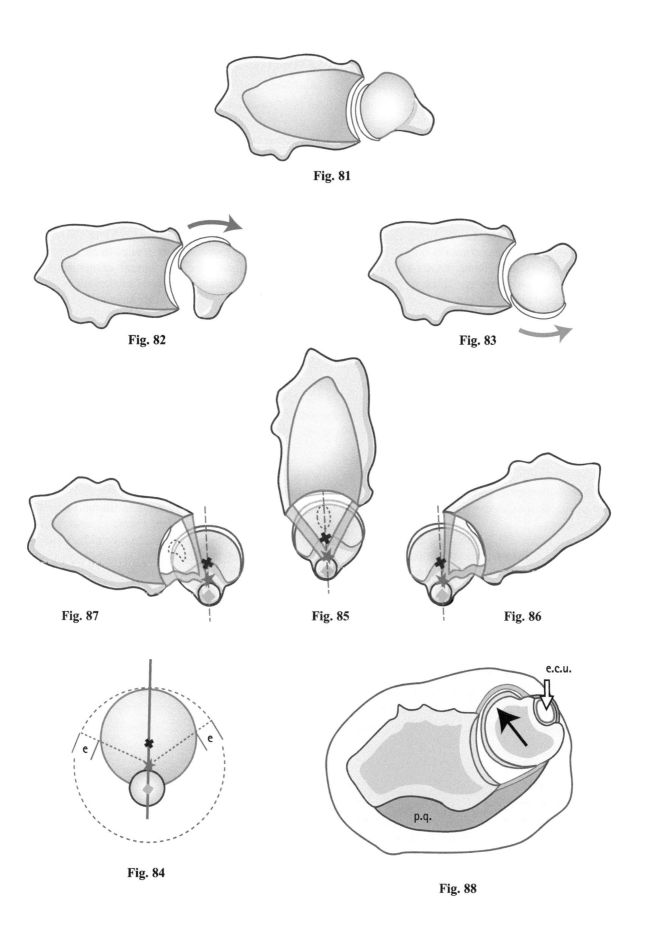

Fig. 81

Fig. 82

Fig. 83

Fig. 87

Fig. 85

Fig. 86

Fig. 84

e.c.u.

p.q.

Fig. 88

The axis of pronation-supination

So far we have discussed the function of the inferior radio-ulnar joint in isolation, but it is easy to understand that there is a **functional coupling of the inferior and superior radio-ulnar joints**, which are **mechanically linked**, since one joint needs the other in order to function. This functional coupling depends on the coupling of the axes of the joints and the coupling of their articular congruence. The two radio-ulnar joints are **coaxial**; they can function normally only when their axes of movement (Fig. 89) are collinear (XX′) and coincide with the hinge of pronation-supination, which runs centrally through the ulnar and radial heads. For example, a door (Fig. 90) cannot be opened easily unless the axes of its hinges are perfectly aligned (a), i.e. collinear. If, as a result of unforgivably bad workmanship, axes 1 and 2 were not collinear (b), the door could not be opened unless it were cut into two independent pieces that could be opened separately. The same reasoning applies to these two joints when the axes are not properly aligned following a badly reduced fracture of one or the other of the bones of the forearm. The **loss of collinearity of the axes** impairs pronation-supination.

When the radius moves relative to the ulna around the common axis XX′ of the two joints (Fig. 89), its path lies along a segment of a conical surface (C), which is concave posteriorly and has its base inferiorly and its apex at the centre of the capitulum humeri.

Supposing that the ulna stays put, pronation-supination is due to the rotation of the radial shaft (red cross) around the axis of the inferior radio-ulnar joint, which is collinear with that of the superior radio-ulnar joint. In this situation the axis of pronation-supination coincides with the hinge of pronation-supination.

If pronation-supination occurs around an axis passing through the thumb, the radius rotates around the styloid process (Fig. 91) of the ulna around an axis that does not coincide with the hinge of pronation-supination. As a result, the inferior end of the ulna moves along a half-circle inferiorly and laterally and then superiorly and laterally, all the while staying parallel to itself. The vertical component of this movement can easily be explained by a concurrent movement of extension and then of flexion at the humero-ulnar joint. Its lateral component used to be explained by a concurrent lateral movement at the elbow, but it is difficult to imagine how a movement of such a range (nearly twice the width of the wrist) could occur in such a tight hinge joint as the humero-ulnar joint. Recently H.C. Djbay has proposed a more mechanical and intellectually satisfying explanation. It is the concurrent lateral rotation (l.r.) of the humerus on its long axis that displaces the head laterally (Fig. 92), while the radius rotates on itself (Fig. 93) around a centre of rotation (Fig. 94) lying right in the middle of the radial head. This theory, implying the existence of a lateral rotation in the scapulo-thoracic 'joint', could be verified by measuring the action potentials of the rotator muscles of the humerus during pronation-supination.

It is worth noting that this change of orientation of the radius should cause the axis of the hand to tilt medially (Fig. 95, red arrow). However, because of the normal *cubitus valgus* (Fig. 96), the axis of the elbow joint is slightly oblique inferiorly and medially, so that the hinge of pronation-supination comes to lie in a longitudinal plane. Thus pronation of the radius brings back the axis of the hand to lie exactly in that longitudinal plane (black arrow).

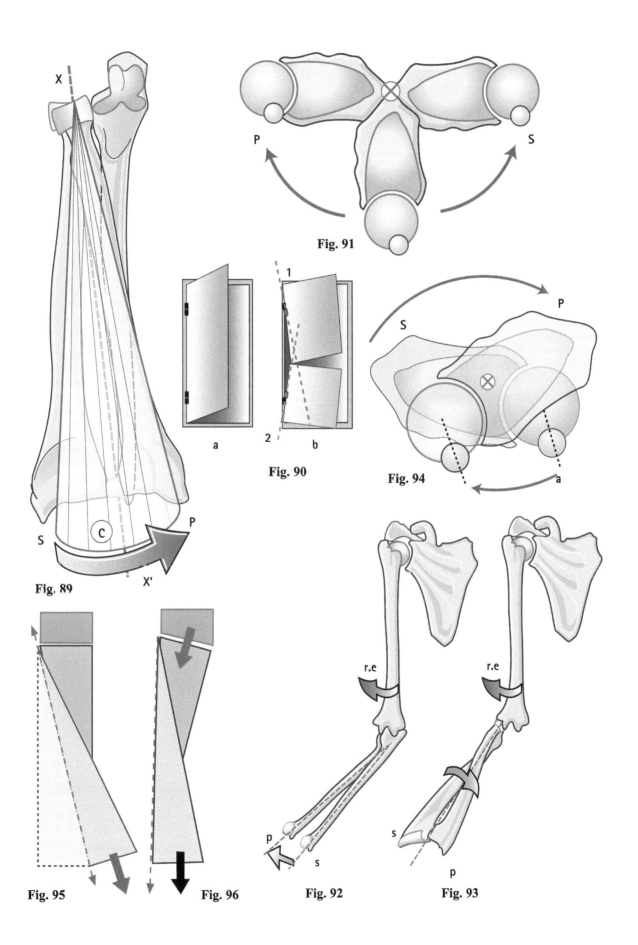

Fig. 89

Fig. 90

Fig. 91

Fig. 94

Fig. 92

Fig. 93

Fig. 95

Fig. 96

If this hypothesis could be confirmed with accurate radiographic and electromyographic studies, the lateral rotation of the humerus should range from 5° to 20° and should occur only during pronation-supination with the elbow flexed at 90°. When the elbow is fully extended, the ulna is held fixed by the olecranon fitting snugly into its fossa and, if the elbow is tightly immobilized, it becomes clear that no pronation occurs while full supination is still possible. This loss of pronation is offset by medial rotation of the humerus. Thus during elbow extension there is a 'point of transition' where there is no associated rotation of the humerus. Pronation is also limited to 45° when the elbow is flexed. The humerus then appears to be unable to rotate on its long axis, and so the lateral displacement of the ulnar head must be explained by a lateral movement in the humero-radial joint.

Between these two extreme cases previously discussed, the axis of pronation-supination passes through the ulnar or radial end of the wrist. In the **usual movement of pronation-supination, centred on the dynamic tripod of prehension** (Fig. 97), the axis is intermediate in location and lies along a **third path** (Fig. 89), which passes through the lower end of the radius (red cross, Fig. 98) near the ulnar notch. The radius rotates on itself for nearly 180°, and the ulna is displaced without rotation along an arc of a circle with the same centre, a displacement made up of a component of extension (ext) and a component of lateral movement (lat). The centre of the ulnar head shifts from position O to position O' while undergoing **circumferential spin** on the axis OO'.

Pronation-supination now becomes a **complex movement** (Fig. 99) with an axis ZZ', which cannot be physically represented in space and is quite distinct from the hinge of pronation-supination. This hinge, dragged along from axis X to axis Y by the ulnar head, traces out the surface of a segment of a cone (see Fig. 89), concave anteriorly in this case.

In sum, there is not a single movement of pronation-supination but a series of such movements, the most common occurring around an axis that passes through the radius and around which both bones 'rotate', as in a **ballet**. The axis of pronation-supination, generally distinct from the hinge of pronation-supination, is **variable and cannot be physically defined in space**.

The fact that this axis cannot be physically represented in space and is not fixed does not mean that it does not exist; by the same token the axis of rotation of the Earth would not exist either.

From the fact that pronation-supination is a movement of rotation it can be deduced with certainty that its axis exists in reality though it cannot be physically defined, that it rarely coincides with the hinge of pronation-supination, and that its position relative to the bones of the forearm depends on the type and the stage of pronation-supination performed.

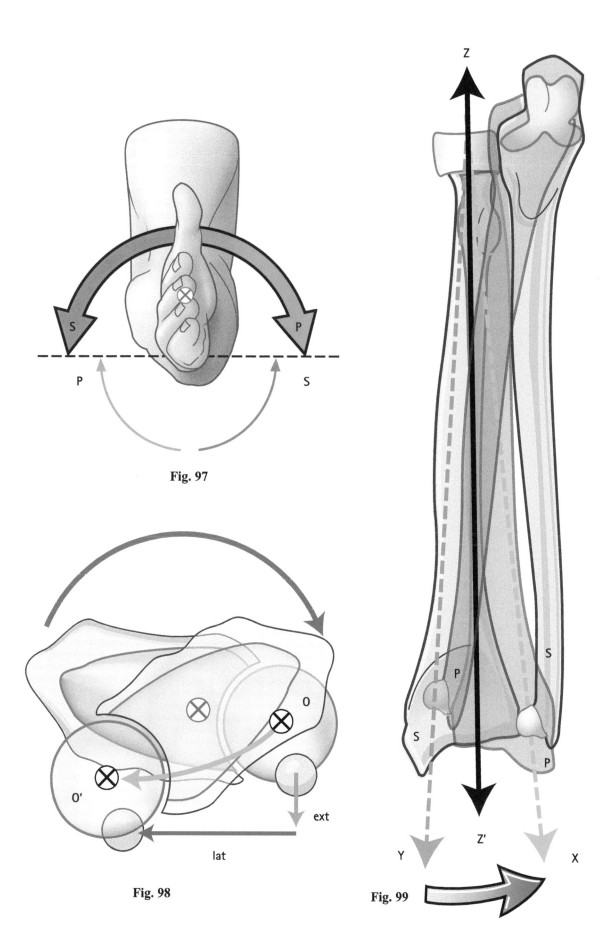

Fig. 97

Fig. 98

Fig. 99

The co-congruence of the two radio-ulnar joints

The functional coupling of the radio-ulnar joints also depends on their articular co-congruence. Thus the position of maximal stability for both joints is attained at the same degree of pronation-supination (Fig. 100). In other words, when the ulnar head (Fig. 101) is in contact with the ulnar notch of the radius at its highest point (h), the same applies to the radial head (i) relative to the radial notch of the ulna (Fig. 102). The planes of symmetry (Fig. 100) of the ulnar notch of the radius (un) and of the radial head (rh), passing through the highest points on their peripheral surfaces, form a solid angle open medially and anteriorly (red arrow). This **angle of torsion of the radius is equal to that of the ulna**, which is correspondingly measured between the ulnar head and the radial notch of the ulna (not shown).

This angle can vary from person to person, as can be observed by looking at the distal end of the ulna along its long axis.

In the intermediate position (Fig. 103) congruence is perfect if the two angles of torsion are identical, i.e. when the ulnar head is in contact with the ulnar notch of the radius by its greatest diameter and the radial head is in contact with the radial notch of the ulna, also by its greatest diameter.

But if the angles of torsion of the two bones are not identical, pronation-supination can be speeded up or delayed. Thus when pronation is speeded up (Fig. 104), the radial head contacts the ulnar notch by its short diameter. Likewise, when supination is delayed (Fig. 105), the radial head can contact the ulnar notch in an inappropriate position.

Thus congruence of the two radio-ulnar joints is attained when the angles of torsion of both bones are equal and therefore congruence may not always be attainable. A large statistical study would no doubt help to establish the full spectrum of these variations in the angles of torsion.

In practice these observations suggest that, during the reduction of a fracture of the shaft of one or the other of these two bones, the rotational discrepancy of the fragments must be reduced with precision, even if the angle of torsion is not restored, which will upset the pronation-supination mechanism.

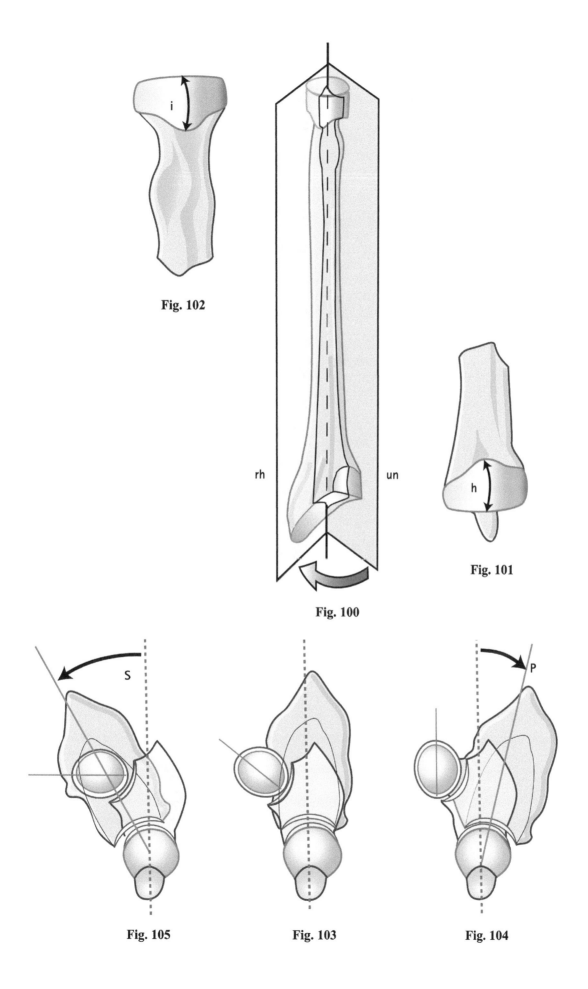

Fig. 102

Fig. 101

rh   un

Fig. 100

Fig. 105   Fig. 103   Fig. 104

The muscles of pronation and supination

To understand the mode of action of these muscles, the shape of the radius must be analysed mechanically (Fig. 106). The radius comprises **three segments**, which together give it roughly the shape of a **crank** (c):

1) The **neck** (the upper segment running obliquely, distally and medially) forms an obtuse angle with

2) the intermediate segment (the upper half of the shaft running obliquely, distally and laterally); the apex (arrow 1) of this obtuse angle, open laterally, coincides with the **radial tuberosity** where the biceps are inserted. These two segments make up the '**supinator bend**' of the radius.

3) The intermediate segment joins the lower segment, which runs obliquely, distally and medially, at an obtuse angle whose apex (arrow 2) coincides with the site of insertion of the *pronator teres*. These two segments make up the '**pronator bend**' of the radius.

Note that the 'radial crank' is tilted at an angle to its axis (c). In fact, this axis XX' (red dashed line) is the axis of pronation-supination and passes through both ends of the arms of the crank and not through the arms themselves. Thus the apices of the two 'bends' lie on either side of this axis.

The axis XX' is shared by both radio-ulnar joints, and this common axis is essential for pronation-supination, provided the bones are not fractured simultaneously or separately. To move this crank two mechanisms are available (Fig. 107):

1) to **unwind a cord** coiled around one of its arms (arrow 1)
2) to **pull on the apex** of one of the bends (arrow 2).

These mechanisms form the basis of the mode of action of the rotator muscles. The muscles of pronation-supination are **four** in number and fall into two groups. There is for each of these movements:

1) a short flat muscle (arrow 1), which acts by 'unwinding'
2) a long muscle inserted into the apex of one of the 'bends' (arrow 2).

Motor muscles of supination

(Fig. 108, anterior view; Figs 111 and 112, the right inferior segment seen from above)

1) The **supinator** (1), wound around the radial neck (Fig. 111) and inserted into the supinator fossa of the ulna, acts by 'unwinding'.

2) The **biceps** (2), inserted into the apex of the 'supinator bend' on the radial tuberosity (Fig. 112), acts by pulling on the superior angle of the crank and attains maximal efficiency when the elbow is flexed at 90°. It is the most powerful muscle of pronation-supination (Fig. 108); hence one turns a **screwdriver by supinating the forearm** with the elbow flexed.

Motor muscles of pronation (Figs 109 and 110)

1) The **pronator quadratus** (4), wrapped around the inferior end of the ulna, acts by 'unwinding', so that the ulna 'unwinds' around the radius (Fig. 109).

2) The **pronator teres** (3), inserted into the apex of the 'pronator bend', acts by traction; its action is weak, especially when the elbow is extended.

The pronator muscles are less powerful than the supinators, so that to unscrew a jammed screw, one must take advantage of the movement of pronation produced by abduction at the elbow. The *brachioradialis*, despite its French name of long supinator, is not a supinator but a **flexor of the elbow**. It can supinate only from the position of complete pronation to that of zero rotation. Paradoxically, it becomes a pronator only from the position of complete supination to that of zero rotation.

There is only one nerve for pronation – the median nerve. Two nerves are necessary for supination: the radial nerve for the supinator and the musculo-cutaneous nerve for the biceps. Thus the function of pronation is more easily lost than that of supination.

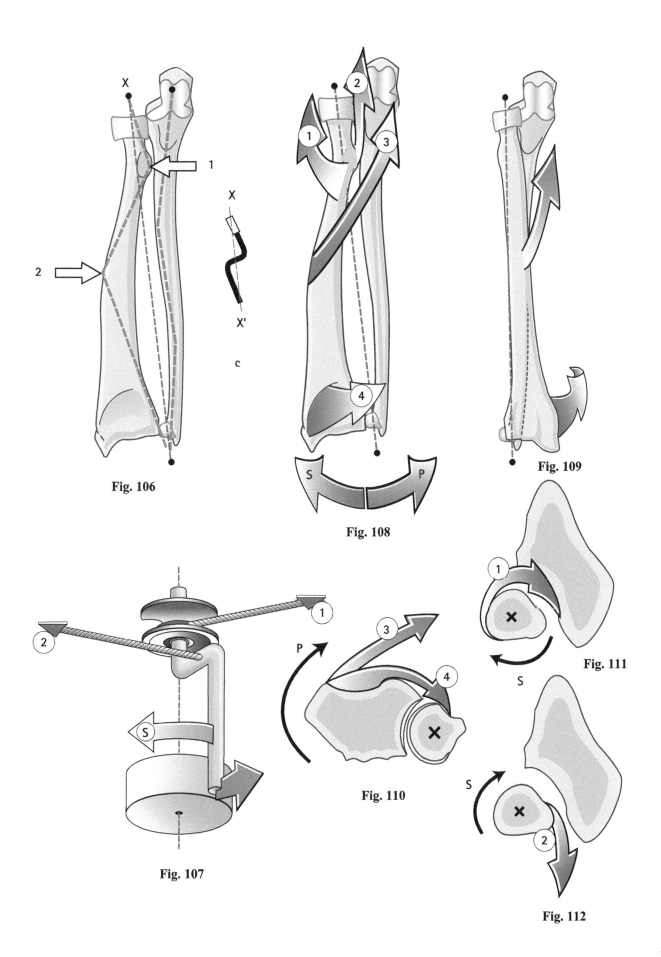

Fig. 106

Fig. 107

Fig. 108

Fig. 109

Fig. 110

Fig. 111

Fig. 112

Why does the forearm have two bones?

In all terrestrial vertebrates starting from our ancestor on earth, the tetrapod, which had just left the sea, the forearm and the leg have two bones each. This segment is called the **zeugopod**. This is a fact, but very few anatomists have answered the question: Why two bones?

Any attempt to provide a logical explanation must resort to the *reductio ad absurdum* and imagine a fictional biomechanical model of the forearm to help explore how it could perform all its actions with only one bone, an **UlRadius**.

To grasp objects the arm must be able to adopt many varied positions, and this implies that the articular complex from the shoulder must have **seven degrees of freedom**; not one more, not one less! Three degrees of freedom are needed to allow the upper limb to be placed anywhere in space, one degree is needed at the elbow for the hand to be moved away from or towards the shoulder and the mouth, and **three degrees** are needed at the wrist for orientation of the hand. The logical solution then would have been to place a spherical ball-and-socket joint like the shoulder at the distal end of the UlRadius. Let us then imagine the biomechanical consequences of such a structure. At first there are two possibilities, depending on whether the spherical component of this joint is distal (Fig. 113) and forms part of the wrist, or is proximal (Fig. 114) at the distal end of the UlRadius. Would the first solution impose fewer complications on the structure of the wrist? Let us, however, look at the second solution. A ball-and-socket joint at the distal end of the UlRadius is clearly a disadvantage. Rotation, involving the two articular surfaces and taking place in a very tight space, generates shearing stresses in all the structures that bridge the joint, including the tendons (Fig. 115). The diagram of the wrist in perspective (a) shows that any rotation of the distal articular surface will shorten these bridging structures by a distance (r). A superior cross-section (b) shows that rotation in both directions (c) and (d) forces the tendon to follow a longer path, thus provoking relative shortening associated with pseudo-contraction of the muscle, which is difficult to offset, especially if the hand is moved laterally (Fig. 117) from the straight position (Fig. 116). The blood vessels face a similar mechanical problem, which is easily understood from the view taken in perspective (Fig. 118). The arteries also undergo relative shortening, which is combined with twisting but is more readily offset because of their corkscrew nature at rest. In the solution with two bones (Fig. 119) the radial artery is dragged over its whole length during rotation of the radius without itself undergoing rotation or shortening.

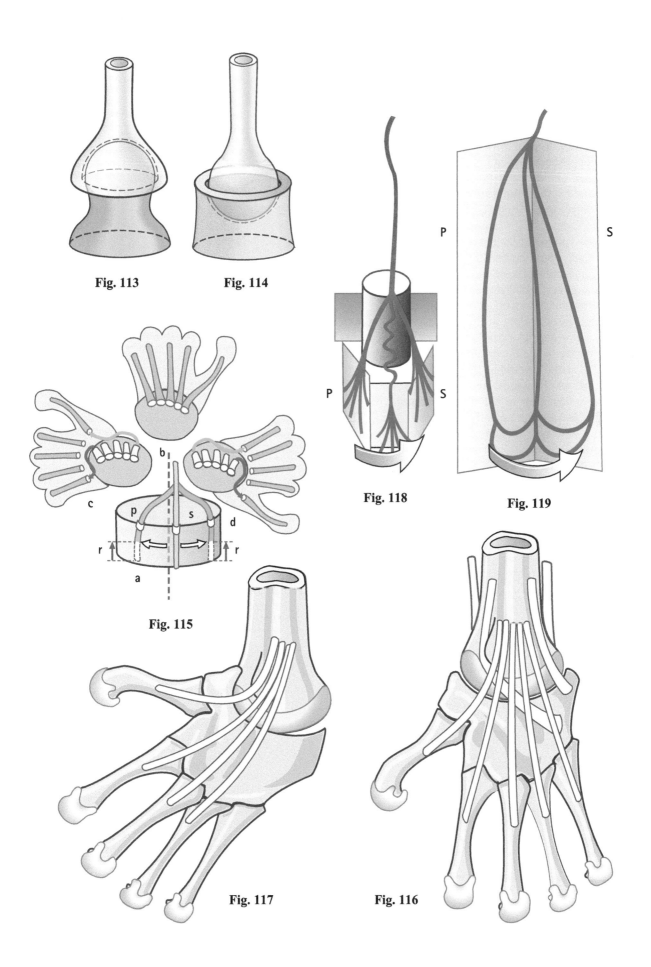

Fig. 113

Fig. 114

Fig. 115

Fig. 118

Fig. 119

Fig. 117

Fig. 116

137

The problems linked to the relative shortening of the tendons preclude the placement of **powerful extensors and flexors of the hand** in the forearm. Therefore these muscles **extrinsic** to the hand should now be located **in the hand as intrinsic muscles** with serious if not catastrophic consequences, since the strength of a muscle is proportional to its volume. One can only imagine the equivalent mass of flexor muscles in the palm of the hand (Fig. 121) to realize that **the hand would become almost useless** for grasping an object with the palm, which in the normal hand (Fig. 120) can accommodate a relatively large object.

The shape and the volume of the hand would be vastly altered (Fig. 122); the hand would be transformed into a 'battledore-hand' (a-b), i.e. huge, cumbersome and deprived almost entirely of its functional and aesthetic value (c-d).

Such a structure would have an effect on that of the whole body because of the increased weight of the extremity of the upper limb (Fig. 123, half « normal » man). The **barycentre or partial centre of gravity** of the upper limb, normally lying close to the elbow (blue arrow), would be displaced distally **close to the wrist** (red arrow). This increase in the moment of force generated in the upper limb would require **strengthening of the scapular girdle** and consequently of the lower limb. This would result in a new type of human being as shown in the composite diagram, where the left side is normal, while the right side has become modified by the simple transformation of the wrist into a ball-and-socket joint. This is a different picture from the human being we know (Fig. 126)!

Since the UlRadius solution is not workable, the two-bone solution is the only viable one, with splitting of the UlRadius into the ulna and the radius. The question now centres on the **arrangement of the bones** (Fig. 124). Their arrangement in series is not practical (a), since the poorly integrated interlocked joint would be too weak and would not allow one to lift a piano or even a knapsack! The only solution left is a side-to-side

parallel arrangement with two possibilities: one anterior to the other (b) and one lateral to the other (c). If the radius lies anterior to the ulna (b), flexion at the elbow is likely to be limited. The more practical solution is to have the radius in the same plane as the ulna but lateral to it, since this takes advantage of the *cubitus valgus*, i.e. the carrying angle of the forearm. The **two-bone solution** indisputably makes the architecture of the elbow and wrist more complicated by bringing in **two additional joints**, i.e. the radio-ulnar joints, but it solves some problems, notably that of the vessels, which are no longer twisted over a short distance, and also that of the nerves. More important, it solves the muscle problem; the **strong muscles** can now be placed in the forearm as **extrinsic muscles** of the hand, and the **intrinsic muscles** of the hand, weak and light, can now become **muscles of precision**. The muscles attached to the radius **rotate simultaneously with it** and change in length without any 'parasitic' effect on the fingers during rotation of the wrist. The few flexor muscles attached to the ulna also rotate along their entire length, cancelling any 'parasitic' effect on the fingers.

The appearance of two bones in the intermediate segment of the four limbs goes back 400 million years (Fig. 126) to the mid-Devonian period, when our remote ancestor (an obscure fish, the Eusthenopteron) left the sea following a change in its pectoral fins and became a four-legged animal like the modern lizard or crocodile. The rays of its fins were progressively reorganized (a-b-c), as follows: the proximal single ray became the humerus (h), the subsequent two rays became the radius (r) and ulna (u), and the distal rays gave rise to the wrist bones and the five fingers. Since that time, the **prototype of the terrestrial vertebrate has always had two bones in the forearm and in the leg**, i.e., the **zeugopod**. Later, among the more advanced vertebrates, pronation-supination became increasingly important and attained its maximal efficiency among the primates and finally in Homo sapiens (Fig. 126).

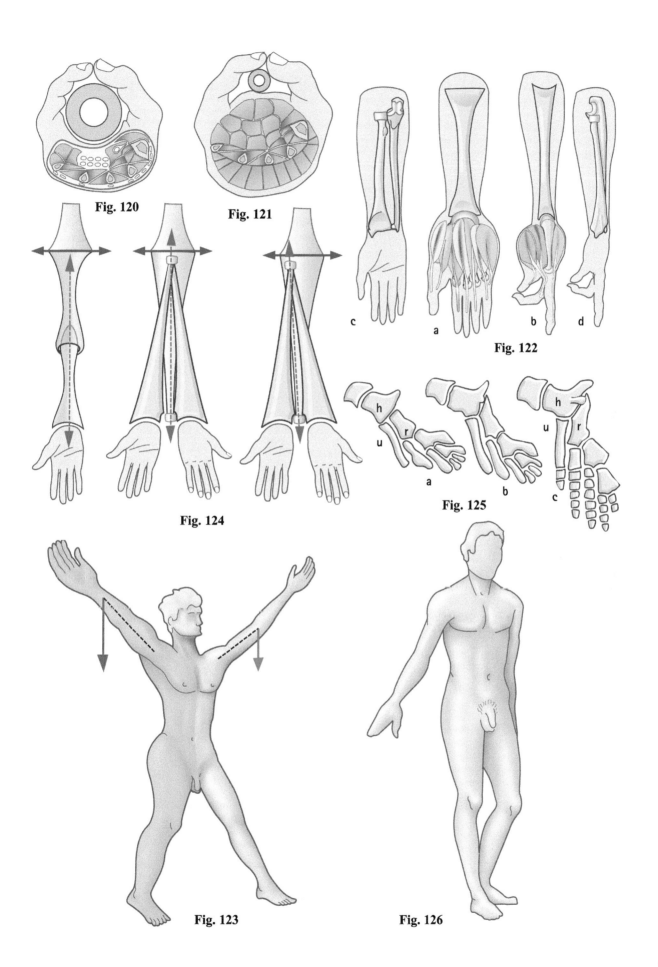

Fig. 120

Fig. 121

Fig. 122

Fig. 124

Fig. 125

Fig. 123

Fig. 126

Mechanical disturbances of pronation and supination

Fractures of the two bones of the forearm
(Figs 127 and 128, inspired by Merle d'Aubigné)

The displacement of the fragments varies with the level of the fracture lines and is determined by the resultant muscular pull:

- If the fracture line lies in the **upper third of the radius** (Fig. 127), the two separate fragments are acted upon by antagonistic muscles, i.e. the supinators acting on the upper fragment and the pronators on the lower fragment. Thus the gap between the fragments due to the rotation of one fragment relative to the other will be maximal with the upper fragment in extreme supination and the lower fragment in maximal pronation.

- If the fracture line lies in the **middle of the radial shaft** (Fig. 128), the gap is less marked, since the pronation of the lower fragment is due only to the pronator quadratus and the supination of the upper fragment is attenuated by the pronator teres. The gap is then reduced to half the maximum.

Therefore reduction of the fracture must aim not only at correcting the angular displacement but also at restoring the normal curvatures of these bones, especially of the radius, as follows:

- The curvature in the sagittal plane, concave anteriorly. If it is flattened or reversed, the range of pronation will be curtailed.

- The curvature in the coronal plane, essentially the 'pronator bend'. If it is not properly restored, the range of pronation will be limited by the decreased efficiency of the pronator teres.

Dislocations of the radio-ulnar joints

These rarely occur on their own because of the mechanical linkage between the two bones, and are usually associated with a fracture.

Dislocation of the inferior radio-ulnar joint

This is often combined with a proximal fracture of the radial shaft (blue arrow), i.e. the so-called **Galezzi's fracture** (Fig. 129). It is difficult to treat because of the persistent instability of the dislocated joint.

Dislocation of the superior radio-ulnar joint

This has some similarity with the previous and consists of anterior dislocation of the radial head (red arrow) associated with a fracture of the ulnar shaft (**Monteggia's fracture**) (Fig. 130), produced by direct trauma, e.g. a blow from a club or a truncheon. It is essential to reposition the radial head, which is rendered unstable by the pull of the biceps (B), and to repair the annular ligament.

Consequences of the relative shortening of the radius

The function of the radio-ulnar joint can be disrupted by a relative shortening of the radius due to any of the following:

- inadequate growth after an **unrecognized fracture in childhood** (Fig. 132)
- congenital malformation of the radius, as in **Madelung's disease** (Fig. 131)
- fracture of the distal radius, the most common type being the **Colles' fracture**, which predominantly afflicts the elderly. It produces a true dislocation of the inferior radio-ulnar joint in the coronal and sagittal planes, as follows:
  - **In the coronal plane**, the distal end of the radius is tilted laterally (Fig. 133), causing a widening of the articular interspace inferiorly. The pull on the articular disc (Fig. 134) often uproots the ulnar styloid process as it snaps at its base. This is the **Gérard-Marchant fracture.** The separation (diastasis) of the articular surfaces is made worse by a more or less extensive rupture of the interosseous membrane and of the medial ligament of the wrist joint.
  - **In the sagittal plane** the posterior tilt (not shown) of the fragment of the radial epiphysis interferes with pronation-supination.

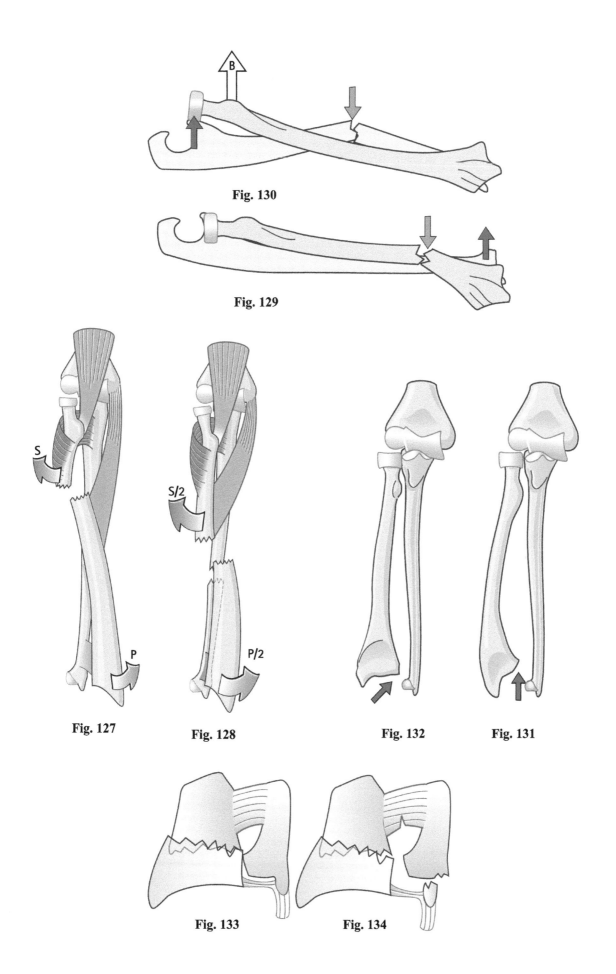

Fig. 130

Fig. 129

Fig. 127

Fig. 128

Fig. 132

Fig. 131

Fig. 133

Fig. 134

In the normal state (Fig. 135) the axes of the radial and ulnar articular surfaces coincide. When the two bones are separated (a) one can see that the articular surfaces are congruent. When the bones are brought together (b) the surfaces fit snugly one into the other.

When the distal epiphyseal fragment of the radius is tilted posteriorly (Fig. 136, a) the axes of the ulnar and radial articular surfaces form a solid angle open inferiorly and posteriorly with loss of congruence of the surfaces, as shown in diagram (b), where only the surfaces and their axes are included. Permanent dislocations of the inferior radio-ulnar joint often cause serious problems with pronation-supination, which can be treated by simple resection of the ulnar head (**Moore-Darrach's operation**) or by a definitive arthrodesis (immobilization) combined with a segmental resection of the ulnar shaft above the fracture in order to normalize pronation-supination (**M. Kapandji-L. Sauvé's operation**, Fig. 137).

Functional disturbances of the inferior radio-ulnar joint can also result from disturbances in the superior radio-ulnar joint, i.e. in the **Essex-Lopresti syndrome** (Fig. 138). Relative shortening of the radius can follow **resection of the radial head** after a comminuted fracture (a), **excessive wear and tear of the articular surfaces of the radio-humeral joint** (b), or a fracture of the radial neck with impaction into the head (c). It results in superior dislocation of the inferior radio-ulnar joint (d), with an abnormal inferior overshoot of the ulnar head, which can be measured by using the **ulnar variance index**. Only the anterior fibres (pink) of the interosseous membrane (Fig. 139) can check the ascent of the radius. If these fibres are torn or inadequate, there follows dislocation of the inferior radio-ulnar joint, i.e. the Essex-Lopresti syndrome, which is difficult to treat.

Our knowledge of the functional disturbances of the inferior radio-ulnar joint is in a state of flux, but one can conclude that fractures of the distal end of the radius (the most frequent) need to be well treated from the start.

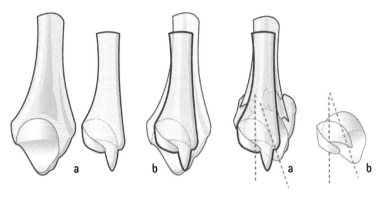

Fig. 135   **Fig. 136**

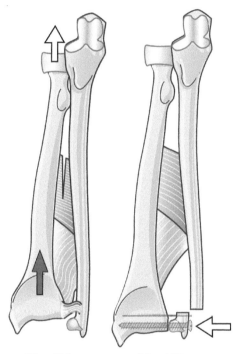

Fig. 139   **Fig. 137**

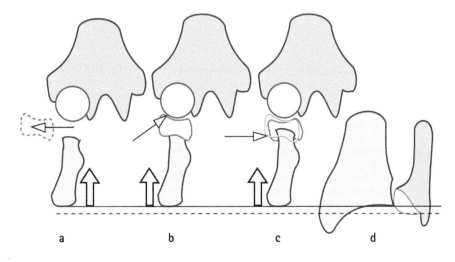

Fig. 138

The position of function and compensatory movements

'**One supinates with the forearm**', as when one turns a key in a lock (Fig. 140). In fact, when the upper limb hangs down beside the trunk with the elbow flexed, supination can take place only by rotation of the forearm on its long axis at the radio-ulnar joints. This can be called true supination, since the shoulder does not participate in this movement. This explains why paralysis of the movement of supination cannot be easily compensated. There is some compensation, however, since complete paralysis rarely occurs, because the biceps has a different nerve supply (musculo-cutaneous nerve) from the supinator radial nerve.

'**One pronates with the shoulder**' (Fig. 141). On the other hand, during pronation the action of the pronators can be augmented or replaced by abduction of the shoulder. This movement takes place when one empties a saucepan. When the shoulder is abducted at 90°, the hand is normally pronated by 90°.

The position of function of the forearm

For pronation-supination this position lies between these two positions:

- the intermediate position (Fig. 142), e.g. while holding a hammer
- the position of semi-pronation at 30-45° while holding a spoon (Fig. 143) or when writing (Fig. 144).

The position of function corresponds to a state of natural equilibrium between the antagonistic muscle groups so that expenditure of muscular energy is minimal.

The movement of pronation-supination is **essential for carrying food to the mouth**. In fact, when one picks up a piece of food lying on a horizontal plane as on a table or on the ground, grasping takes place with the hand pronated and the elbow extended. To carry it to the mouth the elbow must be bent and the hand supinated to present it to the mouth. The biceps are the ideal muscle for this **feeding movement**, since they are at once a flexor of the elbow and a supinator of the forearm.

Besides, **supination reduces the degree of associated elbow flexion**. If the same object had to be carried to the mouth with the arm pronated, a greater degree of elbow flexion would be required.

The waiter test

As with the shoulder, the overall function of the elbow can be evaluated by the **waiter test**. When a waiter carries a tray above his shoulder (Fig. 145), his elbow is flexed and his wrist is in full extension and pronation. When he lays the tray of glasses down on your table (Fig. 146), he carries out a triple movement of extension at the elbow, flexion at the wrist to the straight position and **above all full supination**. Thus the waiter test allows one to make a diagnosis of full supination, even at a distance by telephone. If you can carry a full glass on a plate without overturning it, you have full supination, an important movement in everyday life, e.g. picking up change at a supermarket checkout or even begging at the church door!

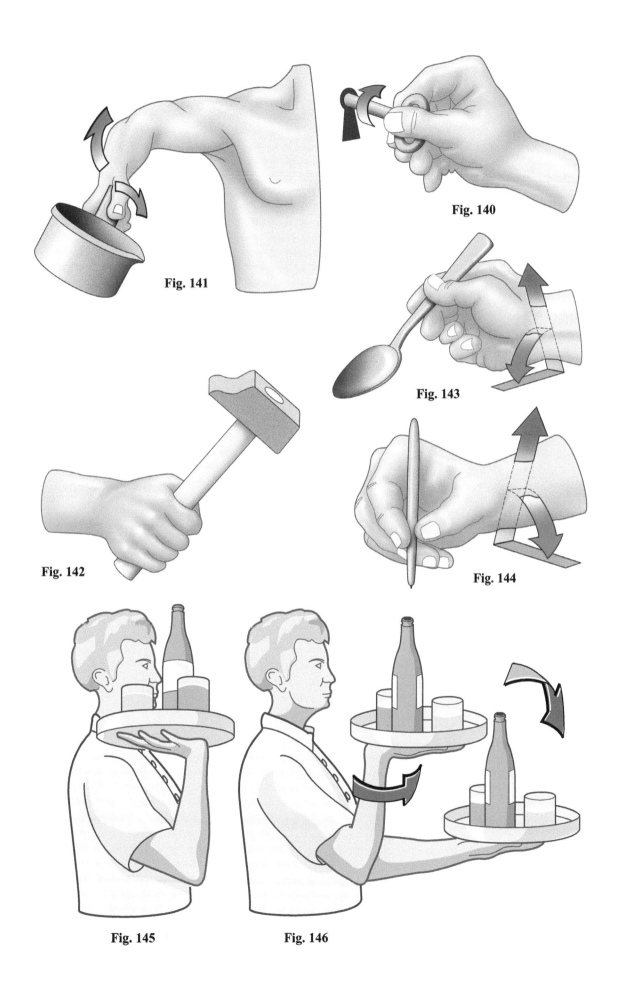

Fig. 140

Fig. 141

Fig. 142

Fig. 143

Fig. 144

Fig. 145

Fig. 146

Chapter 4

THE WRIST

The wrist is the distal joint of the upper limb and allows the hand, which is the effector segment, to assume the optimal position for prehension.

The articular complex of the wrist has two degrees of freedom. When these are combined with pronation-supination, i.e. rotation of the forearm around its long axis, a third degree of freedom is added, and the hand can be oriented at any angle to grasp or hold an object.

The nucleus of the wrist is the carpus, consisting of eight small bones, which over the last 30 years have been extensively studied by anatomists and by hand surgeons who operate daily on the wrist. Thus knowledge of the subject has been completely revamped and provides a better understanding of the very complex functional anatomy of this mechanically disconcerting articular complex, but we still need further study to understand it fully.

The articular complex of the wrist consists in actual fact of two joints, included with the inferior radio-ulnar joint in the same functional unit:

- the **radio-carpal joint** (wrist joint) between the carpal surface of the radius and the proximal row of the carpal bones
- the **mid-carpal joint** between the proximal and distal rows of the carpal bones.

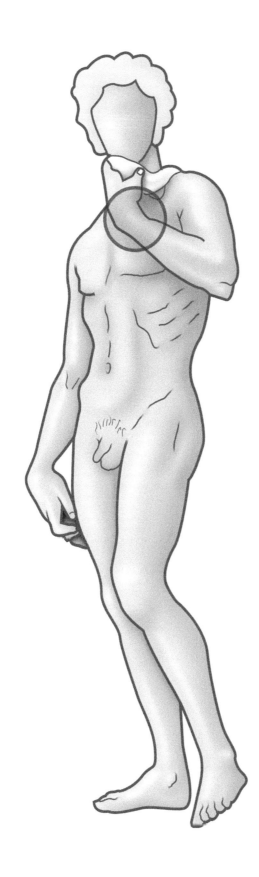

Movements of the wrist

Movements of the wrist (Fig. 1) occur around **two axes** when the hand is in the anatomical position, i.e. when sully supinated and straight, with its axis collinear with that of the forearm:

- **A transverse axis AA′**, lying in a coronal plane (C) and controlling the movements of **flexion-extension** in the sagittal plane (S):
  - **Flexion** (arrow 1): the anterior (palmar) surface of the hand moves towards the anterior aspect of the forearm.
  - **Extension** (arrow 2): the posterior (dorsal) surface of the hand moves towards the posterior aspect of the forearm. It is better to avoid the terms dorsiflexion, which contradicts the action of the extensor muscles, and even more palmar flexion, which is tautological. These two terms must be **banned** absolutely from the anatomical and medical literature.
- **An antero-posterior axis BB′**, lying in a sagittal plane (S) and controlling movements of **adduction-abduction**, which take place in the coronal plane and are wrongly called ulnar deviation or radial deviation, following the lead of anglophone authors:
  - **Adduction** or ulnar deviation (arrow 3): the hand moves towards the axis of the body, and its medial (palmar) border forms an obtuse angle with the medial border of the forearm.
  - **Abduction** or radial deviation (arrow 4): the hand moves away from the axis of the body, and its lateral (radial) border forms an obtuse angle with the lateral border of the forearm.

In actual fact, the natural movements of the wrist occur most often around oblique axes to produce the following:

- **combined flexion and adduction**
- **combined extension and abduction.**

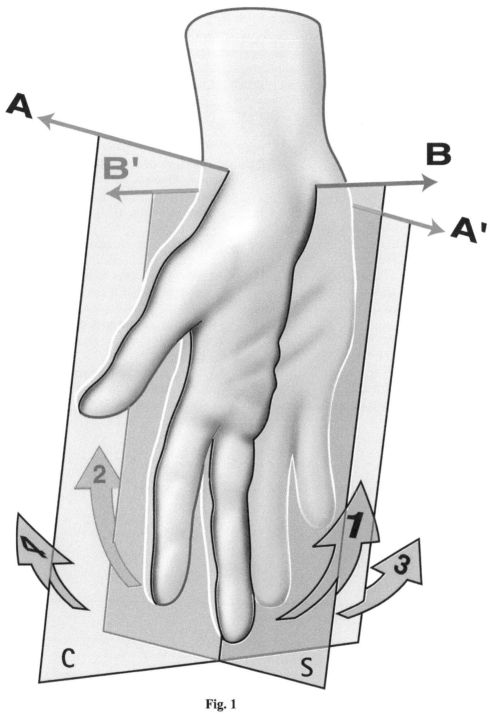

Fig. 1

Range of movements of the wrist

Movements of abduction-adduction

The range of these movements is measured from the **reference position** (Fig. 2), i.e. when the axis of the hand, which is shown diagrammatically as running through the middle finger and the third metacarpal, and the axis of the forearm are collinear.

The range of **abduction** (radial deviation) does not exceed 15° (Fig. 3).

The range of **adduction** (ulnar deviation) is 45° (Fig. 4), when measured as the angle between the reference position and the line joining the middle of the wrist and the tip of the middle finger (dashed blue line).

This range varies, however, being 30° if the axis of the hand is used for measurement and 55° if the axis of the middle finger is used. This is due to the fact that adduction of the hand is combined with adduction of the fingers.

For practical purposes the range of adduction is 45°.

The following points need to be stressed:

- The range of adduction (or ulnar deviation) is 2-3 times that of abduction (or radial deviation).
- The range of adduction is greater in supination than in pronation (Sterling Bunnell), when it falls short of 25-30°.

In general, the range of abduction and adduction is minimal when the wrist is fully flexed or extended, because of the tension developed in the carpal ligaments. It is maximal when the hand is in the reference position or slightly flexed, because the ligaments are relaxed.

Movements of flexion-extension

The range of these movements is measured from the **reference position** (Fig. 5), i.e. when the wrist is straight and the posterior aspect of the hand is in line with the posterior surface of the forearm.

The range of **active flexion** (Fig. 6) is 85°, falling just short of the right angle.

Active extension (Fig. 7) is wrongly called dorsiflexion, which is an oxymoron. It also has a range of 85°, falling short of the right angle.

As in the case of abduction and adduction, the range of these movements depends on the degree of slackness of the carpal ligaments. Flexion and extension are maximal when the hand is neither abducted nor adducted.

Passive movements of flexion-extension

The range of **passive flexion** (Fig. 8) exceeds 90° in pronation, i.e. 100°.

The range of **passive extension** (Fig. 9) exceeds 90°, i.e. 95°, in both pronation and supination.

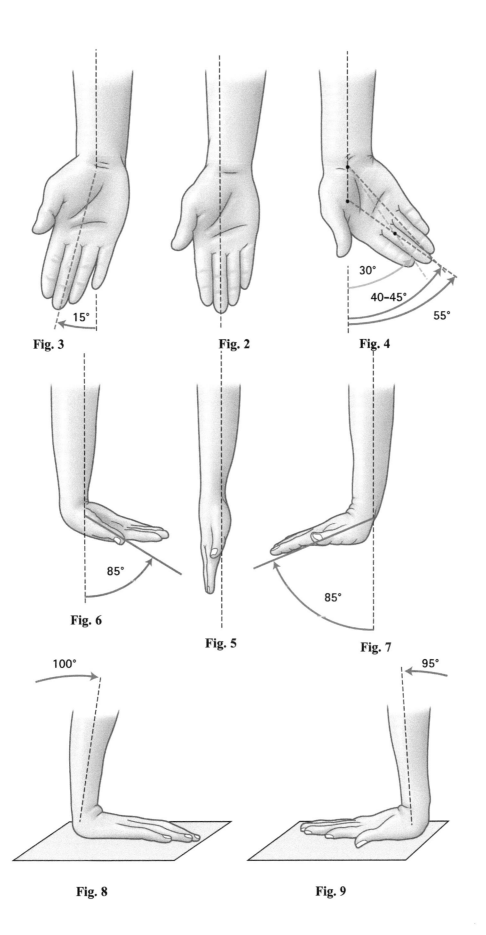

Fig. 3

15°

Fig. 2

Fig. 4

30°

40–45°

55°

Fig. 6

85°

Fig. 5

Fig. 7

85°

100°

Fig. 8

95°

Fig. 9

The movement of circumduction

This is defined as the combination of the movements of flexion-extension with those of adduction-abduction. It is thus a single movement, taking place about the two axes of the wrist joint simultaneously.

When circumduction is at its greatest, the axis of the hand traces in space a conical surface, called the cone of circumduction (Fig. 10), with its apex O at the centre of the wrist and a base defined in the diagram by the points F, R, E and C, which trace the path taken by the tip of the middle finger during maximal circumduction.

This cone is not regular and its base is not circular, because the range of the various elementary movements involved in circumduction is not symmetrical with respect to the axis of the forearm OO'. Since the range of movement is maximal in the sagittal plane FOE and minimal in the coronal plane ROC, the cone is flattened from side to side and its base is an ellipse distorted in space (Fig. 11), with its great axis FE running postero-anteriorly.

This ellipse is distorted medially (Fig. 12) because of the greater range of ulnar deviation. Therefore the axis of the cone of circumduction OA does not coincide with OO' but lies on its ulnar side at an angle of 15°. Besides, the position of the hand in 15° adduction is the position of equilibrium for the muscles controlling ulnar deviation and so is one of the components of the position of function.

In addition to the base of the cone of circumduction (Fig. 11) one can observe the following:
- a coronal section of the cone (Fig. 12), including a position of abduction (R), a position of adduction (C) and the axis of the cone of circumduction OA
- a sagittal section of the cone (Fig. 13) with the position in flexion F and the position in extension E.

Since the range of movements of the wrist is less in pronation than in supination, it follows that the cone of circumduction is less open in pronation. Nevertheless, because of the combined movements of pronation-supination, the 'flattening' of the cone of circumduction can be offset in some measure so that the axis of the hand can lie anywhere within a cone with an angle of aperture of 160-170°.

In addition, as typically occurs in **biaxial universal joints**, i.e. biaxial joints with two degrees of freedom (see the trapezo-metacarpal joint later), a concurrent or successive movement about these axes gives rise to **an automatic rotation**, i.e. **the conjunct rotation of MacConaill**, around the long axis of the mobile segment, i.e. the hand. As a result, the palm comes to lie obliquely with regard to the plane of the anterior aspect of the forearm. This is clear-cut only in the positions of extension-adduction and flexion-adduction. Its functional significance is different when the thumb is involved.

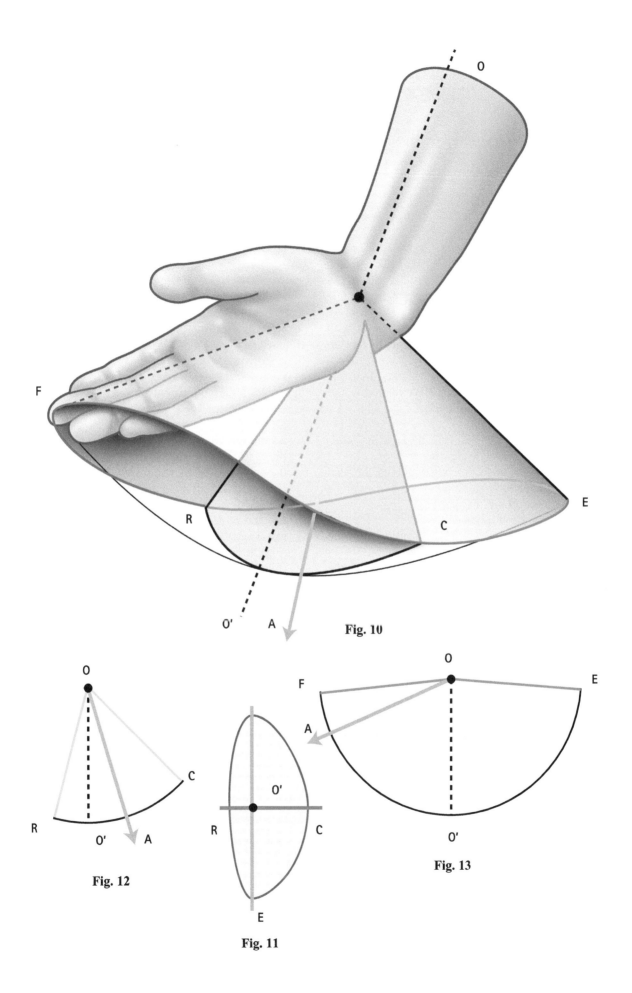

Fig. 10

Fig. 12

Fig. 11

Fig. 13

153

The articular complex of the wrist

This consists of **two joints** (Fig. 14):
1) the **radio-carpal joint** (1) between the distal end of the radius and the proximal row of the carpal bones
2) the **mid-carpal joint** (2), between the proximal and distal rows of the carpal bones.

The radio-carpal joint

This is a **condyloid joint** (Fig. 15). The articular surface of the carpal bones (considered to a first approximation as a single entity) exhibits **two convexities**:
- an **antero-posterior or a sagittal convexity** (arrow 1), with a transverse axis AA′ related to the movements of **flexion and extension**
- a **transverse convexity** (arrow 2), more marked than the former, with an antero-posterior axis BB′, related to the movements of **adduction and abduction**.

In the skeleton:
- The axis AA′ of flexion-extension runs through the interspace between the lunate and the capitate.
- The axis BB′ of abduction-adduction passes through the head of the capitate (not shown).

The **capsular ligaments** fall into two groups:
1) The **collateral ligaments** (Figs 16-18):
   - the **radial collateral ligament** (1), extending from the radial styloid process to the scaphoid
   - the **ulnar collateral ligament** (2), extending from the ulnar styloid process to the triquetrum and the pisiform.

The distal insertions of these ligaments lie more or less at the 'exit point' (red dot) of the axis of flexion and extension (AA′).

2) The **radio-carpal ligaments** (Figs 19-21, lateral views), which will be discussed in greater detail later:
   - The **anterior radio-carpal ligament** or rather the **anterior ligamentous complex** (3) is attached to the anterior edge of the concave distal surface of the radius and the neck of the capitate.
   - The **posterior radio-carpal ligament** or rather the **posterior ligamentous complex** (4) forms a posterior strap for the joint.

Both these ligaments are anchored on the carpus roughly at the 'exit points' (red dots) of the axis of abduction-adduction BB′. If, to a first approximation, the carpus is considered as a monolithic structure, as was thought 30 years ago and is now known to be incorrect (see further discussion later), the **action of the ligaments** of the radio-carpal joint can be broken down as follows:
- **During adduction-abduction** (Figs 16-18, anterior views) the medial and lateral collateral ligaments are active. **During adduction** (Fig. 17) the lateral ligament is stretched and the medial ligament relaxes. **During abduction** (Fig. 18) the opposite occurs, with a negligible contribution from the anterior ligament lying close to the centre of rotation.
- **During flexion-extension** (Figs 19-21, lateral views) the anterior and posterior ligaments are active. From the position of rest (Fig. 19) the posterior ligament is stretched during flexion (Fig. 20) and the anterior ligament is stretched during extension (Fig. 21), while the collateral ligaments are barely involved.

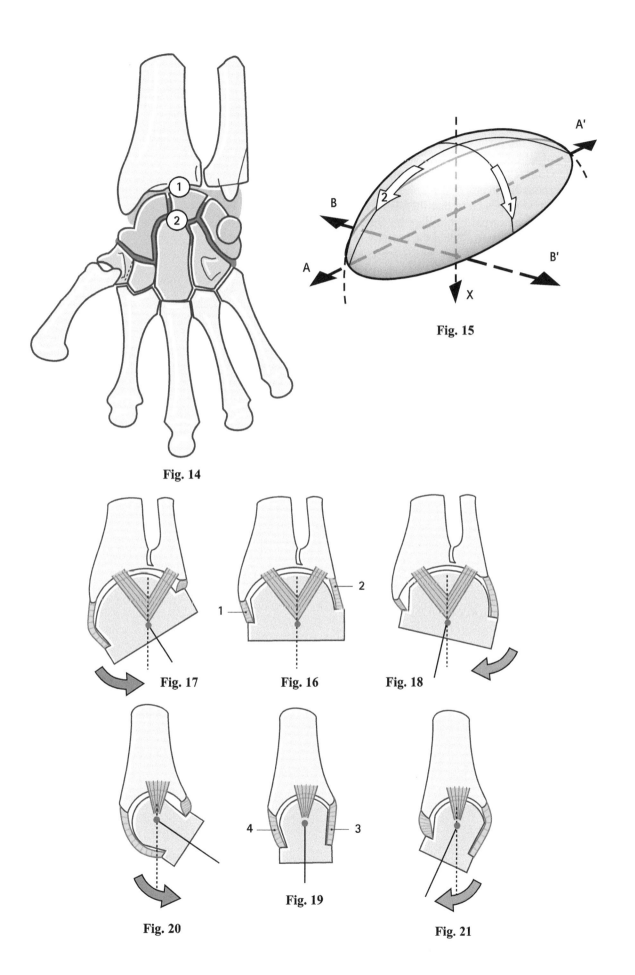

Fig. 14

Fig. 15

Fig. 17

Fig. 16

Fig. 18

Fig. 20

Fig. 19

Fig. 21

155

The articular surfaces of the radio-carpal joint (Figs 22 and 23; the numbers have the same meanings in both) are the proximal row of the carpal bones and its concave antebrachial surface. The **carpal surface** (Fig. 23, anterior view, with the bones pulled apart) consists of the juxtaposed proximal surfaces of the three proximal carpal bones arranged latero-medially, i.e. the **scaphoid** (1), the **lunate** (2) and the **triquetrum** (3), which are linked by interosseous ligaments (the **scapho-lunate** = s.l. and the **lunato-triquetral** = l.t.). Note that the **pisiform** bone (4) and the distal row of the carpal bones, i.e. the **trapezium** (5), the **trapezoid** (6), the **capitate** (7) and the **hamate** (8), do not belong to the radio-carpal joint. These bones are linked by interosseous ligaments (**trapezo-trapezoidal** = t.t., **trapezoido-capitate** = t.c. and **hamato-capitate** = h.c.).

The proximal surfaces of the scaphoid, lunate and triquetrum and their interosseous ligaments are coated with cartilage to form a **continuous articular surface**, i.e. the carpal surface of the radio-carpal joint.

The lower half of Figure 22 (inspired by Testut) shows the distal aspect of the joint, i.e. the articular surfaces of the **scaphoid** (1), the **lunate** (2) and the **triquetrum** (3). The upper half of Figure 22 shows the concave **antebrachial surface** of the joint formed by the following:

- the **distal articular surface of the radius** laterally, concave, cartilage-coated and divided by a blunt crest (9) into two facets corresponding to the scaphoid (10) and the hamate (11)
- the **distal surface of the articular disc** (12) medially, concave and cartilage-coated. Its apex is inserted at the foot of the ulnar styloid process (13) and the ulnar head (14), which overreaches it slightly anteriorly and posteriorly. Its base is occasionally incompletely attached, so that there is a tiny cleft (15) allowing the radio-carpal and the inferior radio-ulnar joints to communicate.

The capsule (16), shown intact posteriorly, binds together these two sets of articular surfaces. The radioscapholunate ligament (17) carries the blood vessels and extends from the anterior border of the distal radial articular surface to the interosseous scapholunate ligament. Its length and its flexibility allow it to follow the carpus as it moves on the radial articular surface.

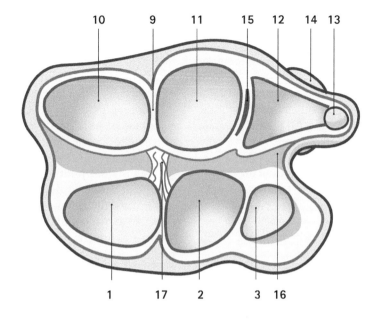

Fig. 22

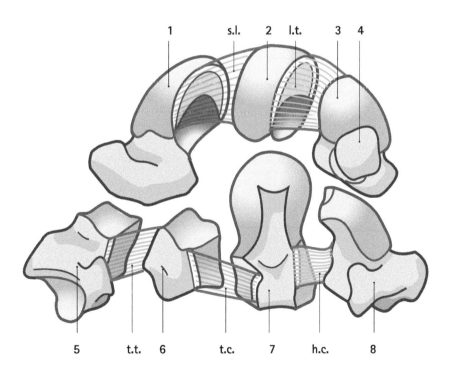

Fig. 23

The mid-carpal joint

This joint (Fig. 24, opened posteriorly (inspired by Testut)), lying between the two rows of carpal bones, consists of the following:

1) the **proximal surface** (postero-inferior view), made up of three bones arranged latero-medially as follows:
   - the **scaphoid**, with two slightly convex surfaces distally, one for the trapezium (1) and the other medially for the trapezoid (2), and a deeply concave (3) medial facet for the capitate
   - the distal surface of the **lunate** (4), with its distal concavity articulating with the head of the capitate
   - the distal surface of the **triquetrum** (5), concave distally and laterally, articulating with the proximal surface of the hamate.

The pisiform bone, in contact with the palmar surface of the triquetrum, does not belong to the mid-carpal joint and is not shown in this diagram.

2) the **distal surface** (postero-superior view), consisting of the following bones latero-medially:
   - the proximal surfaces of the **trapezium** (6) and the **trapezoid** (7)
   - the head of the **capitate** (8) in contact with the scaphoid and the lunate

- the proximal surface of the **hamate** (9), which is mostly in contact with the triquetrum but also has a small facet (10) in contact with the lunate.

If one considers each row of carpal bones as a single structure, then the mid-carpal joint has two parts:

- a **lateral part**, consisting of plane surfaces (trapezium and trapezoid in contact with the base of the scaphoid), i.e. **a plane joint**
- a **medial part**, made up of the surfaces of the head of the capitate and the hamate, convex in all planes and fitting into the concavity offered by the three proximal carpal bones, i.e. **a condyloid joint**.

The **head of the capitate** forms a central hinge, on which the lunate can tilt laterally (Fig. 25), rotate around its long axis (Fig. 26) and above all tilt antero-posteriorly (Fig. 27), i.e. posteriorly (a) into the position of volar intercalated segment instability (VISI) and anteriorly (b) into the position of dorsal intercalated segment instability (DISI) (p. 168).

The distal row of carpal bones forms a relatively rigid structure, whereas the proximal row, which represents an '**intercalated segment**' between the radius and the distal row, can undergo all types of movement, including displacements of one bone relative to another, as a result of the laxity of the ligaments.

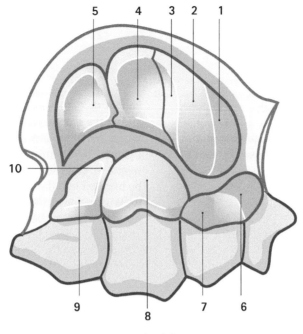

Fig. 24

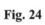

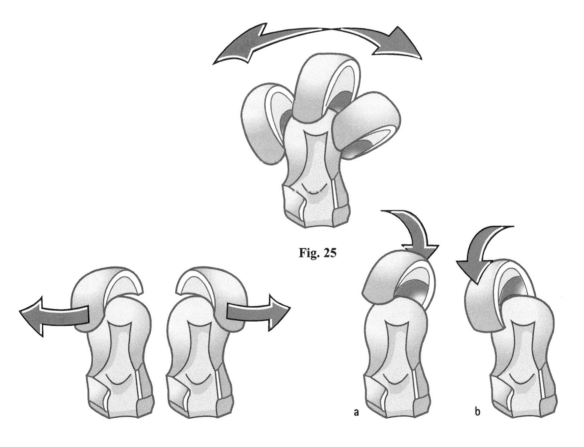

Fig. 25

Fig. 26

a   b

Fig. 27

The ligaments of the radio-carpal and mid-carpal joints

The description of these ligaments is in constant flux, but we feel that N. Kuhlmann's (1978) version offers the best explanation of their role in stabilizing the wrist joint and especially in ensuring its adaptation to the constraints imposed by movements of the wrist.

The Anterior Ligaments

Figure 28 (**anterior view**) shows:
- the two collateral ligaments of the radio-carpal joint
- the anterior radio-carpal ligaments, composed of two bands
- the ligaments of the mid-carpal joint.

The two collateral ligaments of the radio-carpal joint
- The **ulnar collateral ligament**, attached proximally to the ulnar styloid process and intricately admixed with the fibres of the **articular disc** at its apex (1). It then divides into a **posterior stylo-triquetral band** (2) and an **anterior stylo-pisiform band** (3). According to modern authors, this ligament plays a minor role in the physiology of the wrist.
- The **radial collateral ligament**, also made up of two bands attached to the radial styloid process:
  - a **posterior band**, (4), running from the apex of the styloid process to a point just below the lateral aspect of the proximal articular surface of the scaphoid
  - an **anterior band** (5), very thick and strong, extending from the anterior border of the styloid process to the scaphoid tubercle.

The anterior radio-carpal ligaments
These are composed of two bands:
- Laterally, the **anterior radio-lunate band** (6), running obliquely inferiorly and medially from the anterior edge of the radial articular surface to the anterior horn of the lunate; hence its name of **anterior brake of the lunate.** It is supplemented medially by the anterior ulno-lunate ligament (7).
- Medially, the **anterior radio-triquetral band** (8) (recognized by N. Kuhlmann) is attached proximally to the medial half of the anterior edge of the distal surface of the radius and to the anterior border of the ulnar notch of the radius, where its fibres are interwoven with those of the anterior ligament of the inferior radio-ulnar joint (9). This triangular ligament, stout and resistant, runs inferiorly and medially to be inserted into the anterior surface of the triquetrum lateral to its articular surface for the pisiform. It forms the anterior portion of the 'triquetral sling', which will be discussed later.

The ligaments of the mid-carpal joint
- The **radio-capitate ligament** (10), running obliquely distally and medially from the lateral position of the anterior border of the distal surface of the radius to the anterior aspect of the capitate. It lies in the same ligamentous plane as the radio-lunate and the radio-triquetral bands and is thus an anterior ligament for both the radio-carpal and the mid-carpal joints.
- The **lunato-capitate ligament** (12), stretching vertically from the anterior horn of the lunate to the anterior aspect of the neck of the capitate and directly continuous distally with the radio-lunate ligament.
- The **triquetro-capitate ligament** (13), running obliquely inferiorly and laterally from the anterior aspect of the triquetrum to the neck of the capitate, where it forms a true ligamentous relay station with the two previously described ligaments. The anterior aspect of the capitate contains a point of convergence of ligaments (14), i.e. the apex of Poirier's V-shaped space, where the scapho-capitate ligament is also inserted (11).
- The **scapho-trapezial ligament** (15), short but broad and resistant, linking the tubercle of the scaphoid to the anterior aspect of the trapezium above its oblique crest and supplemented medially by the scapho-trapezoidal ligament (16).
- The **triquetro-hamatal ligament** (17), which is in effect the medial ligament of the mid-carpal joint.
- Finally, the **piso-hamate** (18) and the **piso-metacarpal ligaments** (19), the latter also belonging to the carpo-metacarpal joint.

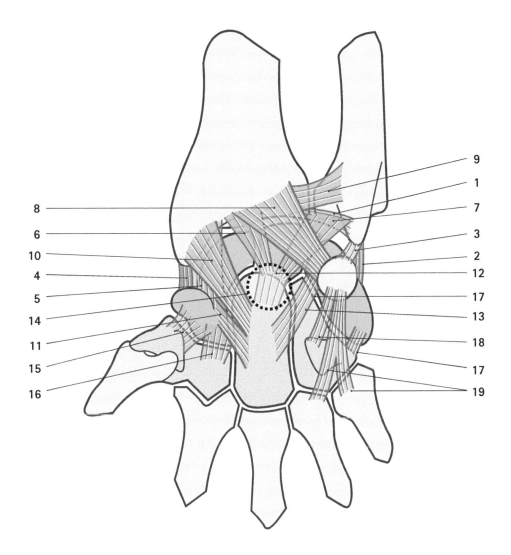

Fig. 28

The Posterior Ligaments

Figure 29 (**posterior view**) shows:

- The posterior band (4) of the radial collateral ligament of the radio-carpal joint.
- The posterior band (2) of the ulnar collateral ligament of the radio-carpal joint, with its fibres interwoven with those of the articular disc (1).
- The posterior ligament of the radio-carpal joint, consisting of the two following bands running obliquely, distally and medially:
  - The **posterior radio-lunate band** (20), called the posterior brake of the lunate.
  - The **posterior radio-triquetral band** (21), with its mode of insertion fairly similar to that of its anterior homologue, including the dovetailing of its fibres with the posterior ligament of the radio-ulnar joint (22) on the posterior border of the ulnar notch of the radius. This band completes the 'triquetral sling'.
- The two transverse posterior straps of the wrist:
  - The **proximal band** (23), running transversely from the posterior aspect of the triquetrum (25) to that of the scaphoid (24) as it relays through the posterior horn of the lunate and sends fibres to the radial collateral ligament and the posterior radio-triquetral ligament.
  - The **distal band** (26), stretching obliquely, laterally and slightly distally from the posterior aspect of the triquetrum to that of the trapezoid (27) and to that of the trapezium (28) along the posterior surface of the capitate.
- The **triquetro-hamate ligament** (30), whose posterior fibres are inserted into the posterior aspect of the triquetrum, and which acts as a relay station for the anterior ligaments.
- Finally, the **posterior scapho-trapezoid ligament** (29).

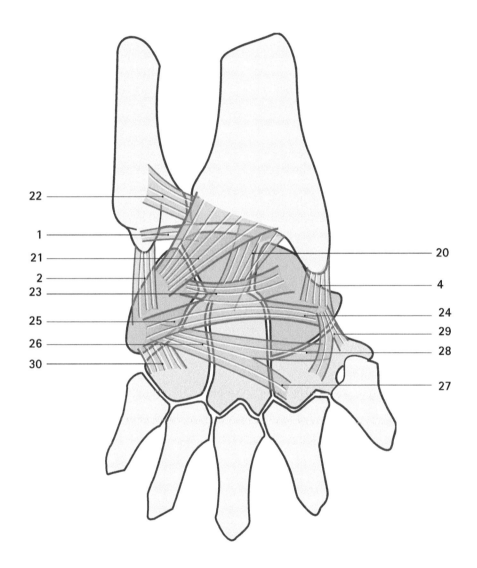

Fig. 29

The stabilizing role of the ligaments

Stabilization in the coronal plane

The prime function of the ligaments of the wrist is to stabilize the wrist in the coronal and sagittal planes.

In the coronal plane (Fig. 30, diagrammatic view from the front) the ligaments are essential because the concave antebrachial surface of the wrist joint faces inferiorly and medially, so that as a whole it can be represented by a plane running obliquely, proximo-distally and proximo-laterally at an angle of 25-30° with the horizontal plane. As a result of the pull of the longitudinal muscles, when the carpus is in the straight position, it **tends to slip proximally and medially** in the direction of the red arrow.

On the other hand, if the carpus is **adducted** to approximately 30° (Fig. 31), the compressive force of the muscles (white arrow) now acts perpendicular to the plane of movement previously mentioned and stabilizes the carpus by bringing back the carpal bones into the centre of the joint. Therefore this position of slight adduction is the natural position of the wrist, i.e. the position of function, coinciding with the position of maximal stability. Conversely (Fig. 32), when the wrist is **abducted**, however slightly, the compressive force of the long muscles accentuates the instability and tends to displace the carpal bones proximally and medially (red arrow).

The ulnar and radial collateral ligaments of the radio-carpal joint, running lengthwise like the muscles themselves, cannot check this dislocating effect. As shown by Kuhlmann, the full brunt is borne by the **two radio-triquetral bands of the anterior and posterior ligaments of the radio-carpal joint** (Fig. 33), as they run obliquely, proximally and laterally and thus keep the carpal bones in position (white arrow) by preventing their medial displacement (red arrow).

Figure 34 (**postero-medial view**) shows the distal end of the radius after removal of the distal end of the ulna. Also seen are the ulnar notch of the radius (1) and the triquetrum (2), flanked by the pisiform (3) after removal of the other carpal bones (not shown here). The triquetrum and the radius are linked by two radio-triquetral ligaments, anterior (4) and posterior (5), which constitute the 'triquetral sling' (described by **N. Kuhlman**), responsible for exerting a permanent proximal and medial pull on the triquetrum. This sling, as we shall see later, plays a vital role in the mechanics of the carpus during abduction.

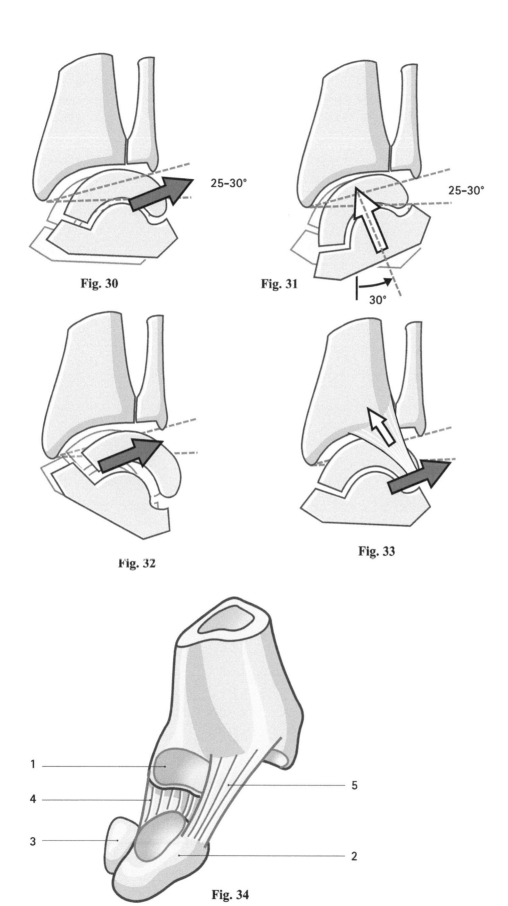

Fig. 30

Fig. 31

Fig. 32

Fig. 33

Fig. 34

Stabilization in the sagittal plane

In the sagittal plane roughly similar events take place.

Because the **concave proximal articular surface of the radio-carpal joint** points distally and anteriorly (Fig. 35, lateral view, where the centre of rotation of the lunato-capitate joint is marked by a black cross), the proximal carpal bones tend to slide proximally and anteriorly in the direction of the red arrow, i.e. in a plane parallel to that of the proximal surface of the joint, at an angle of 20-25° to the horizontal.

When the **wrist is flexed** 30-40° (Fig. 36) the muscular pull (red arrows) tends to displace the carpal bones in a plane perpendicular to the proximal surface of the radio-carpal joint, thus repositioning and stabilizing these bones.

Thus the **role of the ligaments** (Fig. 37) is relatively reduced. The anterior ligaments are relaxed and inactive, whereas the posterior brake of the lunate and the proximal band of the trans-verse carpal ligament are stretched, thus bringing the lunate and the antebrachial surface of the joint closer together (red arrow). **When the wrist is in the straight position** (Fig. 38), the tensions developed in the anterior and posterior ligaments are equal, and as a result the carpal bones are stabilized in contact with the antebrachial surface of the joint.

But **when the wrist is extended** (Fig. 39) the tendency of the carpal bones to escape proximally and anteriorly (red arrow) is reinforced. Under these circumstances, **the ligaments become essential** (Fig. 40), not so much the posterior ones, which are slackened, as the anterior ones, which develop a tension proportional to the degree of extension. Their deep surfaces displace the lunate and the head of the capitate proximally and posteriorly (red arrow), thereby repositioning and stabilizing the proximal row of the carpal bones.

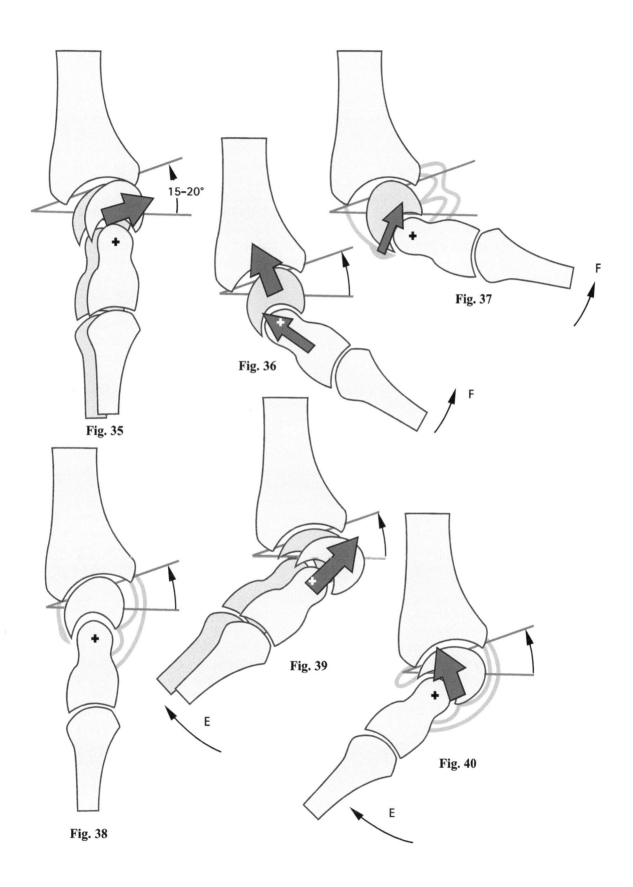

Fig. 35

Fig. 36

Fig. 37

Fig. 38

Fig. 39

Fig. 40

The dynamic properties of the carpus

The lunate pillar

It is known that the carpus is not a fixed structure, and the concept of it as a monolith no longer corresponds to reality. In fact, one must keep in mind a **geometrically variable carpus**, which alters its shape as a result of the **relative movements of the bones**, produced by **bony contacts** and **ligamentous restraints**. These elementary movements have been extensively studied by Kuhlmann, as they occur in the **median pillar** of the lunate and capitate and in the **lateral pillar** of the scaphoid, trapezium and trapezoid.

The dynamic properties of the median pillar depend on the asymmetrical shape of the lunate, which is bulkier and thicker anteriorly than posteriorly. Thus the head of the capitate is capped by a variably shaped lunate, resembling a Phrygian cap (Fig. 41), a Cossack's hat (Fig. 49) or even a turban (Fig. 50); rarely it resembles a symmetrical two-pointed hat (Fig. 44), and in this case it is the head of the capitate that is asymmetrical, with a greater obliquity anteriorly. In about 50% of subjects, the lunate resembles a Phrygian cap as it lies wedge-wise between the capitate and the concave articular surface of the radio-carpal joint. Thus the **effective distance** between these two structures varies with the degree of flexion-extension of the wrist.

When the wrist is straight (Fig. 45), this distance corresponds to the mean thickness of the lunate.

When the wrist is extended (Fig. 46), the distance is less, since it corresponds to the minimal thickness of the lunate.

When the wrist is flexed (Fig. 47), the distance is increased, since it corresponds to the full thickness of the bulkier portion of the lunate.

However, the **obliquity of the antebrachial surface of the wrist joint** is also added to this effective distance and thus can neutralize some of its effects. Thus it is when the wrist is straight that the distance between the centre of the head of the capitate and the antebrachial articular surface of the wrist joint is maximal as measured along the long axis of the radius.

When the wrist is extended (Fig. 46), the proximal 'ascent' of the head of the capitate is partly cancelled by the distal 'descent' of the posterior edge of the proximal surface of the wrist joint.

When the wrist is flexed (Fig. 47), its 'descent' is partly cancelled by the 'ascent' of the anterior border of the proximal surface of the wrist joint. Thus the centre of the head of the capitate lies in both cases roughly at the same level (h), i.e. slightly proximal to its position when the wrist is straight (Fig. 45).

On the other hand, **when the wrist is flexed** (Fig. 47), this centre undergoes an **anterior displacement** (a) equal to more than twice the posterior displacement (p) occurring during extension. As a result, the tensions and moments of force developed by the flexor and extensor muscles of the wrist are inversely related.

Classically, flexion is greater at the radio-carpal (50°) than at the mid-carpal joint (35°) and conversely extension is greater at the mid-carpal (50°) than at the radio-carpal joint (35°). This is certainly true for the extreme ranges of movement, but in movements of small range the degree of flexion and extension is almost equal in both joints.

Because of the **asymmetry of the lunate**, the carpus is very sensitive to the relative location of the lunate in the articular complex. When the wrist is in the straight position (Fig. 48), the lunate is held down securely by the anterior and posterior ligamentous 'brakes'. If then the lunate is tilted anteriorly (Fig. 49) or posteriorly (Fig. 50) without any flexion or extension of the capitate relative to the radius, it can be observed that the centre of the capitate is displaced proximally (e) as well as posteriorly (c) or anteriorly (b) respectively. Hence the localized instability of the lunate, caused by rupture or overstretching of its anterior (Fig. 49) or of its posterior (Fig. 50) ligamentous 'brake', will spread through the capitate to the entire carpus.

The stability of the lunate depends on the intactness of its attachments to the scaphoid and the triquetrum. If its attachment to the scaphoid is broken, it **tilts anteriorly** (Fig. 51) by extension into the radio-carpal joint, causing what the Americans call **DISI** (dorsal intercalated segment instability). If its attachment to the triquetrum is lost, it tilts posteriorly (Fig. 52) by flexion into the radio-carpal joint cavity, causing **VISI** (volar intercalated segment instability). These two terms have become very important in explaining the pathology of the carpus.

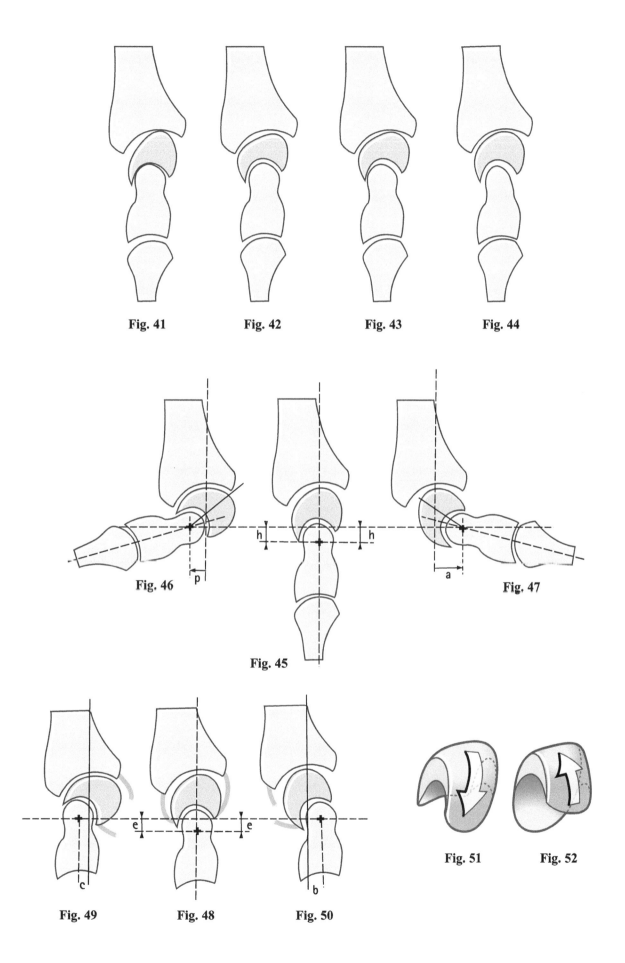

Fig. 41

Fig. 42

Fig. 43

Fig. 44

Fig. 46

Fig. 45

Fig. 47

Fig. 49

Fig. 48

Fig. 50

Fig. 51

Fig. 52

The scaphoid pillar

The dynamic properties of the lateral pillar depend on the shape and spatial orientation of the scaphoid. In Figure 53 (lateral view) the scaphoid is kidney-shaped or bean-shaped, with its proximal rounded end corresponding to the concave distal articular surface of the radius and its distal end forming the tubercle in contact with the trapezoid (not shown) and the trapezium. It lies clearly anterior to the trapezoid and the capitate because **it is the starting-point of antepulsion, i.e. movement of the thumb anterior to the plane of the palm.** Consequently the scaphoid is **jammed obliquely between the radius and the trapezius,** with the degree of obliqueness depending on its shape. Thus the scaphoid can be **kidney-shaped and 'lying down'** (Fig. 53), **bent and 'sitting down'** (Fig. 54) or **mostly straight and 'erect'** (Fig. 55). The 'lying down' scaphoid is the most frequent type and will be shown in the diagrams.

Because of its elongated shape, the scaphoid has a long diameter and a short diameter (Fig. 56), so that contact with the articular surface of the radius and the proximal surface of the trapezium varies with the position of the scaphoid. This underlies the **variations in the effective distance** between these two bones. In the **neutral position** (Fig. 57), i.e. when the wrist is straight, this distance is maximal. Then the scaphoid and the distal surface of the radius are in contact at a and a′, and the scaphoid and the centre of the proximal surface of the trapezium are in contact at b and g. The anterior ligaments, i.e. the radio-scaphoid (pale green) and the scapho-trapezial (dark green) ligaments, are neither stretched nor relaxed.

During extension (Fig. 58) the effective distance is reduced as the scaphoid rises and the trapezium moves posteriorly. Contact between the articular surface of the radius and the scaphoid occurs at c-c′, and between the trapezium and the scaphoid at d-g. The point of contact c′ on the radius is more anterior, while the point of contact d′ on the distal surface of the scaphoid is more posterior. The tension in the anterior ligaments checks these movements.

In flexion (Fig. 59), the distance between the radius and the trapezium is also reduced, but more so than during extension. The scaphoid lies down completely flat and the trapezium slides proximally. The following findings deserve special mention:

1) The **contact points** (e, e′, f and g) move on the articular surfaces of the radius and of the scaphoid (Fig. 60) as follows:
   - **On the radial articular surface** the point of contact in extension (c′) lies anterior to the point of contact in the neutral position (a′) and both of these contact points lie anterior to the contact point in flexion (e′).
   - **On the proximal articular surface of the scaphoid** the contact point (e) in flexion lies anterior, the contact point (c) in extension lies posterior and the contact point (a) in the neutral position lies in between. On the distal articular surface of the scaphoid the contact points have the same relative location, i.e. f for flexion lying anterior, d for extension lying posterior and b for the neutral position lying in between. The important point in terms of disease is that the 'lying down' scaphoid (Fig. 60) exerts maximal pressure on the **posterior part of the radial articular surface** (a′ and e′), which is the seat of incipient osteoarthritis secondary to abnormal scapho-lunate relationships (see later).

2) The **effective diameters of the scaphoid** ab, cd and ef, corresponding to the neutral position, extension and flexion respectively, are almost parallel and almost equal, with cd and ef being nearly parallel, ab and ef being almost equal and cd being slightly shorter. **So the anterior tilt of the scaphoid reduces the 'effective distance' between the radius and the trapezium.**

3) The **displacement of the trapezium relative to the radius** (Fig. 61): in the neutral position (N), in flexion (F) and in extension (E) the locations of the trapezium lie along the arc of a circle concentric with that of the distal surface of the radius, while the trapezium also rotates on itself through an angle virtually equal to the angle subtended by the arc of a circle representing its excursion from F to E. Hence its proximal surface always points towards the centre of the circle C.

So far we have discussed the concurrent movements of the scaphoid and trapezium. Later the isolated movements of the scaphoid will be discussed.

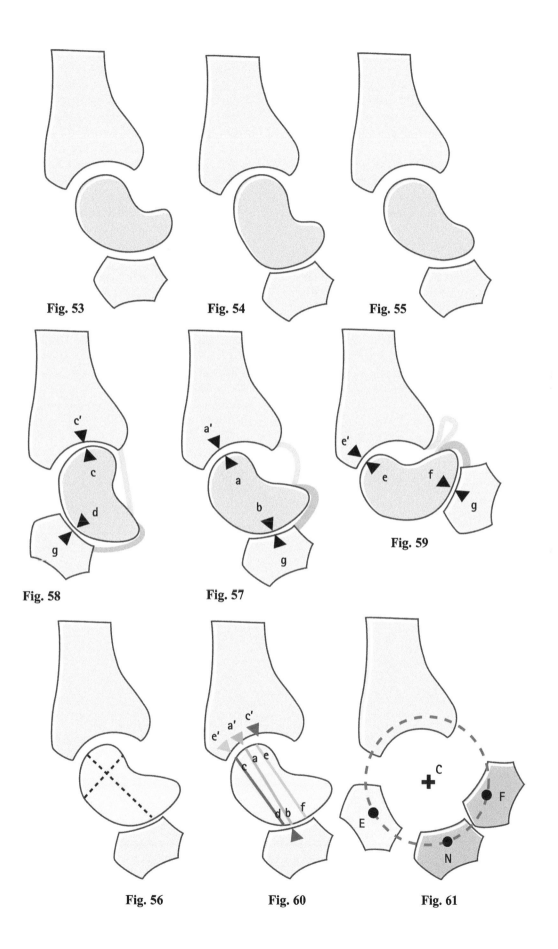

Fig. 53

Fig. 54

Fig. 55

Fig. 58

Fig. 57

Fig. 59

Fig. 56

Fig. 60

Fig. 61

Movements of the scaphoid

Located in the middle of the lateral pillar, the scaphoid is jammed between the trapezium and the trapezoid distally and the articular surface of the radius proximally so that it tends to tilt anteriorly during flexion and **come to lie underneath the radius**.

- The **first stabilizing factor** (Fig. 62) is its attachment to the trapezium by the very important **scapho-trapezial ligament**, to the trapezoid by the **scapho-trapezoidal ligament** and to the capitate by the **scapho-capitate ligament**.
- The **second stabilizing factor** (Fig. 63) is the strong radio-capitate ligament, extending from the anterior border of the radial styloid process at the centre of the relay station of the ligaments to the anterior aspect of the capitate. As it runs obliquely, inferiorly and medially, it forms a tie-like sling along the anterior aspect of the scaphoid in a depression lying between its proximal articular surface and its tubercle. When stretched, this ligament brings back the inferior pole of the scaphoid posteriorly (arrow). More important (Fig. 64, anterior view), when the scaphoid tilts anteriorly to lie down underneath the radius (arrow), the radio-capitate ligament checks this tilting movement.
- The **third stabilizing factor** (Fig. 65) is the tendon of the *palmaris longus*, which runs anterior to the scaphoid in a fibrous tunnel towards its insertion into the anterior surface of the base of the second metacarpal. Figure 66 (lateral view) demonstrates perfectly how contraction of this tendon (green arrow) pulls back the scaphoid posteriorly (red arrow).

The tilting movements of the scaphoid can be represented diagrammatically in the following lateral views:

- **When the scaphoid lies flat in flexion** (Fig. 67) after being pushed by the first two metacarpals (red arrow), its inferior pole slides on the proximal articular surfaces of the trapezium and of the trapezoid (curved red arrow). This movement is controlled by the tension developed in the scapho-trapezial and the scapho-trapezoidal ligaments and also in the radio-capitate ligament (shown as a transparent structure). At the same time, its proximal pole rotates under the concave articular surface of the radius and hits its posterior border. Furthermore, the contraction of the *palmaris longus* pulls it back posteriorly.
- **When the lateral pillar is being stretched** (Fig. 68) by the first two metacarpals (red arrow), the scaphoid rights itself, helped by the contraction of the *palmaris longus*, which checks the elongation of the pillar. Meanwhile its base slides posteriorly on the trapezium and the trapezoid, and its proximal pole goes back into the concavity of the radial articular surface.

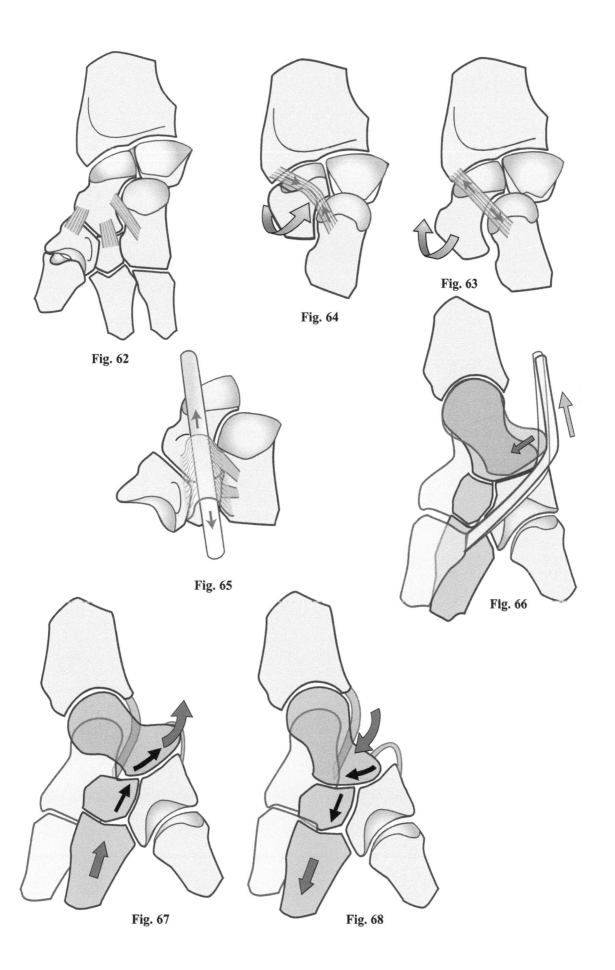

Fig. 62

Fig. 63

Fig. 64

Fig. 65

Fig. 66

Fig. 67

Fig. 68

173

The scaphoid-lunate couple

Kuhlmann divides the movements of flexion-extension of the wrist into four sectors (Fig. 69):

1) The **sector of permanent adaptability I**, extending up to 20°. The elementary movements are small and difficult to recognize, the ligaments stay slack and the pressure on the articular surfaces is minimal. The most common movements take place in this sector, and normal mobility must be restored here after any operation or trauma.

1) The **sector of everyday movements II**, extending to 40°. The ligaments begin to be stretched and intra-articular pressures start to rise. Up to this point, the movements occurring at the wrist and mid-carpal joints have roughly the same range.

1) The **sector of increasing physiological restraints III**, extending up to 80°. The tensions developed in the ligaments and the intra-articular pressures rise to a maximum to achieve eventually the locked or close-packed position of MacConaill.

1) The **sector of pathological restraints IV**, exceeding 80°. From this point onwards, movement can only occur **if ligaments are torn or forcibly overextended**. This event, often clinically undetected, can then lead to instability of the wrist and **secondary fracture or dislocation**, as will be discussed later.

These notions of restraint and locking of the joints are essential for the understanding of the **asynchrony of the locking mechanism** of the lunate and scaphoid pillars during extension of the wrist.

In effect, the **locking of the scaphoid pillar in extension** (Fig. 71), due to maximal stretching of the radio-scaphoid (1) and the scapho-trapezial (2) ligaments and jamming of the scaphoid between the trapezium and the articular surface of the radius, precedes the **locking of the lunate pillar in extension** (Fig. 70), which is due to stretching of the anterior radio-lunate (8) and the lunato-capitate (4) ligaments and also to the **bony impact** of the posterior aspect of the neck of the capitate on the posterior edge of the proximal articular surface of the

wrist joint (black arrow). Thus extension goes on in the lunate pillar when it has already stopped in the scaphoid pillar.

Starting from the **position of flexion** (Fig. 72, lateral view of the lunate and scaphoid together), at first (Fig. 73) the scaphoid and lunate move together during extension and then (Fig. 74) the scaphoid comes to a halt, while the lunate tilts forwards 30° more thanks to the **elasticity of the interosseous scapho-lunate ligament**. Thus the total range (S) of movement of the lunate is 30° greater than that of the scaphoid (s).

This **scapho-lunate ligament** (Fig. 75, diagrammatic view of the medial aspect of the scaphoid), shown here in pink and transparent after it has been excessively stretched (L), links the two adjacent surfaces of the scaphoid and lunate. It is stronger and thicker posteriorly than anteriorly, and its proximal surface is covered by cartilage continuous with that covering the adjacent bones. This ligament is relatively pliable and can be twisted (Fig. 76) along its axis X. Relative to the scaphoid the lunate can move as follows:

- **It can tilt anteriorly**, into the position of dorsal intercalated segment instability (DISI), since the lunate lies posterior to the radius (hence the other term dorsal instability).
- **It can tilt posteriorly**, into the position of volar intercalated segment instability (VISI) because the lunate comes to lie anterior to the radius (hence volar or palmar instability).

In the **normal state** (Fig. 77: the scapholunate angle) the lunate lies neatly side by side with the scaphoid and can move for 30° (Fig. 78). These relative movements can be recognized by the **changes in the scapho-lunar angle**, formed by the contour line of the scaphoid (blue dotted line) and the line running through the two horns of the lunate (red dotted line). This angle is measured between the extreme positions of flexion and extension of the wrist. When the **scapho-lunate ligament is torn** (Fig. 79), the whole of the lunate tilts anteriorly into the DISI position and closes the scapho-lunate angle, which is normally around 60° but can be reduced to 0°, as shown by the two parallel lines in the diagram.

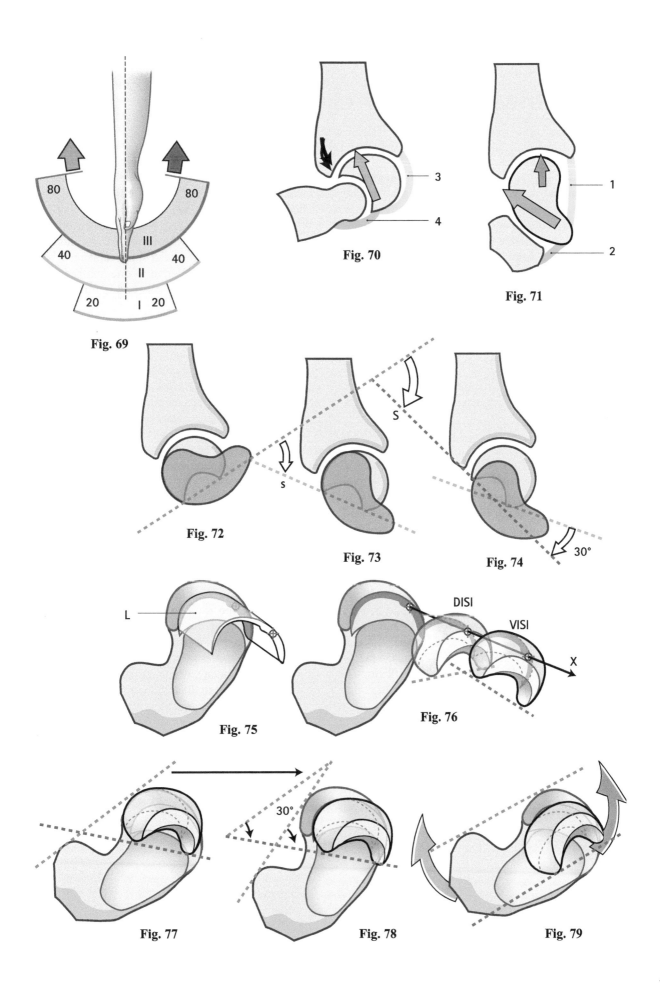

Fig. 69

Fig. 70

Fig. 71

Fig. 72

Fig. 73

Fig. 74

Fig. 75

Fig. 76

Fig. 77

Fig. 78

Fig. 79

175

The geometrically variable carpus

The carpus is a grouping of **eight bones, seven of which contribute to the geometry** of what can be called the 'carpal pillar'. For the last 30 years, the carpus has no longer been viewed as a monolithic complex, and the complicated elementary movements that influence its structure are now well known. It can be thought of as a **bag of walnuts** (Fig. 80) and it is distorted by the pressures exerted during movements of the wrist, but these distortions are not random, as in the case of real walnuts. They are **organized** and **logical**, because the **shape of each bone is** moulded by its movements, which **are directed by the interosseous ligaments**.

Abduction-adduction

It is during these movements that changes in the shape of the bones are the most obvious, as evidenced by a careful study of anterior radiographs.

Abduction

During abduction (Fig. 81) the whole carpus rotates around a centre located in the head of the capitate, while the proximal row of carpal bones (arrow 1) moves proximally and medially so that half of the lunate comes to lie distal to the ulnar head and the triquetrum pulls away from the lunate distally. This displacement of the triquetrum is soon checked by the medial collateral ligament (M) of the radio-carpal joint, and above all by the 'triquetral sling' (S). Thus halted, the triquetrum now acts as a check for the hamate. If abduction goes on, only the distal row of carpal bones can move, as follows:

- The **trapezium** and **trapezoid** move proximally (arrow 2), reducing the effective distance between the trapezium and the radius. Wedged between the trapezium (2) and the radius (3), the scaphoid shortens by 'lying down' into flexion (f) in the radio-carpal joint (Fig. 83) and extension in the mid-carpal joint (e).
- The **capitate** moves distally (arrow 4), increasing the available space for the lunate, which is held in check by the anterior radio-lunate ligament. It tilts posteriorly (Fig. 84) into flexion (f) in the radio-carpal joint and presents its widest diameter. At the same time the capitate moves posteriorly into extension (e) at the mid-carpal joint. As the scaphoid shortens, the capitate and the hamate can slide proximally under the first row of carpal bones (red arrows). The triquetrum, held in check by its three ligaments, 'climbs' over the hamate towards the head of the capitate. When the carpal bones stop moving relative to one another, the **locked or close-packed position is reached in abduction.**

Adduction

During adduction (Fig. 82) the whole carpus starts to rotate but this time the proximal row moves distally and laterally, while the lunate slips completely under the radius, and the trapezium and trapezoid (arrow 1) move distally, thereby increasing the available space for the scaphoid. The latter, pulled distally by the scapho-trapezoidal ligament, rights itself (Fig. 86) anteriorly into extension (e) at the radio-carpal joint and filling the empty space under the radius. Concurrently the trapezium slides anteriorly under the scaphoid into flexion (f) at the mid-carpal joint. As the distal 'descent' of the scaphoid (arrow 2) is checked by the lateral ligament of the radio-carpal joint (E), adduction proceeds in the distal bones, which move relative to the proximal bones (red arrows) as follows:

- The head of the capitate slips under the concave surface of the scaphoid, the lunate slips over the head of the capitate to hit the hamate, and the triquetrum 'descends' distally along the slanting surface of the hamate.
- Meanwhile, the triquetrum rises anteriorly (arrow 3) as it hits the ulnar head (arrow 4), cushioned by the articular disc, thus transmitting stresses from the hand to the forearm.
- The capitate moves proximally (arrow 5), reducing the useful space for the lunate, which, as the anterior radio-lunate ligament slackens, can tilt anteriorly (Fig. 85) with extension (e) at the radio-carpal joint and present its narrowest diameter. At the same time the capitate also moves anteriorly with flexion (f) at the mid-carpal joint.
- When the carpal bones come to a halt, the **locked or close-packed position is reached in adduction.**

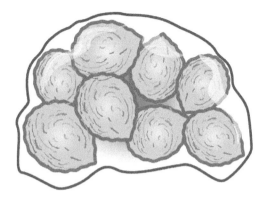

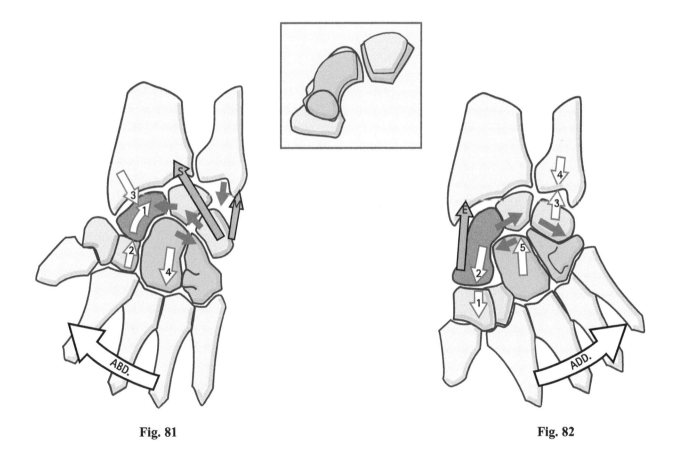

Fig. 80

Fig. 81

Fig. 82

Dynamic properties of the proximal row

If the scaphoid-lunate couple (inset Fig. 80, p. 177) is compared during abduction (dark) and during adduction (light), it is clear that the two bones undergo inverse changes. During abduction the functional surface of the scaphoid decreases and looks like a ring on radiographs, while that of the lunate increases; the converse is true in adduction. These changes result from movements of flexion-extension in the two joints of the carpus as follows:

- **During abduction** (Figs 83 and 84), flexion in the radio-carpal is cancelled by extension in the mid-carpal joint.
- **During adduction** (Figs 85 and 86), conversely, extension in the radio-carpal is offset by flexion in the mid-carpal joint.

Thus one can logically draw the following conclusions:

- **Wrist flexion** is coupled with **abduction at the radio-carpal and with adduction at the mid-carpal joint**.
- **Wrist extension** is coupled with **adduction at the radio-carpal and abduction at the mid-carpal joint**.

Thus the mechanism proposed by Henke is confirmed.

As regards the shape and position of the **proximal pole of the hamate**, statistical radiographic studies have established that it consists mostly (71%) of a small facet in contact with the lunate all the time (Fig. 87) and is better able to transmit stresses, whereas in a minority of cases (29%) its proximal pole is pointed (Fig. 88) and comes into contact with the lunate only during adduction.

To help understand the difficult concept of DISI (Dorsal Intercalated Segment Instability) and VISI (Volar Intercalated Segment Instability) proposed by the Americans, I would like to use the 'Parable of the Three Friends'.

In this story, the three main bones of the proximal row of carpal bones (Fig. 83) – the scaphoid (S), the lunate (L), and the triquetrum (T) – are personified as three friends who are inseparable because they link arms. These three friends are Stephen (S), Lawrence (L) and Tom (T), who are theoretically linked together by their arms, i.e., S to L and L to T. This causes them to move and to take up any position in unison, as, for instance saluting by bending forwards together (Fig. A) and looking at the sky by bending backwards together (Fig. B). This is precisely what happens to the three bones of the proximal row of bones, which move in the same direction. It can happen that our friends get knocked about, so that two of the three bones become severed from each other, as, for example, Stephen from Lawrence or Lawrence from Tom. Then their movements are no longer interdependent.

1. When S and L are severed by rupture of the scapholunate ligament (see previous page), the interdependence between the two bones is lost. Thus, of our three friends, Lawrence and Tom can bend forwards but Stephen can only move backwards. Anatomically speaking, lateral radiographs show that the scaphoid now lies 'horizontally', i.e., it is 'lying down', whereas Lawrence has tilted anteriorly or undergone a movement of extension in the radiocarpal joint simultaneously with a movement of flexion in the mediocarpal joint. This is what American authors describe as 'Dorsal Inclination', i.e., extension of the intercalated segment, i.e., the lunate; hence the acronym DISI. It is the use of their own terminology that makes the term difficult to understand at first sight. The parable of the three friends makes it easier to understand.

2. When L and T are separated (case 2 in Fig. C) because of rupture of the triquetro-lunar ligament, the opposite sequence of events takes place: the lunate and the triquetrum become separated, and Lawrence is not arm-in-arm with Tom (Fig. D). As a result, Stephen and Lawrence are tilted backwards, while Tom is tilted forwards. In the wrist these changes correspond in the radio-carpal joint to flexion of the scaphoid and of the lunate, and in the medio-carpal joint to extension of the triquetrum, which, now untethered from the lunate, can slide forwards on top of the lunate. For the American authors the lunate undergoes 'Volar or palmar Inclination'; hence the VISI, meaning flexion of the intercalated segment, i.e., the lunate in the radiocarpal joint.

We hope that this 'Parable of the Three Friends' has clarified the meaning of the expressions DISI and VISI and will stay with you.

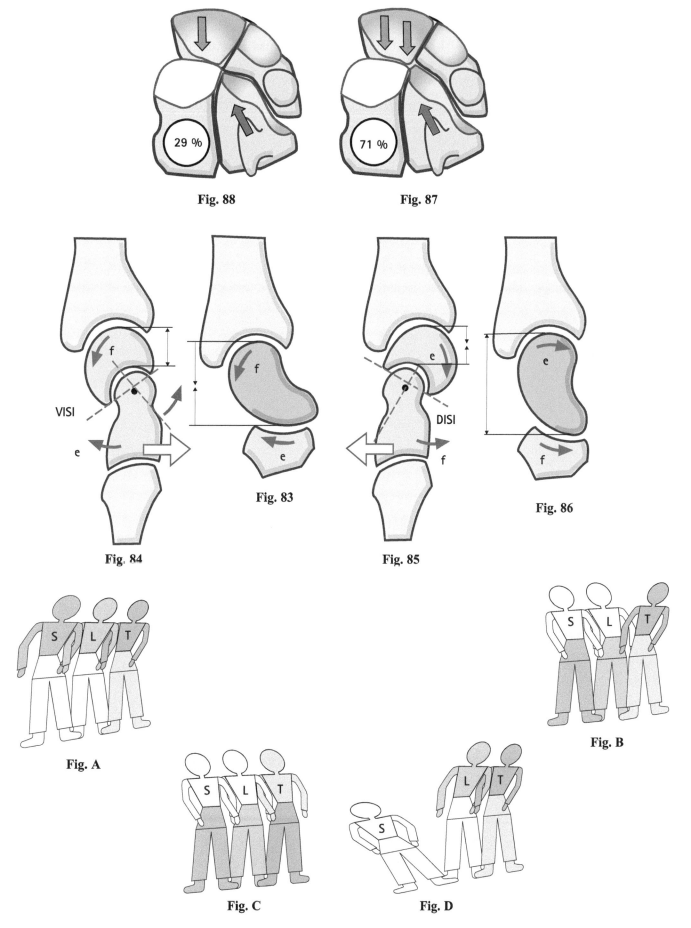

Fig. 88

Fig. 87

VISI

Fig. 84

f

e

Fig. 83

e

DISI

Fig. 85

e

f

Fig. 86

S L T

Fig. A

S L T

Fig. B

S L T

Fig. C

S L T

Fig. D

The intercalated segment

The proximal row of carpal bones is more mobile than the distal row, which can be considered as an almost monolithic structure in practice. It lies between the concave antebrachial surface of the wrist joint and the distal row; hence its name of **intercalated segment**. This row (Fig. 89, anterior view), with no muscle attachments, is held together by interosseous ligaments and is subjected to stresses coming from the well-balanced adjacent structures. When it is compressed as a single structure between the distal row and the articular surface of the radius its three bones tilt anteriorly in flexion in the radio-carpal joint and (Fig. 90, lateral view) stretch the palmar interosseous ligaments (double yellow arrow) and the posterior radio-carpal ligaments (double blue arrow). Moreover, interlinked as they are by the scapho-lunate ligament laterally and the triquetro-lunate ligament medially, these three bones do not undergo exactly the same tilting movement:

- The scaphoid lies down more than the semilunate tilts anteriorly, and it rotates slightly into pronation (blue arrow) on the head of the capitate (Fig. 89).
- The triquetrum slides on the proximal surface of the hamate along a spiral path and rotates slightly into supination (blue arrow).

During these movements the triquetrum is driven by its palmar ligaments (Fig. 91):

- the capito-triquetral ligament, which forms the medial arm of Poirier's V-shaped space (1)
- the triquetro-capitate ligament (2)
- the hamato-triquetral ligament (3).

The movements of the triquetrum (Tri) are essentially guided by the '**triquetral sling**' (Kuhlmann), whose anterior (4) and posterior (5) bands (after removal of the radius) can be seen in the diagram. The sling imparts to the bone a screwing movement on the hamate (Ham) (Fig. 92, lateral view, after removal of the capitate) combining flexion and supination (blue arrow, Fig. 93).

This movement is even more clear-cut during adduction (Fig. 93) as the triquetrum is rotated into supination by its palmar ligaments, particularly the lateral arm of Poirier's V-shaped space (red arrow).

At the same time (see Fig. 82), the gap between the ulnar head and the triquetrum narrows, as does the useful space medially between the triquetrum and the hamate, as a result of the ulnar deviation. On the whole, the height of the medial portion of the carpus is reduced.

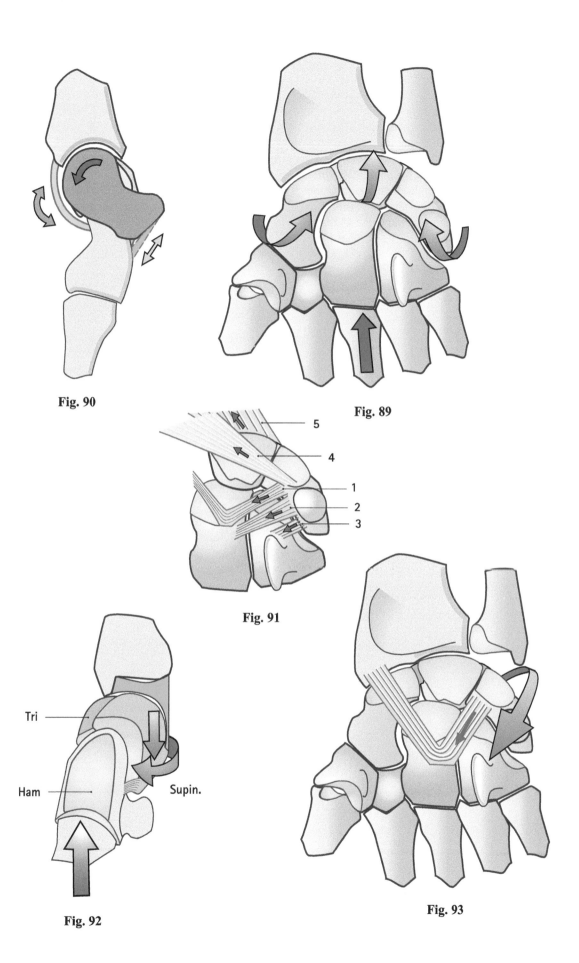

Fig. 90

Fig. 89

Fig. 91

Fig. 92

Fig. 93

181

Dynamic aspects of adduction-abduction

During abduction (Fig. 94), anterior radiographs show that the carpus rotates distal to the proximal articular surface of the wrist joint around a centre located roughly between the lunate and the capitate (star), with the capitate tilting laterally and the lunate (darker) moving medially to come to lie just distal to the inferior radio-ulnar joint. Laterally the scaphoid tilts anteriorly in flexion and loses some of its height; it sinks under the radius and presents its **ring-shaped tubercle**. In reality this rotation occurs around a slightly shifting axis, since globally the carpus is slightly displaced laterally until the scaphoid hits the radial styloid process, which extends farther distally than the ulnar styloid process. As a result, abduction comes to an end before adduction. Medially, the triquetrum moves 15 mm away from the ulnar head. The **range of this movement**, as measured along the axis of the third metacarpal, is 15°.

During adduction (Fig. 95), the capitate tilts medially and the whole of the lunate (darker) moves laterally distal to the radius towards the articular surface of the wrist joint that corresponds to the lunate. Meanwhile the scaphoid moves posteriorly in extension and presents its maximal height with loss of the profile of its concavity. The tapering proximal portion of the hamate comes into contact with the lunate, and the carpus lies neatly centred distal to the radius. The range of this movement, as measured on the third metacarpal, is 30-45°.

The mid-carpal joint contributes to these movements (Figs 96 and 97, anterior view):

- **On the one hand**, movements of adduction and abduction occur in this joint. In full abduction of 15° it would contribute 8°, and in full adduction of 45° it would contribute 15°, so that its total contribution to adduction and abduction would amount to 23°. The range of these movements would be roughly equal in the radio-carpal and the mid-carpal joints (Sterling Bunnell).

- **On the other hand**, the two rows of carpal bones move relative to each other as they rotate around the long axis of the carpus:

  - **During abduction** (Fig. 96) the proximal row rotates in a combined movement of **pronation and flexion** (arrow PF), while the distal row does the opposite, i.e. combining **supination and extension** (arrow SE), which counterbalances the former movement. As the proximal row moves, the scaphoid is displaced slightly and thus can escape or at least delay contact with the radial styloid process, thereby increasing the range of abduction.

  - **During adduction** (Fig. 97) the opposite movements take place. The proximal row rotates in a combined movement of **supination and extension** (arrow SE), while the distal row combines **pronation and flexion** (arrow PF), thus counteracting the movement of the proximal row.

- These movements have a small range and can be recognized only by careful study of radiographs taken in extreme positions.

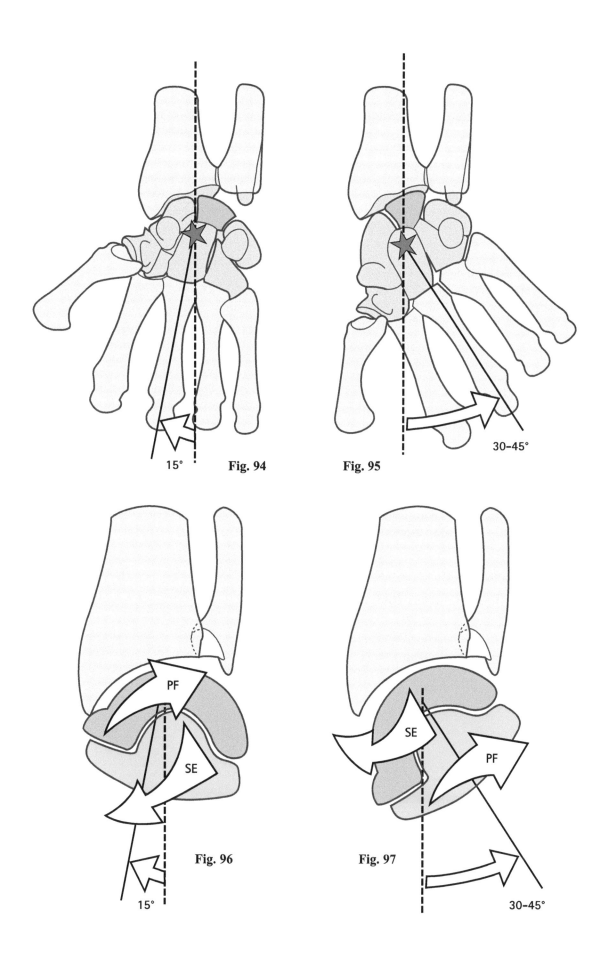

Fig. 94

Fig. 95

15°

30–45°

Fig. 96

Fig. 97

PF

SE

SE

PF

15°

30–45°

Dynamic aspects of flexion-extension

From the previous discussions it is clear that the radiocarpal and mid-carpal joints are **functionally interdependent** in all movements of the wrist.

In the reference position for flexion-extension (Fig. 98, lateral view) the radius (1), the lunate (2), the capitate (3) and the third metacarpal (4) are perfectly aligned along the long axis of the radius. The posterior border of the distal articular surface of the radius extends farther distally than the anterior border. The following two diagrams provide a better understanding of the **individual contributions** of these two joints:

- **During flexion** (Fig. 99) the range of movement is greater in the radio-carpal (50°) than in the mid-carpal joint (35°).
- **During extension** (Fig. 100) the opposite is true, undoubtedly because the posterior margin of the radius hits the carpus sooner. The range is 50° at the mid-carpal and 35° at the radio-carpal joint.

The total range is the same (85°) in both joints, but the maximal ranges of the individual movements are inversely related. A good way to remember this is to note that extension at the radio-carpal joint is checked sooner because the posterior border of the radius extends farther down distally.

Henke's mechanism

In his explanation of wrist movements the German anatomist Henke proposed a theory that seems likely to be confirmed by recent observations. It must be recalled that in biomechanics no axis is really contained in a single reference plane and no axis is stable. In other words, **all axes are mobile**.

Henke defines the **two oblique axes of the wrist** as follows (Fig. 101):

- The **proximal axis** (1) (red), belonging to the radio-carpal joint, is oblique postero-anteriorly and latero-medially.
- The **distal axis** (2) (blue), belonging to the mid-carpal joint, is oblique postero-medially and medio-laterally.

This explains why the movements of flexion and extension are always combined with other movements, such as movements of axial rotation (Figs 102 and 103, r), i.e. pronation or supination, which cancel each other out as follows:

- **During flexion** (Fig. 102, antero-medial view in perspective) the proximal row rotates into pronation (P), thereby producing a composite movement of **flexion/abduction/pronation**, whereas the distal row rotates into supination (S) in a composite movement of **flexion/adduction/supination**. The flexion components are additive, while the adduction/abduction and the pronation/supination components cancel each other.
- **During extension** (Fig. 103, similar view), the proximal row rotates into supination (S), thus producing a composite movement of **extension/adduction/supination**, whereas the distal row rotates into pronation (P), thus providing a composite movement of **extension/abduction/pronation**. The components of extension are additive, while the components of adduction/abduction and pronation/supination cancel each other.

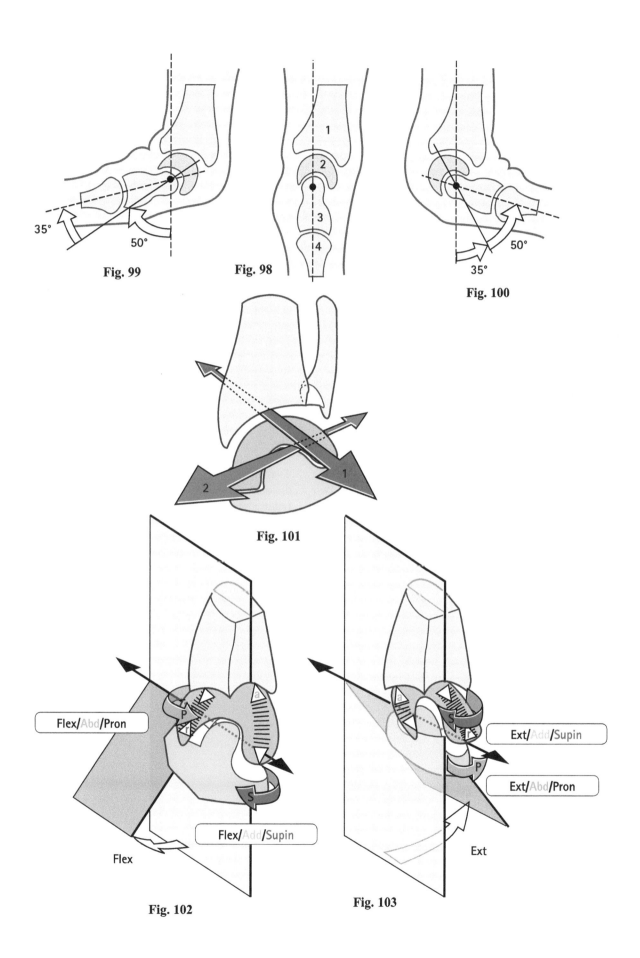

Fig. 99

Fig. 98

Fig. 100

35°

50°

35°

50°

Fig. 101

1

2

Flex/Abd/Pron

Flex/Add/Supin

Flex

Fig. 102

Ext/Add/Supin

Ext/Abd/Pron

Ext

Fig. 103

The transfer of the force couple of pronation-supination

The wrist considered as a universal joint

It is wrong to consider the wrist as a joint concerned only with movements of flexion-extension and of abduction-adduction and to ignore its role in transmitting to the hand the **force couple generated during axial rotation in the forearm** by the motor muscles of pronation and supination. This mistake is quite common, since only the range of the movements of flexion-extension and abduction-adduction are measured, while measurements are rarely made of the **ranges of pronation and supination** and even less of the **force generated during rotation of the hand against resistance**.

As the wrist has **two axes** it must be considered as a **universal joint**. Gerolamo Cardano (1501-1576) invented this type of joint, which at the start was used to hang a compass and protect it from the effects of rolling and pitching on a ship. It is widely used in the automobile industry to transmit a couple of rotation between two non-collinear structures, e.g. between the engine and the front wheels in a car with front-wheel drive.

This joint has **two axes** (Fig. 104), which are shown diagrammatically as a crossbar (inset) and which allow the transfer of the rotation of the primary axis (red arrow) to the secondary axis (blue arrow), regardless of the angle formed by these two axes. In reality as the angle between these two axes exceeds 45°, the couple of rotation is transmitted with increasing difficulty and not at all when the angle reaches 90°. This is exactly the role of the wrist (Fig. 105); it does not contain a crossbar like the one in the diagram, but it has two joints in series, the radio-carpal and the mid-carpal joints, which can easily be dislocated by rotational forces.

This applies to the radio-carpal joint, a **poorly interlocked condyloid joint** (Fig. 106), which allows the proximal carpal bones to slip out of the distal articular surface of the radius (blue and red arrows).

How can the motor power of pronation-supination be transmitted to the hand as it turns a handle against resistance (blue arrow) or as it screws or unscrews a nail? The answer lies in the **role of the ligaments** that connect the two bones of the forearm to the carpus and unite the carpal bones among themselves.

- Figure 107 (**anterior view of the carpus**) shows how the ligaments that run obliquely, proximally and laterally will rotate the carpus into supination and will resist passive pronation of the carpus.
- Figure 108 (**posterior view of the carpus**) shows how the ligaments that run obliquely in the opposite direction will resist passive supination and rotate the carpus into pronation.

The **interosseous ligaments of the carpus** (Fig. 109) prevent dislocation during pronation and supination, particularly as regards the proximal bones (Figs 110-111, superior views). The ligaments check the gliding movement of the scaphoid relative to the lunate and also relative to the distal row during pronation (Fig. 110) and supination (Fig. 111).

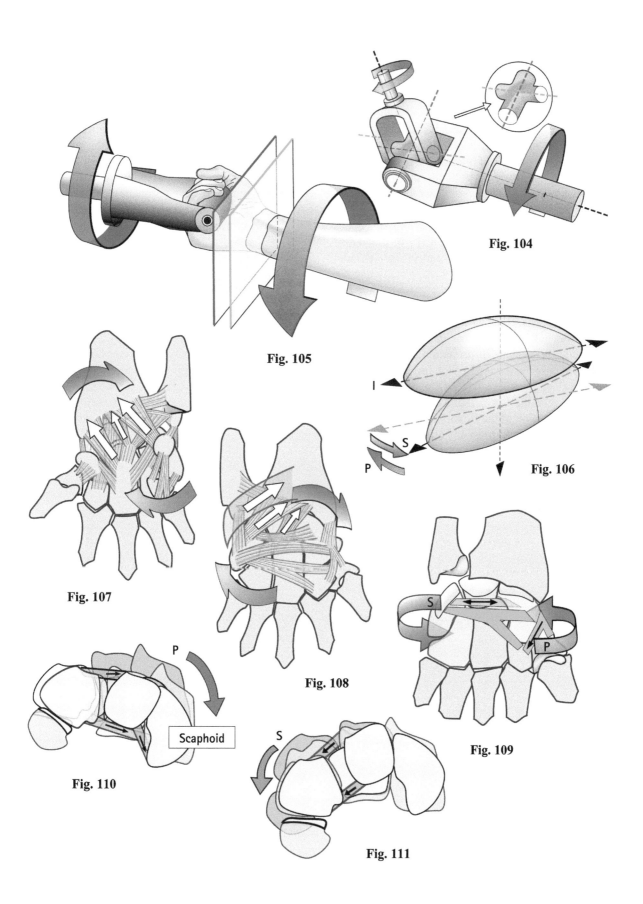

Fig. 104

Fig. 105

Fig. 106

Fig. 107

Fig. 108

Fig. 109

Scaphoid

Fig. 110

Fig. 111

The ligaments cannot by themselves keep the carpus together and transmit the force of the couple of pronation-supination. This has recently been demonstrated (A. Kapandji) in a CT scan study of the wrist using thin slices at 5 mm intervals during pronation and supination of the forearm with or without contraction of the flexor muscles. The serial sections, passing through the distal ends of the two bones of the forearm and through the first and second rows of metacarpal bones, demonstrate the relative movements of these bones and the changes in their spatial orientation.

In the first series of scans, taken with the palm of the hand passively kept stationary, the subject carries out movements of pronation and supination. The 'rotational drift' in the radio-carpal joint is 47°30′ at the level of the forearm (Fig. 112) and 4°30′ at the level of the metacarpus (Fig. 113). Thus, when the flexors are inactive, the rotational drift between the forearm and the hand is 47°30′–4°30′, i.e. 43°.

In the second series of scans, taken when the hand tightly grasps a fixed bar with the help of the flexor muscles, the subject carries out the same movements of pronation and supination. The 'rotational drift' is 25° at the level of the forearm (Fig. 114) and 17° at the level of the metacarpus (Fig. 115). Thus the 'rotational drift' between the forearm and the hand is 25–17°, i.c. 8°. Therefore contraction of the flexors against a resistance has reduced the 'rotational drift' from 43° to 8°, i.e. to less than 20% of what it was when only the ligaments were in play.

The inferior radio-ulnar joint is prone to dislocation during free pronation and supination (Fig. 116), and more so when pronation and supination are 'impeded' by other concurrent active movements (Fig. 117), with an increase in the forces generated. In the proximal row of the carpal bones 'impeded' pronation-supination (Fig. 118) produces a 'rotational drift' of 30° and also alters the anterior concavity of the proximal row by 7° (Fig. 119). Further improvements in 4D in scanning techniques will allow greater refinement in the study of the changes occurring within the wrist during pronation and supination. One thing is already certain, however; it is the contraction of the muscles, particularly of the flexors, that keeps together the articular complex of the wrist. Because the wrist is encased by tendons (Fig. 120, anterior view; Fig. 121, posterior view), the muscles act on the articular complex of the wrist like a clutch, and this action is necessary for the couple of force of pronation-supination to be transmitted from the forearm to the arm.

The concurrent contraction of the extensor carpi ulnaris (Fig. 122) has a positive role to play as it retightens the sling of the annular ligaments and increases the cohesion of the proximal row of carpal bones and of the inferior radio-ulnar joint. Another interesting conclusion is that this mechanism can be studied only in the live subject, because contraction of the muscles is essential for the cohesion of the wrist.

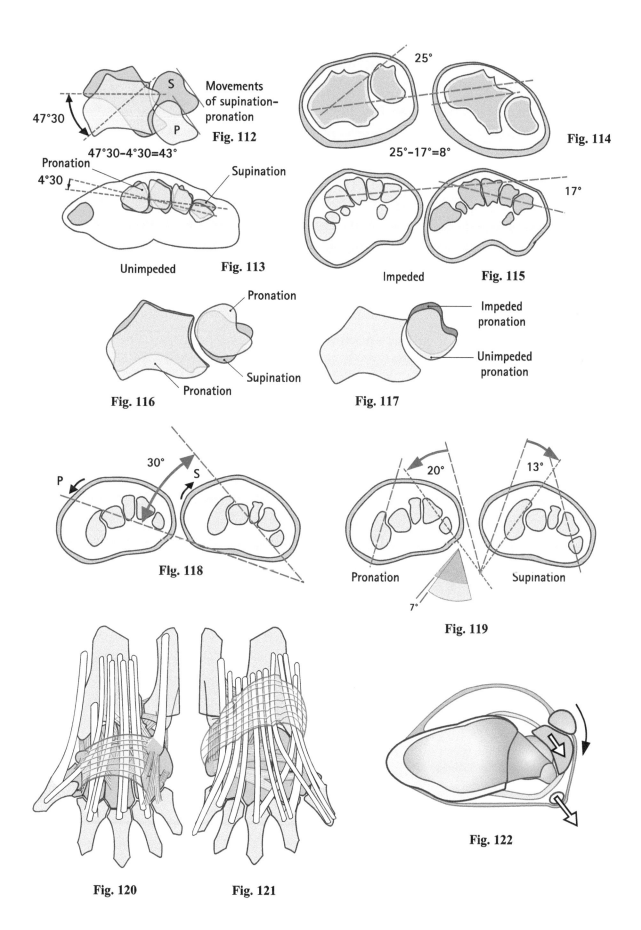

Fig. 112

Movements of supination-pronation

47°30

47°30–4°30=43°

Pronation

4°30

Supination

Unimpeded

Fig. 113

25°

25°–17°=8°

17°

Impeded

Fig. 114

Fig. 115

Pronation

Pronation

Supination

Fig. 116

Impeded pronation

Unimpeded pronation

Fig. 117

30°

P

S

Flg. 118

20°

13°

Pronation

7°

Supination

Fig. 119

Fig. 120

Fig. 121

Fig. 122

Traumatic lesions of the wrist

This scan is taken at the level of the head of the capitate (Fig. 123), flanked laterally by the scaphoid and medially by the proximal extension of the hamate and the adjacent triquetrum and the pisiform. It shows how the concavity of the proximal row of the carpal bones varies, depending on whether the wrist is in pronation or supination. It is greater in supination than in pronation because its borders are brought closer together by 3 mm (from 47 mm to 44 mm), while the angle between the scaphoid and the capitate increases posteriorly by 2° and that between the hamate and the triquetrum increases by 7°.

This concavity is maintained (Fig. 124) by the **tension developed in the flexor retinaculum** and by the anterior interosseous ligaments. During surgical treatment of carpal tunnel syndrome (Fig. 125), the flexor retinaculum, which provides the flexor muscles with **the strongest pulley in the body**, is cut and the borders of the concavity spring apart for 3-5 mm. The anterior interosseous ligaments (Fig. 126) are then the only ligaments (black arrow) that prevent the complete flattening of this concavity. Therefore it is better surgically to lengthen the flexor retinaculum than simply to cut it.

The wrist is the joint **most likely to be traumatized**, e.g. falling on the hand when it is abducted and extended. **Forced abduction** is checked by two factors:

1) the resistance of the ligaments attached to the triquetrum
2) the radial styloid process.

Depending on the position of the scaphoid relative to the proximal articular surface of the wrist joint, either the **distal epiphysis of the radius** (Fig. 127) is fractured with detachment of a segment, or the **scaphoid** is fractured in its mid-portion as it hits the radial styloid process (Fig. 128). In other circumstances, the **radial styloid process** is fractured, often with rupture of the scapho-lunate ligament (not shown here), and this may not be diagnosed unless systematically looked for. The component of extension contributes to the fracture of the distal radius in one piece (Fig. 129, sagittal section), which then tilts posteriorly. This same type of trauma can also frequently lead to the detachment of a **third postero-medial fragment** (Fig. 130, transverse section), thus compromising the inferior radioulnar joint.

In yet other circumstances, the movement of extension tears the anterior ligamentous attachments of the capitate (Fig. 131), which is then displaced behind the lunate still in place, i.e. the **retro-lunate dislocation of the wrist**. This dislocation (Fig. 132) crushes the posterior horn of the lunate and can tear its posterior attachments (Fig. 133), causing its anterior dislocation. The lunate then rotates on itself for 180°, while the head of the capitate replaces the lunate distal to the proximal surface of the wrist joint. This is known as the **peri-lunate dislocation of the wrist**, which is difficult to diagnose radiologically unless one takes strictly lateral views and above all three-quarter views.

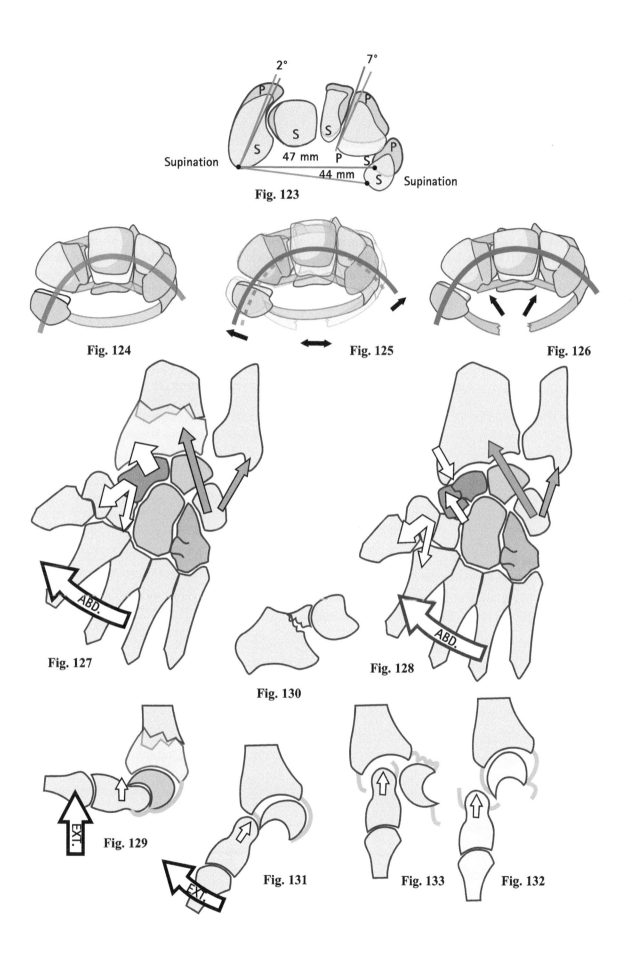

Fig. 123

Fig. 124

Fig. 125

Fig. 126

Fig. 127

Fig. 128

Fig. 130

Fig. 129

Fig. 131

Fig. 133

Fig. 132

The motor muscles of the wrist

The tendons of the motor muscles of the wrist encase the wrist joint and belong to the extrinsic muscles of the fingers and the muscles of the wrist, only one of which (the *flexor carpi ulnaris*) is inserted into the proximal row of carpal bones, i.e. the pisiform.

Figure 134 (**anterior view of the wrist**) shows the following:

- the **flexor carpi radialis** (1), which runs in a special groove deep to the *flexor retinaculum* but separate from the carpal tunnel and is inserted into the anterior surface of the base of the second metacarpal and to a lesser degree into the trapezium and the base of the third metacarpal
- the **palmaris longus** (2), less powerful, which is inserted vertically into the *flexor retinaculum* and also sends four pretendinous bands of fibres into the apex of the palmar aponeurosis
- the **flexor carpi ulnaris** (3), which passes anterior to the ulnar styloid process and is inserted mainly into the proximal surface of the pisiform and also into the flexor retinaculum, the horn of the hamate and the bases of the fourth and fifth metacarpals.

A **posterior view of the wrist** shows the following (Fig. 135):

- the **extensor carpi ulnaris** (4), which passes anterior to the ulnar styloid process in a very strong fibrous sheath and is inserted into the posterior aspect of the base of the fifth metacarpal
- the **extensor radialis brevis** (5) and the **extensor carpi radialis longus** (6), which run along the upper part of the 'anatomical snuffbox' and are inserted respectively into the base of the third metacarpal (6) and the base of the second metacarpal (5).

A view of the medial border of the wrist (Fig. 136) shows the following:

- the **flexor carpi ulnaris** (3), whose efficiency as a wrist muscle is increased by the lever arm of the pisiform
- the **extensor carpi ulnaris** (4).

These two tendons lie on either side of the ulnar styloid process.

A view of the posterior border of the wrist (Fig. 137) shows the following:

- the **extensor carpi radialis longus** (6) and the **extensor carpi radialis brevis** (5)
- the **abductor pollicis longus** (7), inserted into the lateral aspect of the base of the first metacarpal
- the **extensor pollicis brevis** (8), inserted into the dorsal surface of the base of the first phalanx of the thumb
- the **extensor pollicis longus** (9), inserted into the dorsal surface of the base of the second phalanx of the thumb.

The radial muscles (*extensores carpi radialis*) and the long muscles of the thumb encase the radial styloid process. The **anatomical snuffbox** is bounded posteriorly by the tendon of the *extensor pollicis longus* and anteriorly by those of the *abductor pollicis longus* and the *extensor pollicis brevis*.

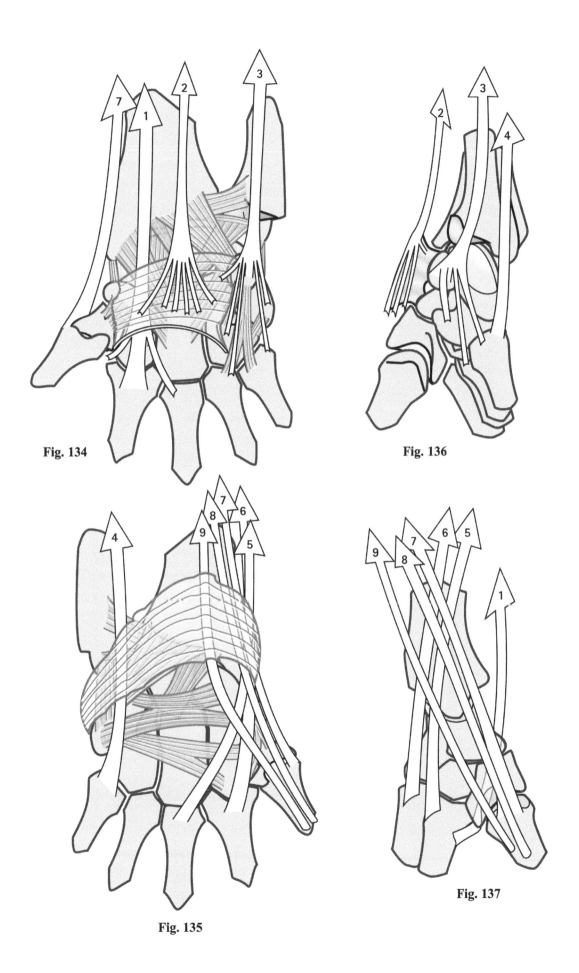

Fig. 134

Fig. 136

Fig. 135

Fig. 137

Actions of the muscles of the wrist

The motor muscles of the wrist fall into **four groups**, defined functionally in relation to the axes of the wrist (Fig. 138, transverse section):

- Axis AA′ of **flexion-extension** (red arrows)
- Axis BB′ of **adduction-abduction** (blue arrows).

This diagram shows the distal aspect of a coronal section through the right wrist so that B is anterior, B′ posterior, A′ lateral and A medial. The tendons correspond to the motor muscles of the wrist and of the fingers (Fig. 139). (The labelling of the muscles of the fingers is given in detail later in the text.)

Group I lies in the antero-medial quadrant and consists of the **flexor carpi ulnaris** (1), which simultaneously flexes the wrist, as it lies anterior to the axis AA′ and the fifth metacarpal via its tendinous expansion, and also adducts the hand, as it lies medial to the axis BB′. It is also helped by the **extensor digiti minimi** (10). The left hand of someone playing the violin illustrates this combined movement of flexion and adduction.

Group II lies in the postero-medial quadrant and consists of the **extensor carpi ulnaris** (6), which simultaneously extends the wrist, as it lies posterior to the axis AA′, and adducts the hand, as it lies medial to the axis BB′.

Group III lies in the antero-lateral quadrant and contains the **flexor carpi radialis** (2) and the **palmaris longus** (3), which flex the wrist, as they lie anterior to the axis AA′, and abduct the hand, as they lie lateral to the axis BB′. Also included on the lateral border of the wrist overlying the radial styloid process are the **abductor pollicis longus** (9) and the **extensor pollicis brevis** (10).

Group IV lies in the postero-lateral quadrant and contains the **extensor carpi radialis longus** (4) and the **extensor carpi radialis brevis** (5), which extend the wrist, as they lie posterior to the axis AA′, and abduct the hand, as they lie lateral to the axis BB′. Also included are the muscles coursing over the dorsal aspect of the distal end of the radius, i.e., the **extensor digitorum** (9) and the **extensor indicis** (1).

According to this theory, none of the muscles of the wrist has a single action. Thus to perform a pure movement two groups of muscles must be activated so as to cancel one component as follows in line with the antagonism-synergism principle:

- **flexion** (Flex): group I (FCU) and Group III (FCR + PL)
- **extension** (Ext): Group II (ECU) and Group IV (the radial extensors)
- **adduction** (Add): Group I (FCU) and Group II (ECU)
- **abduction** (Abd): Group III (PL) and Group IV (the radial extensors).

Thus are defined the movements of the wrist in the four planes of reference, **but its natural movements take place in an oblique plane**:

- flexion-adduction
- extension-abduction.

Furthermore, the electrical stimulation experiments of Duchenne de Boulogne (1867) have revealed the following facts:

- Only the *extensor carpi radialis longus* (4) extends and abducts. The *extensor carpi radialis brevis* is exclusively an extensor; hence its physiological importance.
- The *palmaris longus* is a direct flexor, as is the *flexor carpi radialis longus*, which also flexes the second carpometacarpal joint while pronating the hand. The *flexor carpi radialis*, when driven electrically, does not produce abduction, and it contracts during radial deviation at the wrist to counterbalance the extensor component of the *extensor carpi radialis longus*, which is the main abductor muscle.
- The motor muscles of the fingers, i.e. *flexor digitorum superficialis* (12), *flexor digitorum profundus* (7) and, to a lesser degree, *flexor pollicis longus* (13) can move the wrist under certain conditions.
- The flexors of the fingers flex the wrist only if flexion of the fingers is prevented before these muscles have fully contracted.

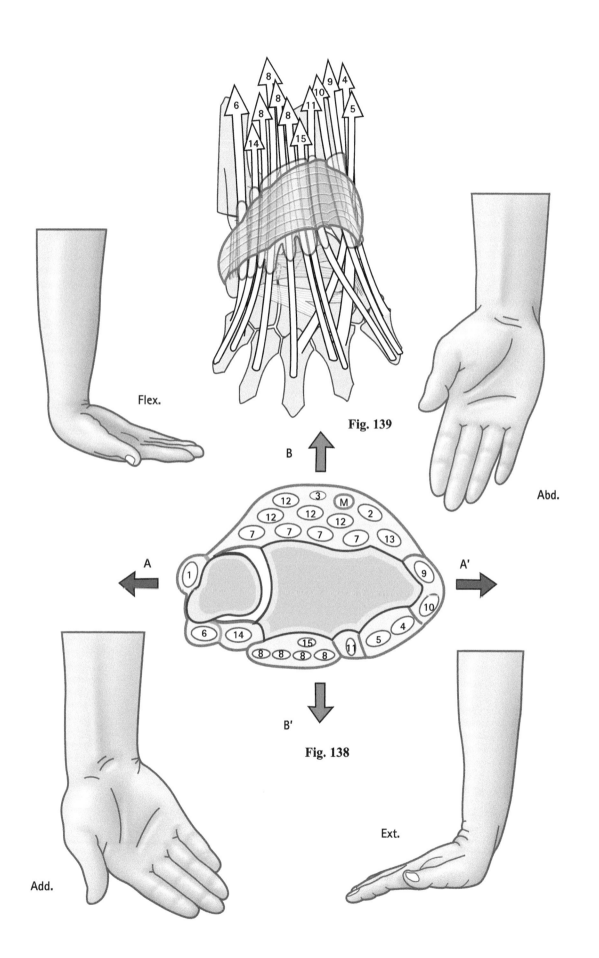

Flex.

Abd.

Fig. 139

B

A

A'

B'

Add.

Ext.

Fig. 138

If the hand holds a large object like a bottle, the flexors of the fingers can contribute to flexion of the wrist.

Likewise, the extensors of the fingers (8), with the help of the *extensor digiti minimi* (14) and of the *extensor indicis* (15), contribute to wrist extension if the fist is clenched:

- The **abductor pollicis longus** (9) and the **extensor pollicis brevis** (10) abduct the wrist unless their action is counterbalanced by that of the *extensor carpi ulnaris*. If the latter contracts simultaneously, isolated thumb abduction is produced by the *abductor pollicis longus*. The synergistic action of the *extensor carpi ulnaris* is therefore essential for abduction of the thumb and in this sense this muscle can be called a 'stabilizer' of the wrist.
- The **extensor pollicis longus** (11), which produces thumb extension and retropulsion, can also cause abduction and extension of the wrist when the *flexor carpi ulnaris* is inactive.
- Another stabilizer of the wrist is the **extensor carpi radialis longus** (4), which is essential for maintaining the hand in the neutral position, and its paralysis causes permanent ulnar deviation.

The synergistic and stabilizing action of the muscles of the wrist (Fig. 140)

The extensor muscles of the wrist act synergistically with the flexors of the fingers:

- During extension of the wrist (a), improperly called dorsiflexion, the fingers are automatically flexed and, to extend the fingers in this position, a voluntary movement is required.

- Moreover, it is when the wrist is extended that the flexors can act with maximum efficiency, because the flexor tendons are then relatively shorter than when the wrist is straight and even more so when the wrist is flexed. The strength of the digital flexors, measured by a dynamometer when the wrist is flexed, is only a quarter of what it is when the wrist is extended.

The flexor muscles of the wrist act synergistically with the extensors of the fingers:

- When the wrist is flexed (b), extension of the proximal phalanx follows automatically. A voluntary movement is needed to flex the fingers towards the palm, and this flexion is weak. Contraction of the digital flexors limits flexion of the wrist, and the range of wrist flexion can be increased by 10° by extending the fingers.

This delicate balance of muscle action can easily be upset. A deformity resulting from an unreduced Colles' fracture changes the orientation of the antebrachial surface of the wrist joint and, by stretching the extensors of the wrist, interferes with the efficiency of the digital flexors.

The functional position of the wrist

This (Fig. 141) corresponds to the position of maximal efficiency of the motor muscles of the fingers, especially of the flexors. This position is defined by:

- slight extension (dorsiflexion) of the wrist to 40-45°
- slight adduction (ulnar deviation) to 15°.

It is in this position of the wrist that the hand is best configured for its function of prehension.

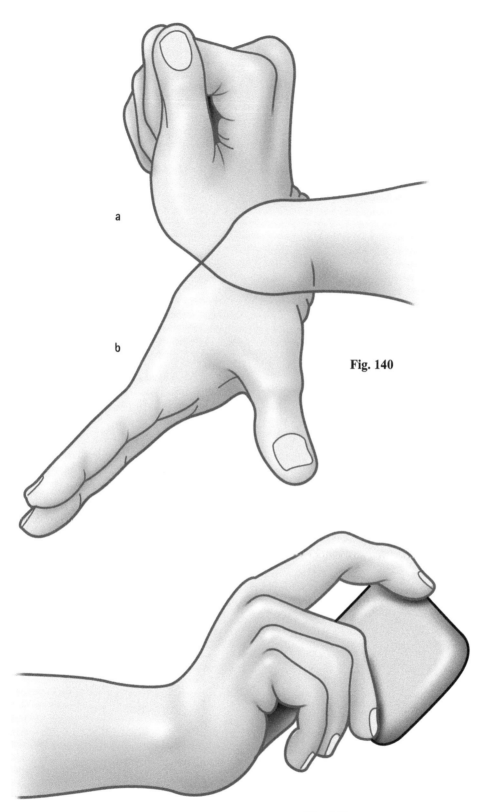

a

b

Fig. 140

Fig. 141

Chapter 5

THE HAND

The human hand is a remarkable instrument, capable of performing countless actions thanks to its essential function: **prehension**.

Prehension is found in all forms of 'hands', from the pincers of the lobster to the hand of the ape, but it attains perfection only in humans. This is due **to a special movement of the thumb**, which brings it into contact with every other finger*. **Opposition of the thumb**, despite what is often written about it, is not a human prerogative; it is also present in the great apes but its range is more limited than in man. On the other hand, some quadrimanual apes have four hands, as indicated by their name, and so have four thumbs.

From the functional point of view, the hand is the effector extremity of the upper limb, which **supports it mechanically** and allows it to adopt the most favourable position for any given action. The hand, however, is not only a motor organ but is also a very sensitive and accurate **sensory receptor** that feeds back information essential for its own performance. Finally, it lets the cerebral cortex know how bulky and how far away objects are and is thus responsible for the development of visual appreciation. **Without the hand our vision of the world would be flat and lacking in contrast.**

The hand can also express mental states and feelings. In this way, with the help of gestures, it can create a language, which has the advantage of being international and universal, just like facial expressions.

More critical than the fact that the thumb is opposable is the **hand-brain couple**. The brain directs the hand and in turn the hand has modified the human brain. The hand therefore forms with the brain an **inseparable interacting functional couple**, and this close interaction is responsible for **man's fearsome ability to alter nature at will** for better or for worse and to dominate other species. This is a serious responsibility.

* This chapter is more easily understood by constructing the mechanical model (see end of the book).

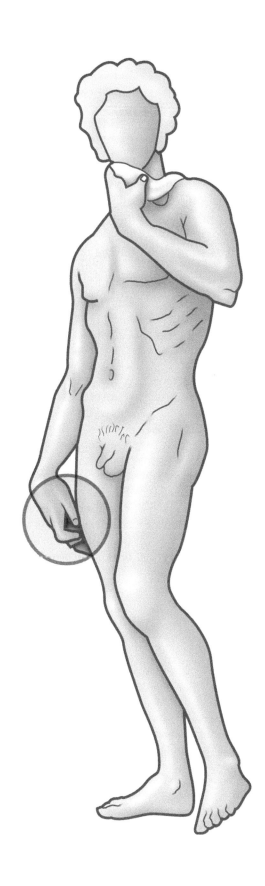

The prehensile ability of the hand

The human hand owes its prehensile ability to its architecture, which allows it to close down on itself either when the fist is clenched or when the hand is wrapped around an object.

When the hand is opened wide (Fig. 1, anterior view), the **palm** is revealed (1), lying distal to the wrist (9) and articulating with the five fingers. This anterior aspect of the hand is called the **palmar surface**. The palm is hollow centrally, and this allows it to receive objects of different sizes. It is bounded on either side by **two convex eminences or projections**, i.e. laterally by the larger **thenar eminence** (4) at the base of the thumb, and medially by the less prominent **hypo-thenar eminence** (7), which forms the medial (ulnar) border of the hand (27) and gives attachment distally to the shortest finger (the **little finger** or **pinkie**), separated from the ring finger by the fourth inter-digital cleft (13).

The palm is criss-crossed by the palmar creases, which vary from person to person and form the basis of the pseudo-science of palmistry. Their pseudo-scientific names will be given here along with their anatomic names, as follows:
- The **distal palmar crease** (2) or 'head line' is the most distal and stands at the medial border of the palm.
- The **middle palmar crease** (3) or 'heart line' is proximal to the former and starts at the lateral border of the palm.
- The **proximal palmar crease** (5) or 'life line' is the most proximal and lies on the medial border of the thenar emi-nence. As it runs obliquely, it forms the floor of the **palmar gutter**.

There is also a less obvious crease, which runs lengthwise along the medial border of the hypo-thenar eminence and can be brought out by closing the palm transversely. It is the **hypothe-nar crease** or the 'luck line' and is the most variable of all four creases. Contraction of a superficial muscle, the *palmaris brevis*, brings out a dimple (8) at the medial border of the hypothenar eminence.

The description of these creases is not given gratuitously, since they are important landmarks on the palm. Their hollowness is due to their fibrous attachments to the deep structures and ensures that the palm remains hollow in all positions of the hand. Surgically these creases provide landmarks for deeper structures and must never be cut perpendicularly to prevent the formation of retractile adhesions that can limit the function of the hand.

The five fingers fall into two groups: **four long fingers and one short finger** (the thumb). The long fingers have different lengths. The longest, the **middle finger**, lies in the centre; the next in length is the **index finger**, the most lateral; the next is the **ring finger**, medial to the middle finger; and the shortest and most medial is the **little finger** (the pinkie). These long fingers have **three creases** on their palmar aspects, indicating the presence of three phalanges:
1) The **distal interphalangeal crease** (17) is usually single, lies slightly distal to the distal interphalangeal (DIP) joint and bounds the pulp proximally (18). The dorsal surface of the third phalanx is filled by a nail, which is surrounded by an overhanging nail fold (37) and develops from the nail matrix (38), located under the skin between the base of the nail and the distal dorsal crease.
2) The **proximal interphalangeal crease** (14) is always double, lies at the same level as the underlying joint and bounds the second phalanx (16) proximally.
3) The **digito-palmar crease** (12), single or double, lies at the junction of the finger and the palm, proximal to the inter-phalangeal joint, and bounds the first phalanx (15) proximally.

These creases, just like their palmar counterparts, tether the skin.

The **thumb**, a short finger, is unique and lies **proximal** to the other fingers. It is attached to the **palmar aspect of the lateral (radial) border of the palm**. It has only **two phalanges**, and **one metacarpal** (Fig. 3, 32), the first metacarpal, which is more mobile than the others and functions like a phalanx. It has two palmar creases. The **single interphalangeal crease** (23) borders proximally the second phalanx, which corresponds to the pulp (22) and lies slightly distal to the interphalangeal joint. The **metacarpo-phalangeal crease** is always double (20 and 21) and lies proximal to the interphalangeal joint.

The **heel of the thenar eminence** (6) corresponds to the tubercle of the scaphoid.

Proximally the junction between the palm and the wrist bears multiple transverse creases, i.e. the **creases of flexion of the wrist** (9), which lie distal to the radio-carpal joint. At the wrist can be seen the prominent tendon of the *flexor carpi radialis* (10), which forms the medial border of the **palpation site of the radial artery** (11).

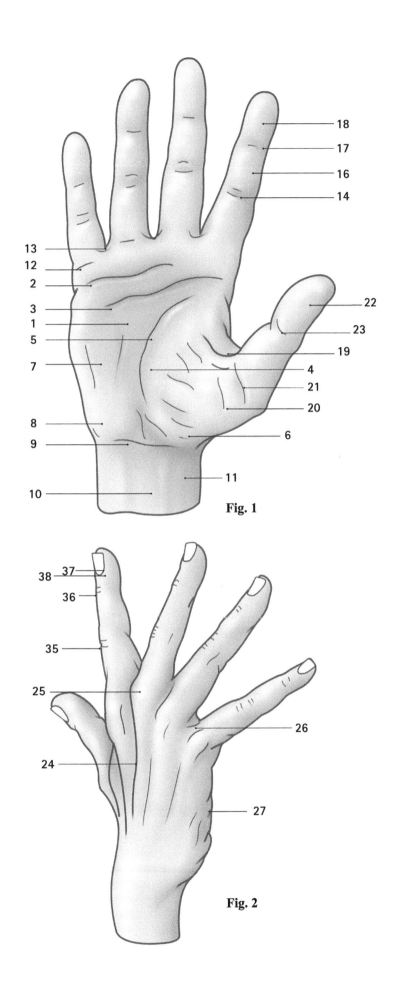

18
17
16
14

13
12
2
3
1
5
7

22
23
19
4
21
20

8
9

6

11

10

Fig. 1

38 37
36

35

25

24

26

27

Fig. 2

When the hand gets ready to grip an object (Fig. 3, lateral view) the long fingers are stretched by the extensors, and the degree of extension decreases from the index to the little finger, while the thumb is extended and abducted because of the depth of the first **interdigital cleft** (19). The **metacarpophalangeal joint** (33) stands out slightly, unlike the **trapezo-metacarpal joint** (31). Proximally lies the **anatomical snuffbox** (28), bounded by the tendon of the **extensor pollicis longus** (30). At the lateral border of the wrist lies the **radial styloid process** (29), and at the postero-medial border lies the projection **of the ulnar head** (34), which disappears during supination.

When the hand gets ready to grip an object (Fig. 2, **medial view**) it twists on itself with distortion of the palm, caused by the displacement of the meta-carpals, which is more marked latero-medially, especially for the fifth metacarpal. The **bases of the interdigital clefts** (26) are more prominent on their palmar surfaces. The **heads of the meta-carpals** (25) and the **extensors** (24) stand out. The **proximal** (35) **and the distal** (36) **inter-phalangeal creases** are always well defined. Between the distal interphalangeal crease and the proximal edge of the nail lies the nail matrix (38) buried under the skin.

When the hand is in use the importance of the five fingers varies. The hand is made up of three zones (Fig. 4):

1) The **zone of prehension I**, the **thumb**, which is clearly the most important functionally because it can be opposed to the other fingers. Its loss virtually destroys the functional capacity of the hand and therefore any risk to the thumb must be avoided, e.g. the wearing of a ring, which can lead to a catastrophic avulsion of the thumb if the ring is accidentally caught.

2) The **zone of prehension II**, made up of the **middle finger** and, more important, of the **index**; these are essential for the **bidigital** grip (thumb/index), i.e. the grip of precision, and for the **tridigital grip** (thumb/index/middle finger), used as a means of feeding by more than half of the world's population.

3) The **zone of prehension III** on the medial (ulnar) side of the hand consists of the **ring finger** and the **little finger**, which are essential to ensure the strength of a **full palmar grip** or of any **firm grip**. It is used **in power grips**, e.g. when gripping tool handles, and is absolutely indispensable.

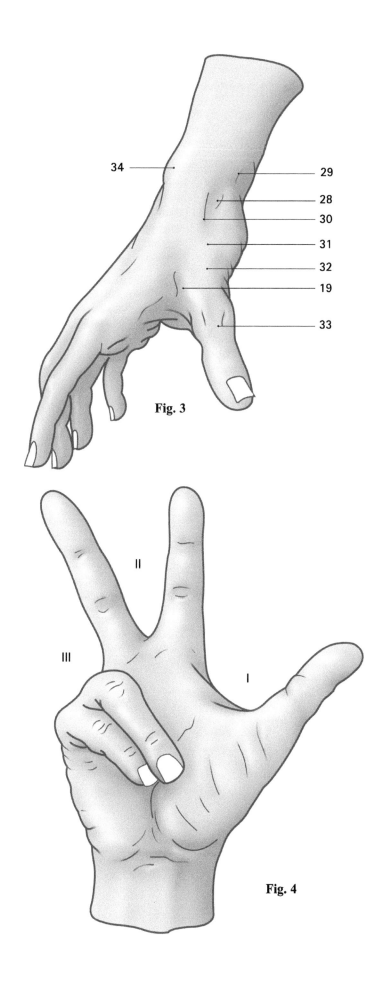

34 ——————— 29

28

30

31

32

19

33

Fig. 3

II

III

I

Fig. 4

The architecture of the hand

The hand can change its shape to grasp objects.

On a **flat surface**, e.g. a glass pane (Fig. 5), **the hand spreads out and becomes flattened** as it makes contact (Fig. 6) at the thenar eminence (1), the hypothenar eminence (2), the metacarpal heads (3) and the palmar surface of the phalanges (4). Only the infero-lateral aspect of the palm does not touch the glass.

When it needs to grip a large object, **the hand becomes hollow**, with the formation of three arches running in **three different directions**:

1) **Transversely** (Fig. 7), the **carpal arch** XOY (blue) corresponds to the concavity of the wrist and is continuous distally with the **metacarpal arch** formed by the metacarpal heads. The long axis of the carpal gutter (blue) crosses the lunate, the capitate and the third metacarpal.

2) **Longitudinally**, the **carpo-metacarpo-phalangeal arches** fan out from the wrist and are formed for each finger by the corresponding metacarpal bone and phalanges. These arches are concave on the palmar surface and the **keystone of each arch lies at the level of the metacarpophalangeal joint**, so that any muscular imbalance at this point interferes with the concavity of the arch. The two most important longitudinal arches are these:

   – the **arch of the middle finger OD3** (Fig. 7), which is collinear with the axis of the carpal gutter
   – the **arch of the index finger OD2** (Fig. 8), which most often interacts with that of the thumb.

3) **Obliquely** (Figs 7-9), the **opposition or diagonal arches** consist of the following:

   – The **most important** is the one linking the thumb and the index finger (D1-D2).
   – The **most extreme** (Figs. 7-9) is that linking the thumb to the little finger (D1-D5).

As a whole, when the hand becomes hollow (Fig. 8), it forms an anteriorly concave gutter, whose borders bear these three landmarks:

1) the thumb (D1), which alone forms the lateral border
2) the index finger (D2) and the little finger (D5), which form the medial border
3) across these two borders of the gutter lie the **four oblique arches of opposition**.

This **palmar gutter**, which runs obliquely at all levels (shown by the large blue arrow inside the palm, Figs 8 and 9), is crossed by the various opposition arches.

It stretches from the base of the hypothenar eminence (Fig. 7, X) – where the pisiform bone can be palpated – to the second metacarpal head (Fig. 7, Z) and corresponds to the palmar crease known as the 'life line'. This is also the direction taken by a cylindrical object, e.g. the handle of a tool, when gripped by the hand.

Conversely, when the fingers are maximally separated (Fig. 10), the hand is flattened and the greatest distance between the pulp of the thumb and that of the little finger is called the **span**. A pianist must have a span of at least an octave.

Finally it is impossible not to notice that in all its positions a **normal healthy hand** has a **harmonious architecture** (Fig. 11) with well-defined **structural elements**, shown here as spirals linking the homologous joints and converging to a focal point (star). These are very useful to painters and draughtsmen as well as to surgeons, who use them to differentiate between a normal and an abnormal hand, whose disorganized architecture is obvious. **Thus the structurally and functionally normal coincides with the aesthetically pleasing.**

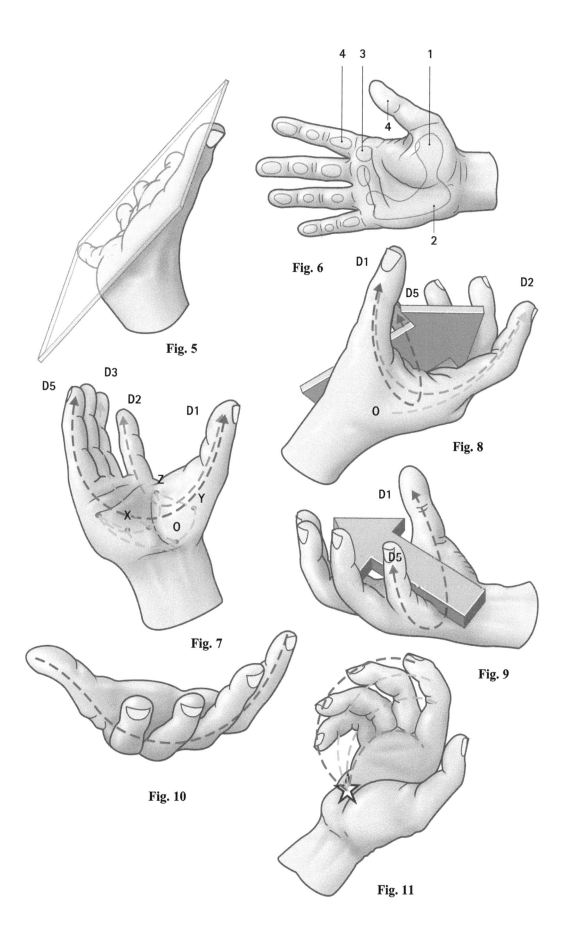

Fig. 5

Fig. 6

Fig. 7

Fig. 8

Fig. 9

Fig. 10

Fig. 11

205

When the fingers are voluntarily spread out (Fig. 12), the axes of the five fingers converge towards the base of the thenar eminence overlying the easily palpated tubercle of the scaphoid. In the hand the movements of the fingers in the **coronal plane**, i.e. **adduction and abduction**, are referred not to the plane of symmetry of the body but to the long axis of the hand, which runs through the **third metacarpal bone and the middle finger**. Therefore the movements of the fingers should be called separation instead of abduction (Fig. 12), and approximation instead of adduction (Fig. 13). During these movements the middle finger is almost stationary but it is possible to abduct and adduct this finger voluntarily, i.e. with respect to the axis of the body.
When the fingers are voluntarily brought together (Fig. 15), their axes are not parallel but converge towards a point lying far distal to the hand. This is due to the fact that the fingers are not cylindrical but taper distally towards their pulps.

When the fingers are allowed to assume a **natural position** (Fig. 14), i.e. a position from which they can be both approximated and separated, they lie a short distance away from one another but their axes do not meet at one point. In the example given, the last three fingers are parallel and the first three fingers diverge from one another, while the middle finger represents the axis of the hand and also the 'zone of transition'.
When the fist is clenched while the distal inter-phalangeal joints are still extended (Fig. 13), the axes of the two distal phalanges of the four fingers and the axis of the thumb (discounting its terminal phalanx) converge at a point corresponding to the 'radial pulse'. Note that in this situation the axis of the index is parallel to the long axis of the hand, while the axes of the other fingers become progressively more oblique the farther they are from the index. The reason for this arrangement and its usefulness will be discussed later.

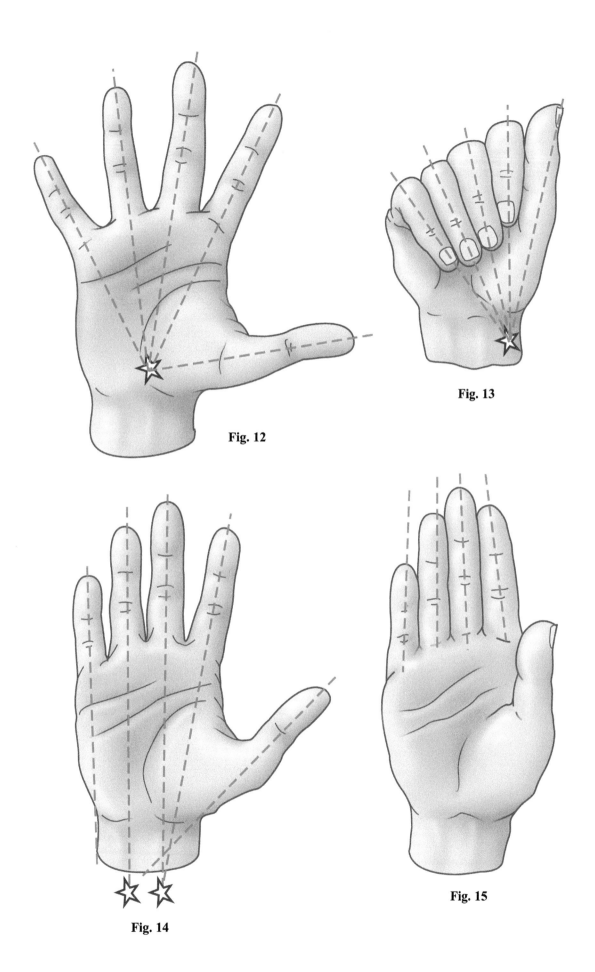

Fig. 12

Fig. 13

Fig. 14

Fig. 15

The carpus

This forms a gutter, which is **concave on the anterior (palmar) side** and is transformed into a **tunnel** by the **flexor retinaculum**, inserted on either side of the gutter.

This gutter arrangement is well seen when one examines the skeleton of the hand with the wrist in hyperextension (Fig. 16) or when one examines radiographs of the hand taken along an axis collinear with that of the carpal tunnel. Its two borders consist of the following:

1) laterally, the tubercle of the scaphoid (1) and the crest of the trapezium (2)
2) medially, the pisiform (3) and the hook of the hamate (4).

(These numbers label the same structures in the other diagrams.)

In the transverse direction, the gutter arrangement is confirmed by **two horizontal sections** as follows:

1) The first section (Fig. 17) passes through the **proximal row of the carpal bones** (Fig. 19, level A) and shows, latero-medially, the scaphoid (1), the head of the capitate (5) encased by the two horns of the lunate, the triquetrum (7) and the pisiform (3).
2) The second section (Fig. 18), passing through the **distal row** (Fig. 19, level B), shows, latero-medially, the trapezium (2), the trapezoid (6), the capitate (5) and the hamate (4). In the distal section (Fig. 18), the *flexor retinaculum* is shown as dashed lines (green).

During hollowing of the palm, the carpal tunnel also deepens because of the small movements occurring at the various inter-carpal joints. These movements are initiated by the thenar (arrow X) and the hypothenar (arrow Y) muscles, whose attachments from the *flexor retinaculum* stretch the ligament (Fig. 18) and bring closer the two borders of the tunnel (dotted lines).

In the longitudinal direction, the carpus (Fig. 19) can also be viewed as made up of **three columns** (Fig. 20):

1) The **lateral column** (a) is the most important, as it includes the **column of the thumb** (Destot), made up of the scaphoid, the trapezium and the first metacarpal. From the scaphoid also springs the column of the index, consisting of the trapezoid and the second metacarpal.
2) The **intermediate column** (b) consists of the lunate, the capitate and the third metacarpal, and forms the axis of the hand (as previously shown).
3) The **medial column** (c), ending in the last two fingers, consists of the triquetrum and the hamate, which articulates with the fourth and fifth metacarpals. The pisiform is 'pulled back' over the triquetrum and does not transmit any forces. It is the site of insertion of the flexor carpi ulnaris and acts as a lever for its action.

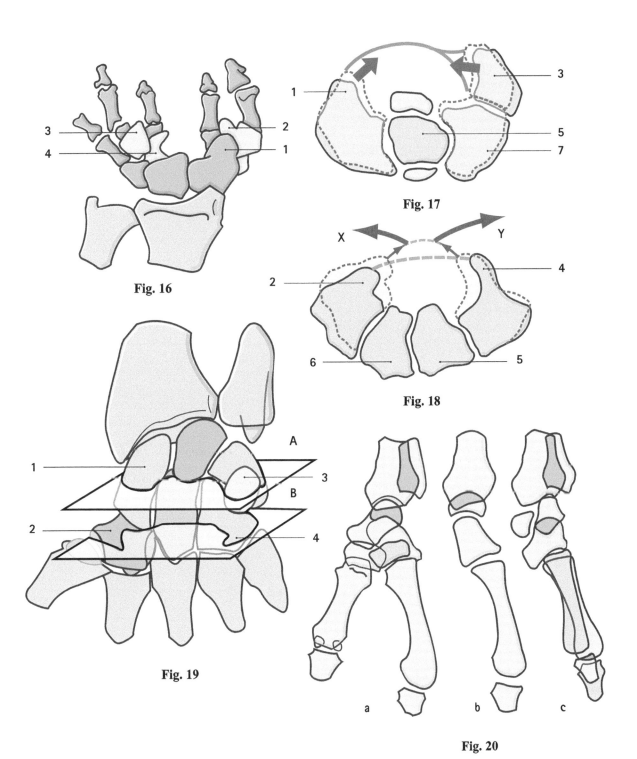

Fig. 16

Fig. 17

Fig. 18

Fig. 19

Fig. 20

The hollowing of the palm

This is due essentially to the movements of the last four meta-carpals (the first one being ignored at present) relative to the carpus. These movements, occurring at the carpo-metacarpal joints, consist of short movements of flexion and extension, as typical of plane joints, but their range increases from the second to the fifth metacarpal:

- When the **hand is flat** (Fig. 22, seen head-on), the heads of the last four metacarpals lie on a straight line (AB).
- When the **palm hollows**, the heads of the last three meta-carpals move anteriorly to A′, i.e. in flexion (Fig. 21, lateral view), and the more so as the last finger is approached. Then the metacarpal heads lie on a curved line A′B, which corresponds to the transverse metacarpal arch.

Two points need to be made:

- The second metacarpal head (B) does not move appreciably, and the flexion-extension movements at the trapezoid-second metacarpal joint are also negligible.
- However, the fifth metacarpal head (A), which is the most mobile (Fig. 22), moves not only anteriorly but also slightly laterally to position (A′).

This brings us to the analysis of the **fifth carpometacarpal joint between the hamate and the fifth metacarpal**. It is a saddle joint (Fig. 24) with slightly cylindrical surfaces. Its axis is oblique in two planes, thus explaining why the metacarpal head moves laterally:

- Figure 23 (distal surface of the distal row of carpal bones) shows that the axis XX′ of the medial facet of the hamate is clearly oblique lateromedially and postero-anteriorly (red dotted line).
- Hence any movement about this axis must logically carry the fifth metacarpal head anteriorly and laterally.
- The axis XX′ of this joint is not quite perpendicular to the long axis OA of the metacarpal but forms an acute angle XOA with it (Fig. 24). This orientation of the axis also explains why the fifth metacarpal head moves laterally according to the following geometrical principles:
- Figure 25 explains the phenomenon of **conical rotation.** When a segment OA of the straight line OZ rotates around an axis YY′ perpendicular to it, it will describe an arc of a circle in the plane P to reach OA″.
- If this same segment OA turns about an oblique axis XX′, it will move **not in the same plane but along a segment of a cone with apex O tangential to P**. After the same degree of rotation as above, point A is now in position A′ at the base of the cone. This point A′ no longer lies in the plane P but in front of it (as shown in the diagram). If one mentally combines this geometrical reasoning with the diagram of the joint (Fig. 24), it becomes clear why the fifth metacarpal head A leaves the sagittal plane P and moves slightly lateral to it.

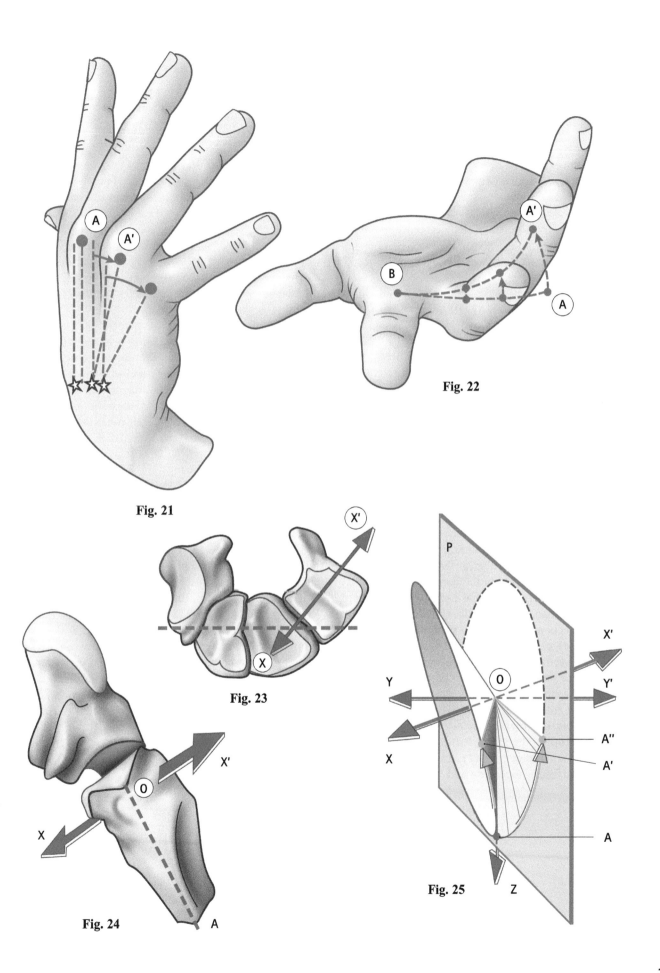

Fig. 21

Fig. 22

Fig. 23

Fig. 24

Fig. 25

The metacarpo-phalangeal (MP) joints

These joints are of the **condyloid type** (Fig. 26, MP joint opened on its posterior aspect) with **two degrees of freedom:**

1) **flexion-extension** in a sagittal plane about the transverse axis YY′ (red)
2) **lateral inclinations** in the coronal plane about the antero-posterior axis XX′ (blue).

They have **two articular surfaces:**

1) The **metacarpal head A** is a biconvex articular surface, broader anteriorly than posteriorly.
2) The **base of the proximal phalanx** B contains a biconcave articular surface, which is much smaller in surface area than the head of the metacarpal. This surface is extended anteriorly by the **fibrocartilaginous palmar plate** (2), which can be considered as a back-up for the articular surface. It is attached to the anterior surface of the base of the phalanx with a small cleft (3), which functions like a **hinge**.

In fact, in Figure 27 (sagittal cut during **extension**), the deep cartilaginous surface of the **palmar plate** (2) is in contact with the metacarpal head. During **flexion** (Fig. 28), the plate **moves past the metacarpal head** and turns upon the hinge-like cleft (3) to **glide along the palmar surface of the metacarpal.** It is clear that if the fibrocartilaginous palmar plate were replaced by a bony plate firmly attached to the base of the phalanx, flexion would be checked earlier by bony contact. Therefore the plate reconciles two apparently contradictory requirements; it increases the area of the articular surface and avoids any movement-limiting contact between the bones.

There is also, however, another essential condition for freedom of movement, i.e. a certain degree of 'slack' in the capsule and in the synovium. This is provided by the **posterior** (4) and the **anterior** (5) **recesses** of the capsule, and **the depth of the anterior recess is essential for the gliding movement of the palmar plate.** On the posterior surface of the base of the phalanx is inserted the deep band (6) of the extensor tendon.

On either side of the joint there are **two types** of ligament:

1) a **ligament joining the metacarpal to the palmar plate** (p. 216) and controlling the movements of the latter
2) a **collateral ligament,** shown cut (1) in Figure 26, keeping the articular surfaces together and restraining their movements.

Since their metacarpal insertion (A) does not lie at the centre of curvature of the metacarpal head (Fig. 29) but **slightly posteriorly, they are slackened in extension and stretched in flexion.** The length is indicated by the double arrow representing the degree of tension developed.

This state of affairs makes lateral movements difficult, **if not impossible**, when the MP joint is **flexed.** On the contrary, during extension, **lateral movements can occur** with a range of 20-30° on each side. One of the collateral ligaments is stretched, while the other is slackened (Fig. 32).

The **range of flexion** (Fig. 29) is close to 90°, being just at 90° for the index finger and **increasing progressively towards the fifth finger** (Fig. 43, p. 221). Moreover, the isolated flexion of the finger (the middle finger here) is checked by the tension developed in the **interdigital palmar ligament** (Fig. 44, p. 221). The range of **active extension varies with the subject** and can reach 30-40° (Fig. 45, p. 221). **Passive extension** can reach up to 90° in subjects with hyperlaxity of the ligaments (Fig. 46, p. 221). When flexion of the four segments of the digital complex formed by the metacarpal and the three phalanges is studied, its curling path (Fig. 30) follows a **logarithmic spiral,** as shown by the American surgeon Littler. This spiral, also called **equiangular,** is generated by the successive interlocking of **golden rectangles,** which are so called because the ratio of their length to their width is 1.618, known as the **golden number.** This number, ϕ (pronounced phi and known since Plato), possesses certain esoteric features; hence its name of 'divine proportion'. It is derived from the **Fibonacci sequence** (Fibonacci was an Italian mathematician, 1180-1250), where each number is the sum of the two preceding numbers, i.e. 1, 2, 3, 5, 8, 13 etc. From the 25th number onwards the ratio between two successive numbers is constant, i.e. 1.618. (Try it on your computer!)

This simply means that the lengths of the four bony components of the digital complex are related in this way. In practice, this relationship is a necessary condition for the phalanges to roll up as the finger curls.

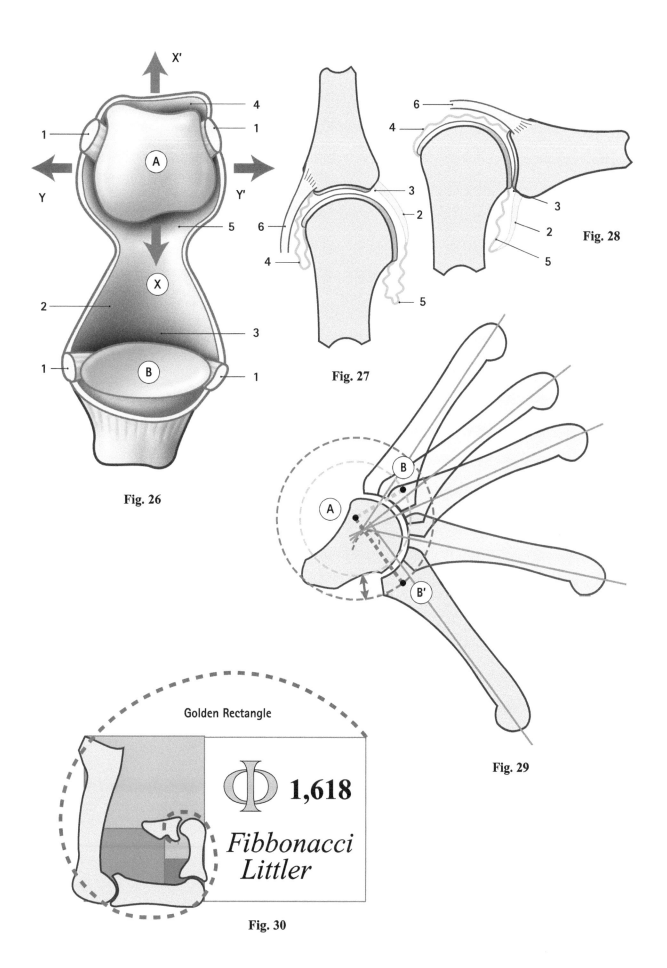

Fig. 26

Fig. 27

Fig. 28

Fig. 29

Golden Rectangle

Φ **1,618**

*Fibbonacci
Littler*

Fig. 30

When the MP joint is straight, a position wrongly termed extension (Fig. 31, coronal section), the collateral ligaments are relaxed and in equilibrium, allowing **lateral** movements to occur (Fig. 32). One ligament is stretched while the other is slackened. The **interossei** initiate these movements. Conversely, during flexion, the tension developed in the lateral ligaments stabilizes the joint.

Another important consequence of this state of affairs is that the MP joints **must never be immobilized in extension** for fear of producing almost irreversible stiffness. The slack collateral ligaments can shorten in extension but cannot do so in flexion, as they are maximally stretched.

The **shape of the metacarpal heads** and the length and direction of the ligaments are critical in influencing at once the obliquity of flexion of the fingers (see later) and their ulnar deviations in rheumatoid arthritis (according to Tubiana).

The **head of the second metacarpal** (Fig. 33, inferior view of the right side) is clearly asymmetrical, being significantly swollen antero-medially and flattened laterally. The medial collateral ligament is thicker and longer than the lateral, which is inserted more posteriorly.

The **head of the third metacarpal** (Fig. 34) is similarly asymmetrical but its asymmetry is less marked. Its ligaments are similar.

The **head of the fourth metacarpal** (Fig. 35) is more symmetrical, with a similar palmar swelling on each side. Its ligaments are similar in thickness and obliquity, with the lateral being slightly longer.

The **head of the fifth metacarpal** (Fig. 36) shows a pattern of asymmetry opposite to that of the second and third metacarpals. Its ligaments are similar to those of the fourth.

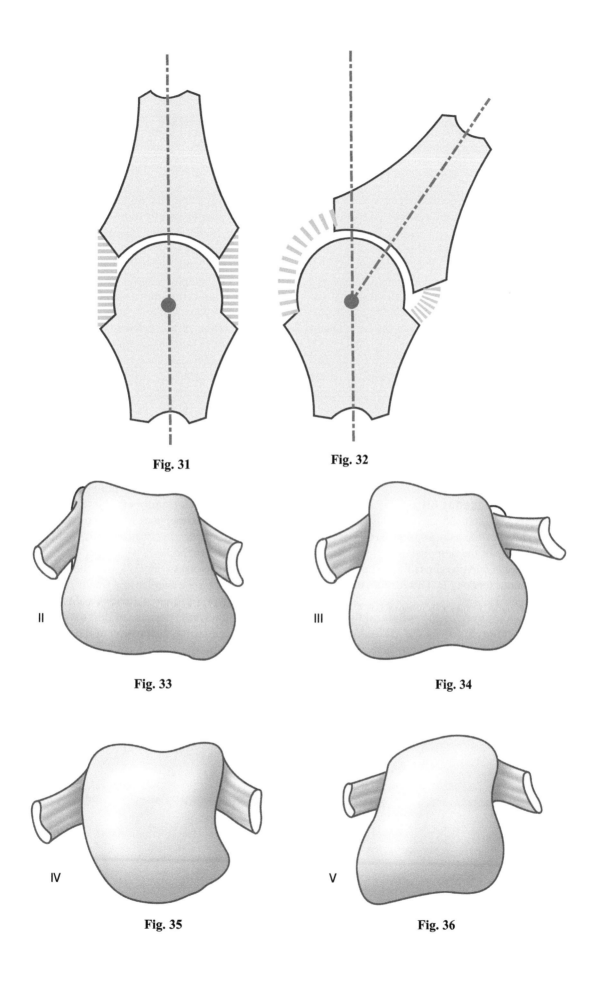

Fig. 31

Fig. 32

Fig. 33

Fig. 34

Fig. 35

Fig. 36

The ligamentous complex of the metacarpo-phalangeal (MP) joints

The collateral ligaments of the MP joints belong to a complex **ligamentous system**, which holds and 'centres' the tendons of the extensors and flexors.

Figure 37 (a **postero-lateral and lateral view of the joint**) also shows the tendons encasing the MP joint posteriorly and anteriorly between the metacarpal M and the first phalanx P1:

- The **extensor digitorum** (1), on the dorsal surface of the capsule, sends a **deep expansion** (a) to be inserted into the base of the first phalanx. It then divides into the **central slip** (b) and the **two lateral slips** (c), which receive the insertions of the interossei (not shown here but clearly visible in figures 86 to 88 on page 241). Just before the deep expansion leaves the tendon, small **sagittal bands** (d) become detached from the lateral borders of the muscle and cross the lateral aspects of the joint before gaining insertion into the **deep transverse metacarpal ligament** (4). Thus, during flexion at the joint, the extensor tendon is kept in the axis of movement as it crosses the convex dorsal surfaces of the metacarpal head. This is an unstable position.
- The **flexor digitorum profundus** (2) and the **flexor digitorum superficialis** (3) enter the **metacarpal pulley** (5), which starts at the level of the palmar plate (6) and extends (5′) to the palmar surface of the first phalanx (P1), where the superficialis tendon splits into two slips (3′) just before being pierced by the profundus tendon (2). This is more obvious in the diagrams on page 231.

The **joint capsule** (7) is reinforced by the **collateral ligament**, attached to the **lateral tubercle** (8) of the metacarpal head posterior to the line of the centres of curvature (see above) and composed of three components:

1) a **metacarpo-phalangeal bundle** (9), running obliquely distally and anteriorly towards the base of the first phalanx

2) a **bundle linking the metacarpal and the palmar plate** (10), running anteriorly to insert into the edges of the palmar plate (6), which is thus pressed against the metacarpal head and stabilized

3) a **thinner bundle linking the phalanx to the palmar plate** (11), which helps to 'recall' the plate during extension.

The **deep transverse metacarpal ligament** (4) is attached to the adjacent borders of the palmar plates of the MP joints, so that its fibres span the full width of the hand at the level of these joints. It contributes to the formation of the fibrous tunnels for the interossei (not shown) and lies posterior to the tendon of the lumbrical (see Fig. 42, page 219 and Fig. 88, page 241). The **metacarpal pulley** (5), attached to the lateral borders of the palmar plate, thus literally hangs from the metacarpal head by the ligament linking the metacarpal to the palmar plate (6) and by the palmar plate itself.

This pulley plays an important role **during flexion at the MP joint**:

- **When intact** (Fig. 38), the pulley, whose fibres roll up distally (red arrow), redirects the 'detaching component' of force (white arrow) back towards the metacarpal head. Hence the flexor tendons stay close to the joint and the phalangeal head is stabilized.
- **In disease states** (Fig. 39), e.g. rheumatoid arthritis, when the ligaments are swollen and finally ruptured, this 'detaching component' of force is directed not towards the metacarpal head but towards the base of the first phalanx, causing anterior and proximal dislocation of the metacarpal head, which becomes more prominent.
- **This condition** (Fig. 40) **can to some degree be treated** by excision of the proximal part of the metacarpal pulley but this leads to loss of efficiency of the flexors.

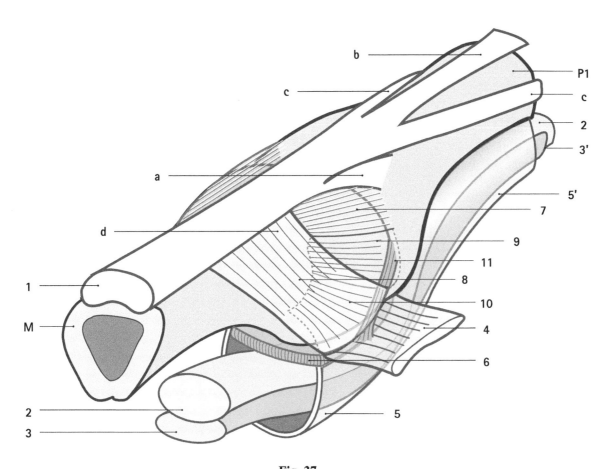

Fig. 37

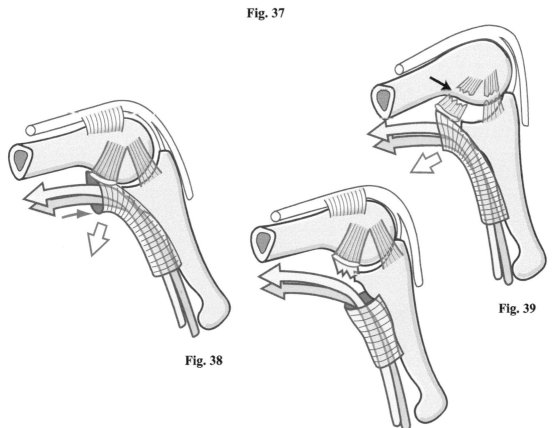

Fig. 38

Fig. 39

Fig. 40

The tendons of the common extensor (Fig. 41), which converge on the dorsal aspect of the wrist, are strongly pulled medially on their ulnar side (white arrows) because of the **angle of divergence** formed by the long axes of the metacarpal and the first phalanx. This angle is greater for the **index finger** (14°) and the **middle finger** (13°) than for the **ring finger** (4°) and for the **little finger** (8°). Only the **radial sagittal band of the extensor tendon**, lying on the radial side, opposes this tendency for the extensor tendon to be displaced medially on the convex dorsal surface of the metacarpal head.

In **rheumatoid arthritis** (Fig. 42, seen at the level of the metacarpal heads), the **collateral ligaments** (10) degenerate and release the **palmar plate** (6), which gives attachment to the **metacarpal pulley** (5), holding the tendons of the *flexor digitorum profundus* (2) and *superficialis* (3). The **radial sagittal band** (d) is also slackened or ruptured, resulting in ulnar displacement of the **extensor tendon** (1) into the **inter-metacarpal gutter**, which normally contains only the **tendons of the interossei** (12) and of the **lumbricals** (13), as they lie anterior and posterior respectively to the **deep transverse metacarpal ligament** (4).

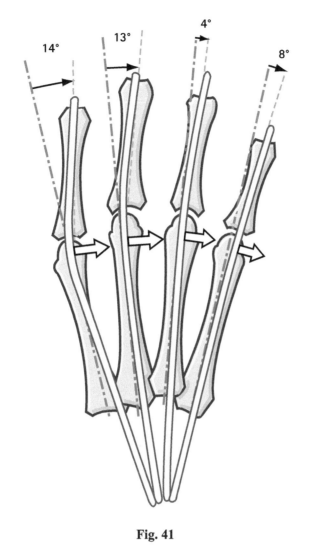

Fig. 41

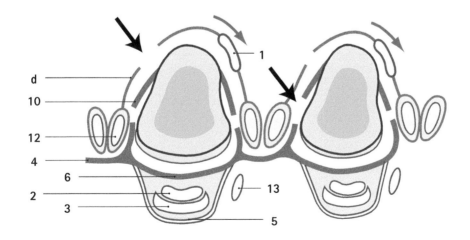

Fig. 42

The range of movements of the metacarpo-phalangeal (MP) joints

Flexion has a range of about 90° (Fig. 43). It falls just short of 90° for the index but increases progressively for the other fingers. Moreover, isolated flexion of one finger (the middle finger here) is checked (Fig. 44) by the tension developed in the palmar interdigital ligament.

The range of active extension varies with the subject and can reach 30-40° (Fig. 45). **Passive extension** can reach 90° in people with very lax ligaments (Fig. 46). Of all the fingers (except the thumb), the **index finger** (Fig. 47) has the greatest range of lateral movements (30°), and, as it is easily moved on its own, the terms abduction (A) and adduction (B) can be used here. The index owes its name to this great mobility (**index = indicator**).

By a combination of various degrees of abduction (A), adduction (B), extension (C) and flexion (D), the index finger (Fig. 48) can perform the **movements of circumduction**, which take place within the **cone of circumduction**. This is defined by its base (ACBD) and its apex (the MP joint). This cone is flattened transversely because of the greater range of the movements of flexion and extension. Its axis (white arrow) corresponds to the **position of equilibrium** or the **position of function**.

Condyloid joints do not normally have a third degree of freedom and do not show axial rotation, and this applies to the MP joints of the four fingers as regards active axial rotation. However, because of the laxity of the ligaments, some **passive axial rotation** is possible with a range of 60° (Roud).

Note that for the index finger the range of passive medial rotation or pronation is much greater (45°) than that of lateral rotation or supination, which is almost zero.

Even if a true active axial rotation is not found at the MP joints, there is **automatic rotation** in the direction of supination, caused by the asymmetry of the metacarpal head and the unequal length and tension of the collateral ligaments. This movement, which is similar to that seen in the interphalangeal joint of the thumb, is greater in the more medial fingers and is maximal for the little finger, where it contributes to the movement of that finger towards the opposing thumb.

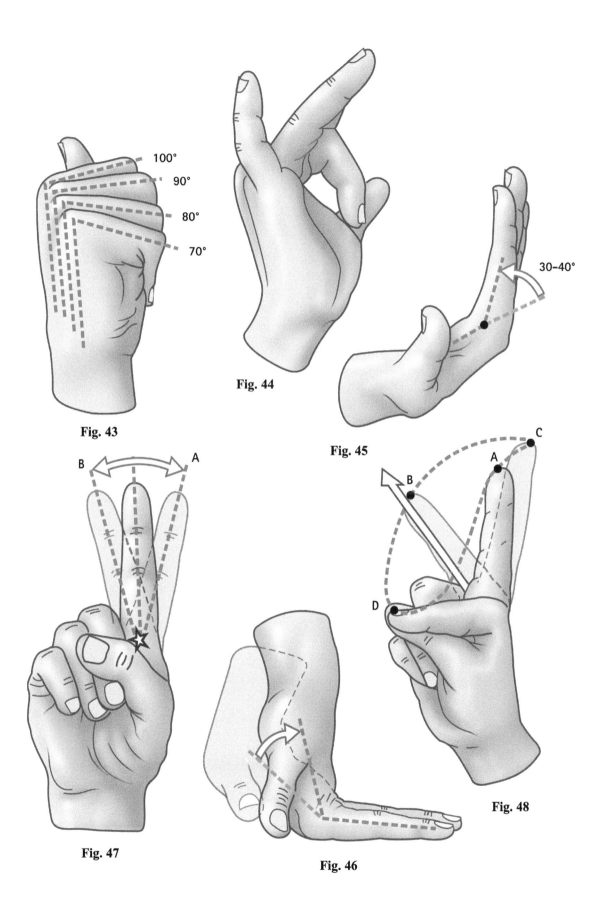

Fig. 43

Fig. 44

Fig. 45

Fig. 46

Fig. 47

Fig. 48

The interphalangeal (IP) joints

These are hinge joints with one degree of freedom:

- The **head of the phalanx** (A) is pulleyshaped (Fig. 50) with only one transverse axis (Fig. 49, XX'), about which flexion and extension take place in the sagittal plane.
- The **base of the immediately distal phalanx** (B) bears two shallow facets, which are in contact with the pulley-shaped head of the proximal phalanx. The shallow crest that separates these two facets comes to rest within the central groove of the pulley. As in the MP joints – and for the same mechanical reasons – the articular surface is widened by the **palmar plate** (2). Note that the numbers have the same meaning as in Figure 53.

During flexion (Fig. 51) the palmar plate glides along the palmar surface of the first phalanx.

Figure 52 (**lateral view**) shows the **collateral ligaments** (1), **the expansions of the extensor tendon** (6) and the **anterior capsular ligaments** (7). **The collateral ligaments are stretched during flexion** to a greater degree than those of the MP joints. The pulley-shaped phalanx (Fig. 50, A) is broader anteriorly, so that the tension in the ligaments is increased and a larger articular surface is available to the head of the distal phalanx. Therefore no lateral movements occur during flexion.

These ligaments are also **stretched in full extension**, which is the **position of absolute lateral stability**. Conversely, they become slack in intermediate positions of flexion, which must never be used during immobilization because of the risk of shortening of the ligaments and stiffening of the joint.

Stiffening in flexion can also be due to **shortening of the 'brakes of extension'**, recently described by anglophone authors

at the level of the proximal interphalangeal (PIP) joints and called the **check rein ligaments** (Fig. 53, PIP joint viewed from the palm and proximally). They consist of a bundle of longitudinal fibres (8), coursing over the palmar surface of the palmar plate (2) on either side of the tendons of the *flexor digitorum profundus* (11) and *superficialis* (12), bridging the ligamentous pulleys of the second (10) and the first (not shown) phalanges, and forming the lateral edge of the **cruciate fibres** (9) of the pulley of the PIP joint. These check rein ligaments prevent hyperextension of the PIP joint and, when they **retract**, cause stiffening of the joint during flexion. They must then be surgically excised.

On the whole, the IP joints, especially the proximal, must be immobilized in a **position close to full extension**.

The **range of flexion** at the PIP joints (Fig. 54) exceeds 90°, so that in flexion P2 and P1 form an acute angle. (In this diagram the phalanges are not seen strictly from the side so that the angles appear obtuse.) As in the case of MP joints, flexion increases in range from the second to the fifth finger to reach a maximum of 135° in the latter.

The **range of flexion** at the DIP joints (Fig. 55) is slightly less than 90°, so that the angle between P2 and P3 remains obtuse. As in the PIP joints, this range increases from the second to the fifth finger to attain a maximum of 90° in the latter.

The **range of active extension** (Fig. 56) at the IP joints is nil at the PIP joints (P) and nil or trivial (5°) at the DIP joints (D).

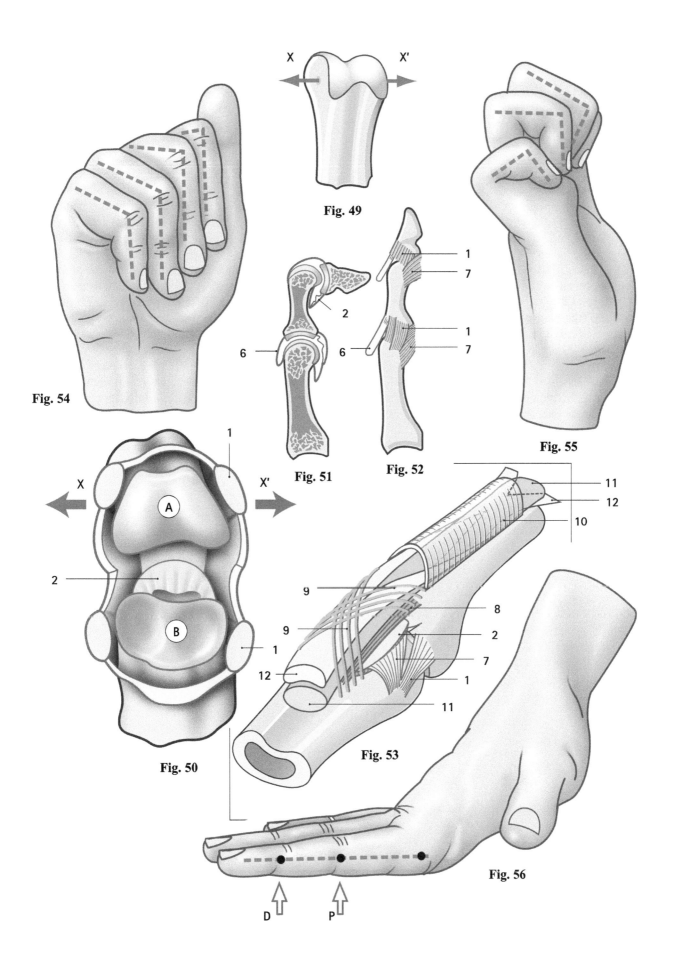

Fig. 49

Fig. 54

Fig. 51

Fig. 52

Fig. 55

Fig. 50

Fig. 53

Fig. 56

223

Passive extension is nil at the PIP joint (Fig. 57) but appreciable (30°) at the DIP joint.

Since the IP joints have only one degree of freedom, there are no active lateral movements, but there are **passive movements** (Fig. 58) in the DIP joint. The PIP joint is very stable laterally, and this explains the problems that arise when one of its collateral ligaments is torn.

The **plane containing the movements of flexion** for each of the last four digits (Fig. 59) deserves special mention:

- The index is flexed in a **strictly sagittal plane** (P) passing near the base of the thenar eminence.
- As shown previously (Fig. 13, p. 207), the axes of the fingers during flexion all converge at a point corresponding to the distal margin of the 'radial pulse'. This can occur only if the last three fingers are flexed not in a sagittal plane like the index finger but in an **increasingly oblique plane latero-medially**.
- The oblique direction of the axes of the little finger and of the ring finger are shown by the blue arrows pointing towards the star. Thanks to the obliquity of their axes of flexion, the more medial fingers **can oppose the thumb, just as the index finger does**.

The diagram in Figure 60 uses strips of cardboard to demonstrate how this type of flexion occurs:

- A narrow piece of cardboard (a) represents the joints of the finger with the metacarpal (M) and the three phalanges (P_1, P_2 and P_3).

- If the fold in the cardboard strip representing the axis of flexion of an IP joint is **perpendicular** XX'' to the long axis of the strip, the phalanx will bend in the sagittal plane (d) and cover the adjacent phalanx exactly.
- If, on the other hand, the fold is **slightly oblique** medially XX', flexion will not occur in the sagittal plane and the flexed phalanx (b) will overshoot the adjacent phalanx laterally.
- Thus only a slight obliquity of the axis of flexion is required, because it is multiplied by a factor of 3 (XX', YY' and ZZ'), so that when the little finger is fully flexed (c), its obliquity brings it into contact with the thumb.
- The same demonstration applies, though to a decreasing extent, to the ring finger and the middle finger.

In real life, the axes of flexion of the MP and IP joints are not fixed or unchanging. They are perpendicular to the joint in full extension and become progressively more oblique during flexion. This change in the orientation of the axis of flexion is due to the **asymmetry of the articular surfaces of the MP** (see above) **and of the IP joints** and also because the **collateral ligaments are stretched differentially**, as will be shown later for the MP and IP joints of the thumb.

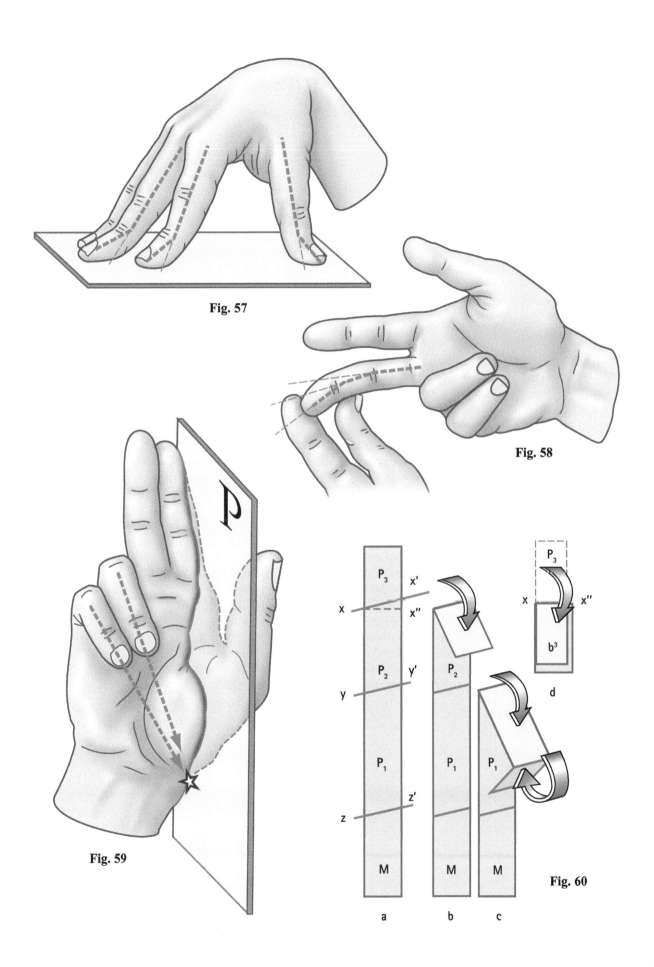

Fig. 57

Fig. 58

Fig. 59

Fig. 60

The tunnels and synovial sheaths of the flexor tendons

During their course through the concave regions of the hand these tendons need to be tethered to the bones by **fibrous sheaths** or else they would, under tension, **take the chordal path** bridging the borders of the concavities. This would mean a relative lengthening of the tendons with respect to the bones and a decrease in their efficiency.

The **first fibro-osseous tunnel** is the **carpal tunnel** (Fig. 62, page 229, inspired by Rouvière), which lets through all the flexor tendons (red arrow) as they pass from the forearm to the hand. The two borders of the tunnel are bridged by the **flexor retinaculum** (FR) (Fig. 61, see-through view of the hand). This combination **creates the most important fibro-osseous pulley in the human body**.

The **section of the carpal tunnel** (Fig. 63, page 229) shows lying in two planes the tendons of the **flexor communis superficialis** (2) and **profundus** (3), as well as the tendon of the **flexor pollicis longus** (4). The tendon of the **flexor carpi radialis** (5) runs through a special compartment of its own before reaching its insertion into the second metacarpal (Fig. 62). Medially the *flexor carpi ulnaris* (FCU) runs outside the tunnel to its insertion into the pisiform. The **median nerve** (Fig. 63, 6) also passes through this tunnel, where it can be compressed by narrowing of the tunnel, unlike the **ulnar nerve** (7), which, with its companion artery, passes through a special tunnel (**Guyon's canal**) anterior to the *flexor retinaculum*.

At the level of the fingers the flexor tendons are tethered by **three arcuate pulleys formed by transverse fibres** (Figs 61 and 64); the **first** (A_1) lies just proximal to the metacarpal head, the **second** (A_3) on the palmar surface of P_1 and the **third** (A_5) on the anterior surface of P_2. Between these arcuate pulleys with transverse fibres the tendons are held down continuously by **oblique and cruciate fibres**, which are less thick and crisscross the joints so as to allow the phalanges to move properly during flexion. These **cruciform pulleys** are A_2 on the palmar aspect of the MP joint and A_4 anterior to the PIP joint. Thus,

along with the slightly concave palmar surface of the phalanges, these pulleys form **true fibro-osseous tunnels** (inset).

The synovial sheaths (Fig. 61) allow the tendons to glide smoothly within their tunnels, a little like the brake linings of a bicycle. Each of the **fingers in the middle** has its own sheath, i.e. the index finger (S_2), the middle finger (S_3) and the ring finger (S_4). These sheaths have the simplest possible structure (Fig. 65, page 229, simplified diagram); the tendon t (only one is shown for simplicity's sake) is surrounded by a **synovial sheath** (partly resected in the diagram), with two layers: a visceral layer (a) in contact with the tendon, and a parietal layer (b) that lines the deep surface of the fibro-osseous tunnel. Between these two layers lies a potential but closed cavity (c) (which is shown here abnormally distended); it contains no air but only a small amount of synovial fluid to facilitate the sliding of one layer on the other. At each end of the sheath the two layers are continuous and form **two peritendinous recesses** (d).

Section A shows this simple arrangement. When the tendon moves in its tunnel, the **visceral layer slides over the parietal layer**, just as the **articulated caterpillar** tracks of an all-terrain vehicle move relative to the ground, i.e. only the upper layer moves relative to the lower layer, which remains in contact with the ground. If an infection develops between the two layers, they become adherent to each other and **the tendon cannot glide in its tunnel**, since it is now 'jammed' like the cable of a rusty brake. As a result of these **tendinous adhesions, the tendon has become functionally useless**.

In some places in the middle portion of the sheath (section B), the two layers are separated by the blood vessels (e) supplying the tendon, forming a **meso-tendon**, i.e. a sort of longitudinal sling (**vinculum tendinis**, f) holding the tendon within its synovial sheath (c). This description is a very simplified version, especially as regards the synovial sheaths, and for further details a textbook of anatomy should be consulted.

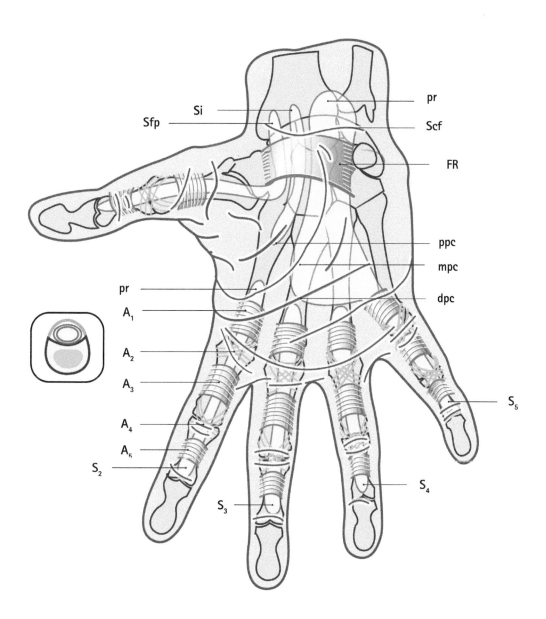

Fig. 61

In the palm of the hand the tendons glide inside **three synovial sheaths** (Fig. 61), which are, latero-medially:

- the **flexor pollicis longus sheath** (Sfp), continuous with the digital sheath of the thumb
- the **intermediate sheath** (Si), investing the **index tendon of the flexor digitorum** without being continuous with its digital sheath
- the **common flexor sheath** (Scf), whose proximal recess (pr) extends back to the anterior surfaces of the wrist. It does not entirely surround the tendons and has the following three prolongations:
    - anteriorly, the **pretendinous recess** (8)
    - posteriorly, the **retro-tendinous recess** (10)
    - the **intertendinous recess** between the superficial and deep tendons (9).

The common flexor sheath merges and communicates with the digital sheath of the fifth finger.

Anatomically it is important to observe the following:

- The synovial sheaths of the flexor tendons start in the forearm proximal to the flexor retinaculum (Fig. 61).
- The sheaths of the three middle fingers extend back to the middle of the palm and their superficial recesses correspond to the **distal palmar crease** (dpc) for the third and fourth fingers and to the **middle palmar crease** (mpc) for the index finger. The **proximal (thenar) palmar crease** (ppc) corresponds to the third ray of the hand in its proximal portion.
- The flexor skin creases (Fig. 64, red arrows) – except for the proximal crease – lie just proximal to the corresponding joints, where the skin is in direct contact with the synovial sheath, **which can be readily infected by an insect bite**.

Note also that the dorsal skin creases (white arrows) lie proximal to their joints.

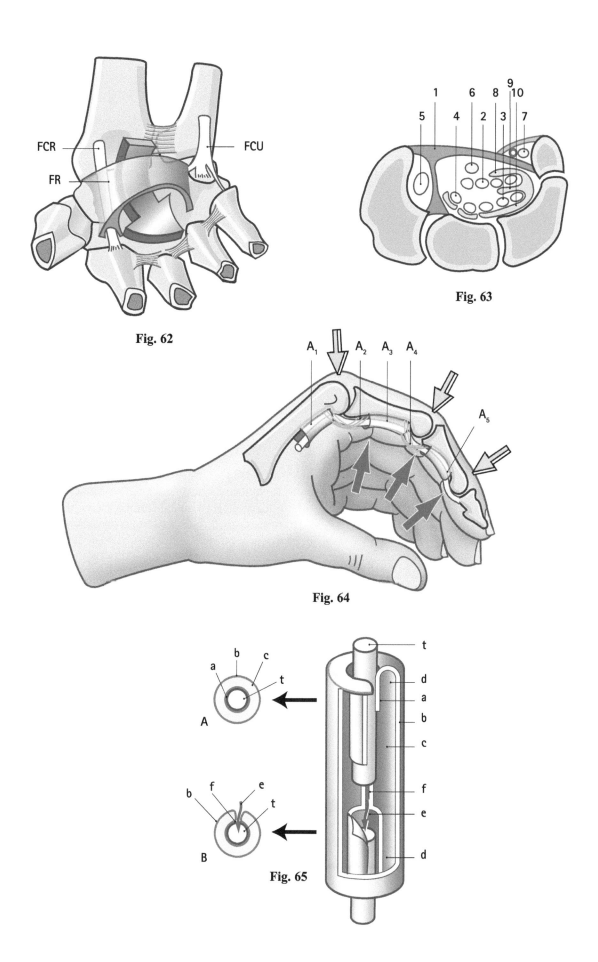

FCR

FCU

FR

Fig. 62

5 1 4 6 2 8 3 9 10 7

Fig. 63

A₁ A₂ A₃ A₄

A₅

Fig. 64

b
a c
t

A

b f e
t

B

t
d
a
b
c

f
e

d

Fig. 65

The tendons of the long flexors of the fingers

The strong and bulky digital flexors lie in the anterior compartment of the forearm and are thus **extrinsic muscles**, since they act on the hand and the fingers via their long tendons, whose insertions are unusual (Fig. 66).

The most superficial muscle, i.e. the **flexor digitorum superficialis** (FDS) (blue in the diagram), is inserted into P_2, and so its insertion is proximal to that of the deep muscle, i.e. the **flexor digitorum profundus** (FDP) (yellow). **Therefore these two tendons must inevitably cross each other in space and must do so symmetrically** to avoid any unwanted component of force. The only solution is for one tendon to perforate the other. Logically one would expect the *profundus* to 'perforate' the *superficialis* since it is inserted distally, and this is exactly what happens. These classic anatomic diagrams demonstrate **how these two tendons cross each other** at the level of metacarpal (M) and of P_1, P_2 and P_3.

The *superficialis* tendon (blue) divides into two slips (Fig. 67) at the level of the MP joint, and these two slips wrap themselves round the *profundus* tendon before reuniting at the PIP joint proximal to their insertion into the sides of P_2. This is further illustrated in Figure 68 and in Figure 69 where the tendon of the flexor digitorum profundus can be seen perforating that of the flexor digitorum superficialis.

A blown-up view (Fig. 70, lateral view) also shows the meso-tendons (**vincula tendinum**), which are synovial partitions that carry the blood supply to the tendons (Lundborg et al.). They fall into two sets:

1) the **first set, related to the FDS**, with two pathways of vascular supply:
   – **proximal (zone A)**, consisting of small longitudinal intratendinous vessels (1) and the vessels coursing down at the proximal end of the synovial sheath (5)

– **distal (zone B)**, consisting of the vessels in the short meso-tendon or **vinculum breve** (3) at the level of the two lateral insertions of the FDS into P_2.

Between these two zones there is an avascular zone (4), located at the division of the FDS tendon.

2) the **second set, related to the flexor digitorum profundus** (FDP), with three pathways of vascular supply:
   – **proximal (zone A)**, consisting of two types of vessel (5 and 6) similar to those of the FDS
   – **intermediate (zone B)**, consisting of vessels running successively through the long meso-tendon or *vinculum longum* (7) and the short meso-tendon or the *vinculum breve* of FDS
   – **distal (zone C)**, consisting of vessels running through the short meso-tendons inserted into P_3 (8).

Thus for the FDP there are **three avascular zones**:
- a short zone (9) between zones A and B
- a short zone (10) between zones B and C
- a peripheral zone (11) 1 mm wide and equal to a quarter of the tendon's diameter. It belongs to what hand surgeons call the **no-man's land** and lies close to the PIP joint.

Hand surgeons must be familiar with the **blood supply of these tendons** if they want to preserve them in optimal condition. Moreover, sutures placed in these avascular zones run a higher risk of giving way.

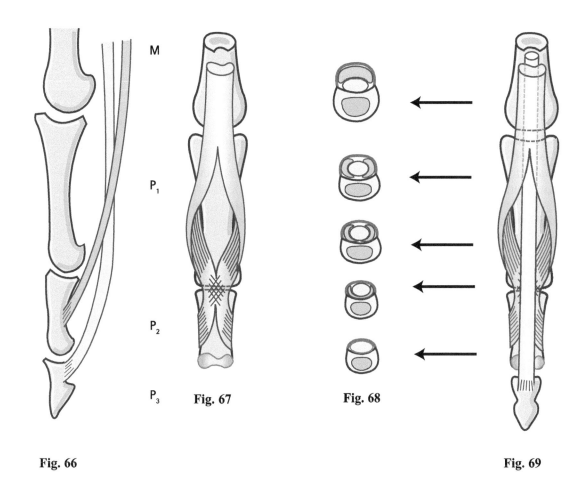

M

P₁

P₂

P₃

Fig. 67

Fig. 68

Fig. 66

Fig. 69

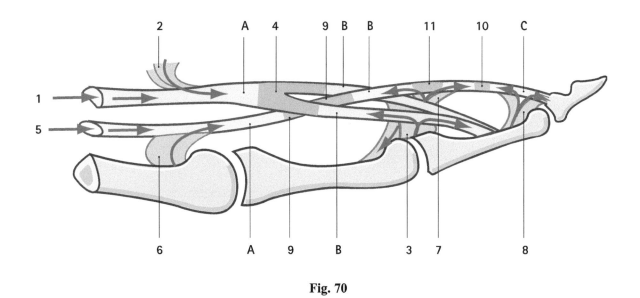

Fig. 70

Theoretically possible is a simpler arrangement where the tendons would not have to cross each other; the tendon inserted on P_2 would be deep and the tendon inserted on P_3 would be superficial. What is the need for the complicated crossing of these tendons? Without being guilty of teleological reasoning, one can be allowed to point out (Fig. 71) that by staying superficial right down to its insertion, the *superficial* tendon forms a greater angle of traction with P_2 than it would by running closer to the bone. **Thus its angle of traction is widened and its efficiency enhanced** (Fig. 74), providing a logical explanation for why the *superficialis* tendon is perforated by the *profundus* and not vice versa. The actions of these two muscles can be deduced from their points of insertion.

- The **flexor digitorum superficialis** (FDS) (Fig. 71) is inserted into P_2 and so flexes the PIP joint. It has little effect on the DIP joint and is a weak flexor of the MP joint only when the PIP joint is fully flexed. Its efficiency is maximal when the MP joint is kept extended by contraction of the *extensor digitorum* (synergistic action). Its angle of traction increases as P_2 is flexed and so does its efficiency.
- The **flexor digitorum profundus** (FDP) (Fig. 72), inserted at the base of P_3, is primarily a flexor of P_3, but this flexion is soon followed by flexion of P_2 because there is no dedicated

extensor to oppose this action. Therefore to measure the strength of the *flexor profundus*, P_2 must be kept extended manually. When P_1 and P_2 are manually flexed to 90° the *profundus* is unable to flex P_3 because it has become too slack for any useful contraction. It works best when P_1 is kept extended by contraction of the *extensor digitorum* (antagonistic-synergistic action). Despite these limitations the FDP is an important muscle, as will be illustrated later.
- The radial extensors (RE) and the *extensor digitorum* (ED) are synergistic with the flexors (Fig. 73).

All these tendons would be ineffectual without pulleys A_1–A_3–A_5 (Fig. 75), which **keep the tendons in contact with the metacarpal and phalangeal bones**. It is easy to understand the **role of these pulleys** (Fig. 76). Compared with its normal position (a), the FDP tendon is artificially lengthened to (b) if pulley A_1 is removed, to (c) if A_3 is removed and to (d) if A_5 is removed. When the tendon 'bowstrings' (d) (i.e. takes a direct path between the two ends of the bony arch), it loses all its power because of its relative lengthening. Fortunately there is still the skin to hold in the tendon! The practical conclusion is that **the pulleys must be maintained as well as possible and must be repaired when they are damaged**.

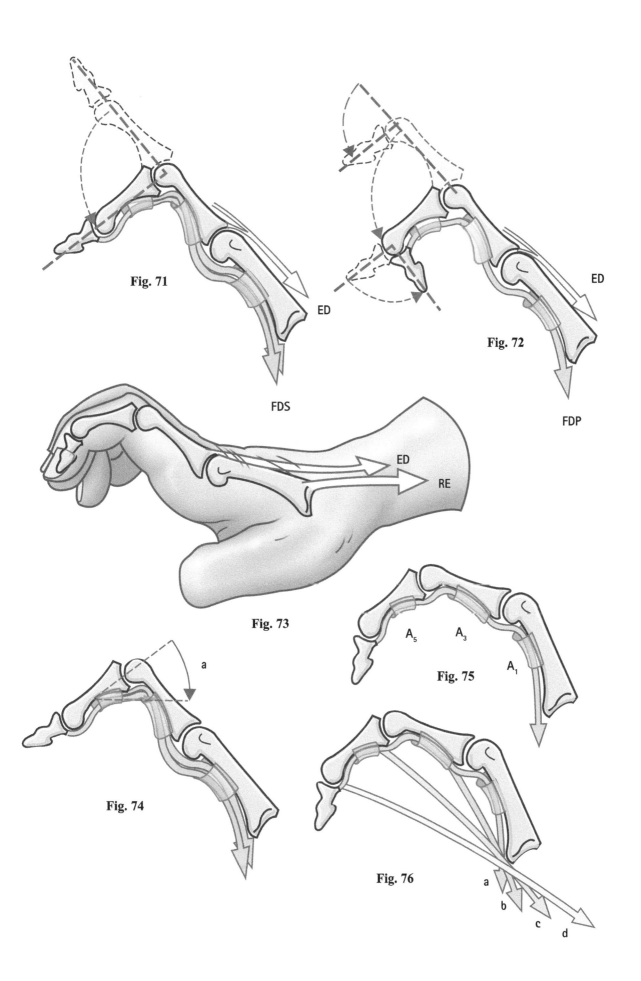

Fig. 71

ED

FDS

Fig. 72

ED

FDP

ED

RE

Fig. 73

A₅ A₃

A₁

Fig. 75

a

Fig. 74

Fig. 76

a

b

c

d

The tendons of the extensor muscles of the fingers

These extensors are mostly **extrinsic muscles of the hand** and they also run inside fibro-osseous tunnels, but, since their course is on the whole convex, the tunnels are fewer than those for the flexors. These tunnels are found only at the wrist, where the tendons become concave outwards during wrist extension. The tunnel at the wrist is formed by the distal ends of the radius and ulna and by the **extensor retinaculum** (Fig. 77) and is **subdivided into six tunnels** containing the following tendons medio-laterally (from left to right in the diagram):

- the extensor carpi ulnaris (1)
- the extensor digiti minimi (2), which joins more distally the tendon of the extensor digitorum for the little finger
- the four tendons of the extensor digitorum (3), accompanied deeply by the tendon of the extensor indicis (3'), which joins distally the tendon of the extensor digitorum for the index finger
- the extensor pollicis longus (4)
- the extensor carpi radialis longus (5) and the extensor carpi radialis brevis (5')
- the extensor pollicis brevis (6) and the abductor pollicis longus (6').

Inside these fibro-osseous tunnels the tendons are invested by **synovial sheaths** (Fig. 78), which extend proximally beyond the *extensor retinaculum* and distally for some distance on the dorsal aspect of the hand.

After the synovial sheaths come to an end, the extensor tendons proceed in a bed of very loose fibro-fatty tissue that lets them slide freely.

Very often, between the extensor tendons of the long fingers, there are tendinous connections, which are very variable in their location and arrangement. They are known by their Latin name of **juncturae tendinum**, which are fibrous bands running in a transverse or oblique direction. In the diagram (Fig. 78), which shows their most frequent orientation, they are represented as red arrows. These bands ensure some measure of interdependence among the fingers during extension depending on their degree of obliquity. For example, it is clear in the diagram that traction on the extensor indicis will have an impact on the ring and middle fingers via the two oblique bands. On the other hand, traction on the extensor of the ring finger will have no effect on the ring finger, whereas it will affect the index finger via a transverse band. It is said that the musician Robert Schumann operated on himself to cut some of these tendinous bands, which interfered with piano playing.

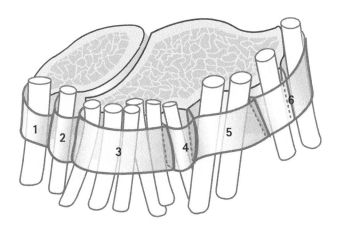

Fig. 77

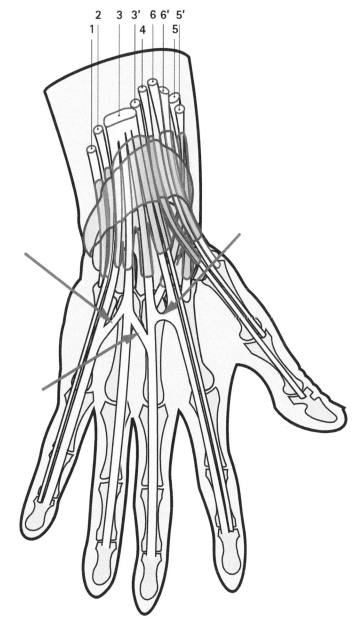

Fig. 78

On the dorsal surface of the hand there are **small intertendinous bands** between the extensor muscles, and they run mostly obliquely and distally between the extensors of the ring finger and those of the middle and index fingers. Their distribution, however, is very variable, and their orientation may change from oblique to transverse so that, **instead of substituting for and helping the function of the extensors**, these bands can impair the independence of the fingers, a serious handicap for pianists. It is rumoured that the famous composer Robert Schumann sectioned one of these bothersome bands himself!

Functionally the **extensor digitorum** is essentially an **extensor of the MP joint**. It is a powerful extensor and active in all positions of the wrist, but its action is facilitated by flexion at the wrist (Fig. 79). It extends P_1 (Figs 80 and 81, the bones of the hand) via the 10-12 mm long extensor expansion (1), which arises from the deep surface of the tendon, crosses the MP joint without blending with its capsular fibres and is inserted at the base of P_1, as shown in Figure 80 (posterior view), where the tendon has been partially resected (4) to reveal the deep expansion (1).

On the other hand, **its action on P_2** via its median band (2) and on P_3 via its two lateral bands (3) depends on the degree of tension in the tendon and consequently on the **position of the wrist** (Fig. 79) and **also on the degree of flexion at the MP joint**:

- This action is appreciable only when the wrist is flexed (A).
- It is partial and weak when the wrist is straight (B).
- It is nil when the wrist is extended (C).

In effect the action of the *extensor digitorum* on P_2 and P_3 depends on the degree of tension in the digital flexors:

- If these flexors are taut because the wrist or the MP joint is extended, the *extensor digitorum* cannot by itself extend the two distal phalanges.
- If, on the other hand, these flexors are relaxed by flexion of the wrist or of the MP joint or are accidentally cut, the *extensor digitorum* can easily extend the last two phalanges.

The tendons of the **extensor indicis** and of the **extensor digiti minimi** behave in the same way as those of the *extensor digitorum* with which they blend. They allow the index and little fingers to be extended singly, e.g. when 'making horns' with the index and little finger, the *'iettatore'* gesture of the Neapolitans.

The accessory movements produced by the extensor tendons of the **index finger** (according to Duchenne de Boulogne) are lateral inclinations (Fig. 82). The *extensor indicis* (A) abducts while the *extensor digitorum* (B) adducts, but only when the interossei are inactivated by flexion of P_2 and P_3 and extension of P_1.

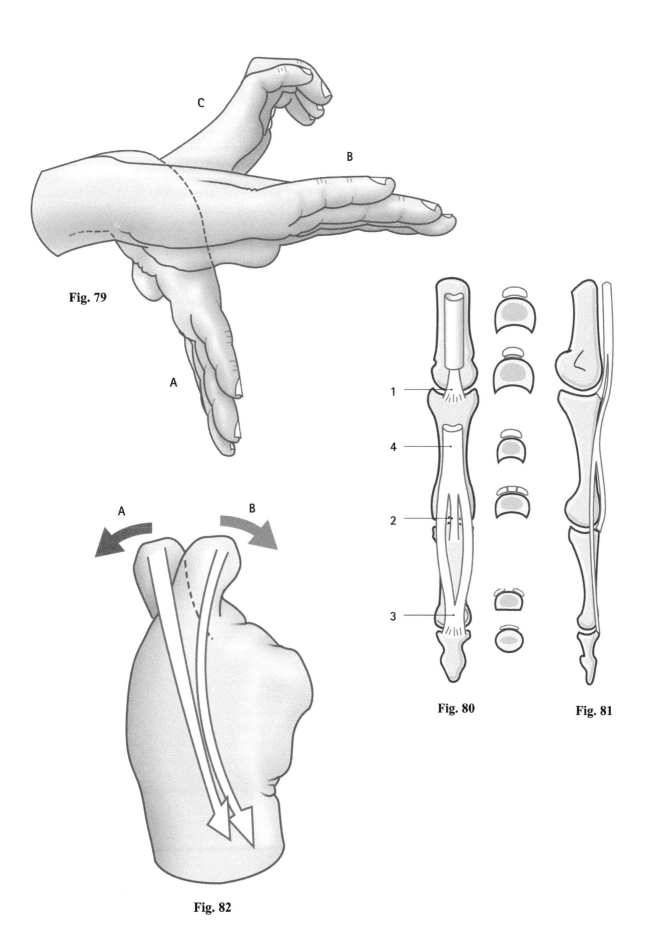

Fig. 79

Fig. 80

Fig. 81

Fig. 82

The interossei and the lumbrical muscles

The **attachments of the interossei** are summarized diagrammatically in Figures 83-85, since we are interested only in the way these insertions influence the actions of the muscles. Functionally the interossei have **two actions at the MP joints: lateral movements** and **flexion-extension**. Their ability to bend the finger to one side or the other depends on the attachment of some of their tendinous insertions into the lateral tuberosity of P_1 (1). Occasionally there is a separate belly of muscle, particularly in the first dorsal interosseus (Winslow).

The direction of the muscle determines the direction of the **lateral movements**:

- When the muscle courses towards the axis of the hand (third finger), e.g. the **dorsal interossei** (Fig. 83, green), it causes separation of the fingers (blue arrows). It is clear that if the second and third interossei contract simultaneously, their opposing actions on the middle finger are cancelled. Abduction of the **little finger** is produced by the **abductor digiti minimi** (Fig. 84, 5), which is equivalent to a posterior interosseus. Abduction of the **thumb** produced by the **abductor pollicis brevis** (6) is of small range and is offset by the **abductor pollicis longus**, which acts on the first metacarpal (M_1).

- When the line of traction of the muscle is directed towards the axis of the hand, e.g. **palmar interossei** (Fig. 84, pink), the muscle pulls the fingers closer together (pink arrow).

The **dorsal interossei** are **bulkier and more powerful** than the palmar interossei, which are thus less efficient in approximating the fingers.

The attachments of the interossei to the metacarpals are shown in detail in Figure 85:

- the attachments of the **dorsal interossei** (green) to two adjacent metacarpals with their tendons running towards the middle finger

- the attachments of the **palmar interossei** (pink) to a single metacarpal, the one farthest away from the middle finger, which receives no interosseus; their tendons are shown running away from the little finger.

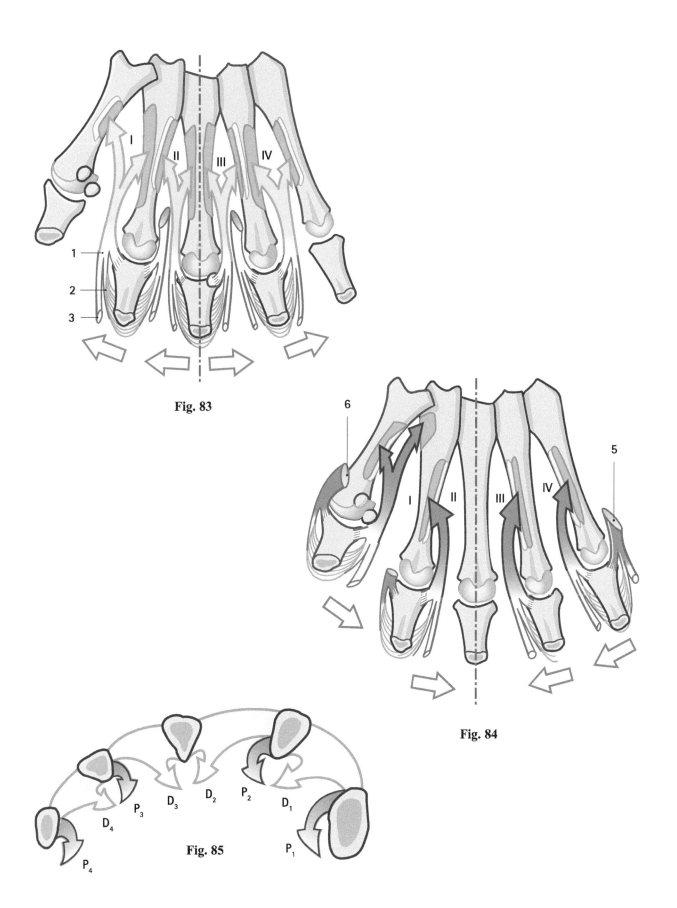

Fig. 83

Fig. 84

Fig. 85

The tendons of the interossei, encased within **fibrous sheaths continuous with the transverse metacarpal ligament**, cannot be dislocated anteriorly during flexion of the MP joints, since they are kept in place by the anteriorly located transverse ligament. The first dorsal interosseus lacks this support and, when its fibrous sheath is damaged in rheumatoid arthritis, its tendon slips anteriorly and **it is changed from an adductor** of the index **into a flexor muscle**.

The actions of the interossei in flexion-extension cannot be understood until the structure of the **dorsal digital expansion** has been described in detail (Figs 86-88).

- The interosseous tendon gives off a **fibrous band**, which passes over the dorsal surface of P_1 to blend with similar fibres from the contralateral muscle and form the **dorsal interosseous expansion** (2). Figure 87 (after removal of the phalanges) shows the deep surface of the dorsal expansion and the interosseous tendon, which, after sending fibres to insert (1) into the lateral tubercle of P_1, now consists of a relatively thick part (2) and a thinner part (2′), whose fibres run obliquely to join the **lateral bands** (7) of the extensor expansion. The thick part (2) slides on the dorsal aspects of P_1 and of the MP joint with an intervening **synovial bursa** (9), distal to which lies the **deep band** (4) of the extensor expansion.

- There is a **third expansion** of the interosseous tendon, i.e. a **thin band** (3), which splits into two groups of fibres before blending with the fibres of the extensor expansion (8) as follows:

- A **triangular band** (10), formed by a few oblique fibres running towards the median band of the extensor expansion. It is extremely important in that it pulls back the fibres of the extensor when the PIP joint is extended. This triangular band is attached distally to the two lateral borders of the median band (15) of the extensor expansion before its insertion into P_2.

- A **second lateral band** (12), formed by fusion of the bulk of the fibres of the third part with the lateral band of the extensor expansion just proximal to the PIP joint. It is inserted with its contralateral homologue into the dorsal surface of the base of P_3.

Note that the lateral band (Fig. 88, 12) does not run posterior but postero-lateral to the PIP joint, where it is tethered to the capsule by a few transverse fibres, i.e. the **capsular expansion** (11).

The **four lumbrical muscles** (Fig. 89), numbered latero-medially, arise from the radial aspects of the flexor tendons of the FDP for the first two and from the edge of the adjacent tendons for the last two. These are the only muscles in the human body that arise from tendons. Their tendons (13) run distally and then curve medially. They are at first separated from the tendons of the interossei (Fig. 88) by the deep transverse metacarpal ligament (14), so that they come to lie in the palmar compartment of the hand. They then blend (Figs 87 and 88) with the third expansion of the interosseous tendon distal to the interosseous expansion.

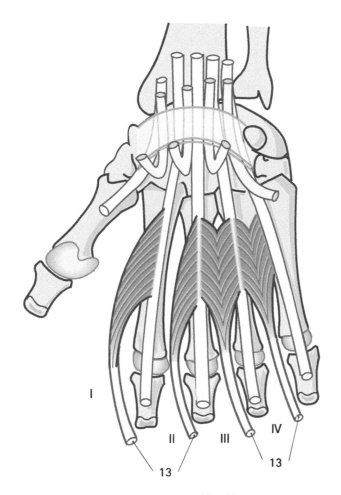

I II III IV

13 13

Fig. 89

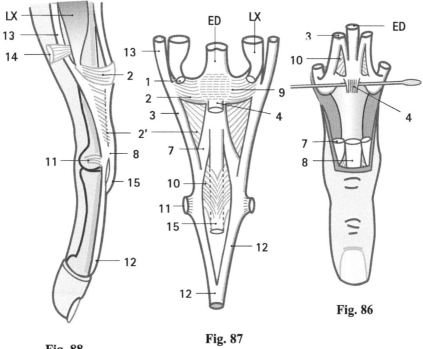

Fig. 88

Fig. 87

Fig. 86

Extension of the fingers

It is produced by the combined action of the *extensor digitorum* (ED), the interossei (IO), the lumbricals (LX) and even to some extent of the *flexor digitorum superficialis* (FDS). These muscles are synergists-antagonists, depending on the position of the MP joint and of the wrist. The **oblique retinacular ligament** contributes purely passively; it also coordinates the movements of the last two phalanges.

Extensor digitorum (ED)

As shown before (p. 236), ED is a true P_1 extensor acting on P_2 and P_3 only when the flexors are relaxed by wrist flexion, MP joint flexion or section of their tendons. On an anatomical model traction on ED completely extends P_1 and incompletely extends P_2 and P_3. The tension developed in the various insertions of ED depends strictly on the degree of flexion of the phalanges:

- Passive flexion of P_3 (Fig. 90) slackens by 3 mm the median band and the deep band so that ED has no more effect on P_1 and P_2 and thus acts directly on P_3.
- Passive flexion of P_2 (Fig. 91):
  - slackens by 3 mm the lateral bands (a) as they 'skid' anteriorly (b) under the pull of the capsular expansion (Fig. 88, 11). During P_2 extension these regain their dorsal position thanks to the elasticity of the triangular band (Fig. 87, 10)
  - slackens by 7-8 mm the deep band (c), which then loses its direct effect on P_1 but ED can still indirectly extend P_1 via P_2 if the latter is stabilized in flexion by FDS, which thus synergizes with ED during MP joint extension (Fig. 92). The components e″ and f″ cancel out, while e′ and f′ add up, producing two components acting on P_1, i.e. an axial component (A) and an extensor component (B), the latter also including part of the action of FDS (R. Tubiana and P Valentin).

The interossei (IO)

They flex P_1 and extend P_2 and P_3, but their actions depend on the degree of flexion of the MP joint and the state of contraction of ED:

- **With the MP joint extended** (Fig. 93) by ED contraction, the extensor hood (a) is pulled over the MP joint towards the dorsum of the metacarpal (Sterling Bunnell). The lateral bands can then be stretched (b) and extend P_2 and P_3.
- **With the MP joint flexed** (Fig. 94) by ED relaxation (a) and contraction of the lumbrical (Lx):
  - the extensor hood slides towards the dorsum of P_1 (b) for 7 mm (Sterling Bunnell)
  - the IO and the lumbrical acting on the extensor expansion strongly flex the MP joint, so that the lateral bands (d), held down by the extensor hood, slacken and can no longer extend P_2 and P_3, the more so as the MP joint is flexed further
  - at this stage ED becomes an efficient extensor of P_2 and P_3.

Thus there is a **synergistic balance** between the extensor actions of ED and IO on P_2 and P_3 (Sterling Bunnell):

- **With the MP joint flexed at 90°** ED is fully active on P_2 and P_3, as are the lumbricals, which retighten the lateral bands (Fig. 96) when IO have become inactive.
- **With the MP joint in the intermediate position**, ED and IO are synergistic.
- **With the MP joint extended** (Figs 93 and 95) ED has no effect on P_2 and P_3, whereas IO are maximally active as they retighten the lateral bands (b).

The lumbricals (LX)

They flex P_1 and extend P_2 and P_3 but, unlike IO, they act whatever the degree of flexion at the MP joint. They are thus extremely valuable for finger movements. They owe their efficiency to two anatomical factors:

- Lying more anteriorly than IO and palmar to the transverse metacarpal ligament, they form a **35° angle of traction with P_1** (Fig. 95) and can therefore flex the MP joint even when it is hyperextended. They are thus the **flexor starters of P_1**, since the IO only act secondarily on the dorsal expansion.
- They are inserted (Fig. 96) into the lateral bands distal to the extensor hood, which does not bind down their tendons; hence **their ability to retighten the extensors of P_2 and P_3**, regardless of the degree of flexion of the MP joint.

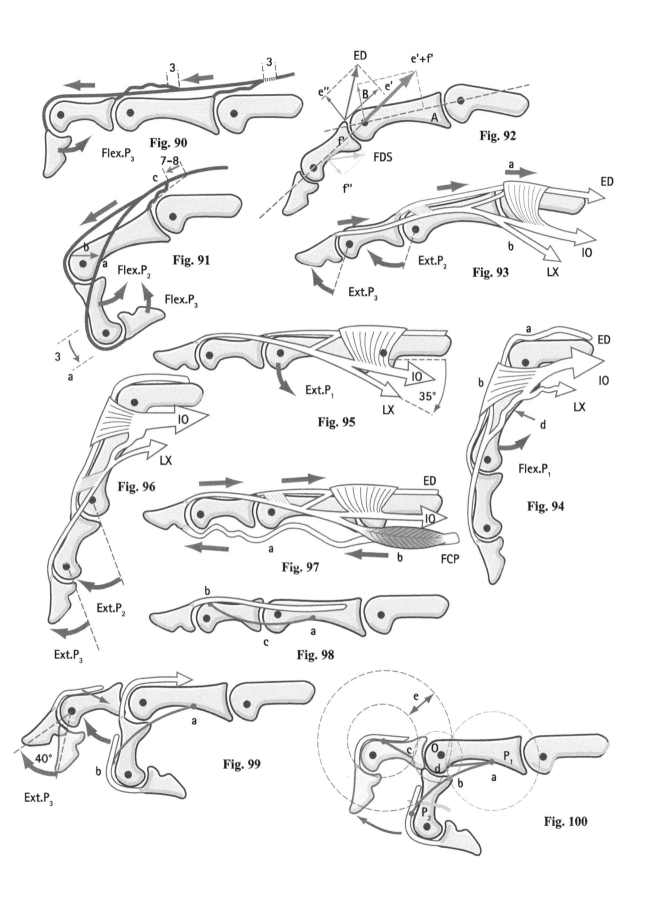

Fig. 90

Flex.P₃

Fig. 91

Flex.P₂

Flex.P₃

Fig. 92

Fig. 93

Ext.P₂

Ext.P₃

Fig. 94

Flex.P₁

Fig. 95

Ext.P₁

Fig. 96

Ext.P₂

Ext.P₃

Fig. 97

Fig. 98

Fig. 99

Ext.P₃

Fig. 100

Eyler, Marquee and Landsmeer have shown that sometimes the interossei have two separate insertions, one for dorsal expansion and the other for lateral expansion:

- According to Recklinghausen, the **lumbricals** (Fig. 97) promote extension of P_2 and P_3 by slackening the distal portion of the FDP tendon (a) from which they arise (b). Because of their **diagonal course**, their contraction functionally displaces the FDP insertion from the palmar to the dorsal aspect of P_3 and thus changes FDP into an extensor like an interosseus. This system is like a transistor that shunts current in one direction or the other, depending on its state of excitation. This **transistor effect** uses a weak muscle (the lumbrical) to shunt the power of a strong flexor muscle (FDP) into the extensor grid. From their numerous **proprioceptive receptors** the lumbricals gather essential information (P. Rabischong) for the coordination of the extensors and flexors as they run transversely from one group to the other.

- The **oblique retinacular ligament** (RL), first described by Landsmeer in 1949, consists of fibres (Fig. 98) arising from the palmar surface of P_1 (a) and blending with the lateral extensor expansion of the *extensor digitorum* before it inserts into P_3. But, more important, its fibres, unlike those of the lateral expansions, run across the PIP joint palmar to its axis (c). Therefore (Fig. 99) extension of the **PIP joint stretches the fibres of RL** and **causes a 40° automatic extension of the DIP joint** with a range equal to half its maximum; in other words, the DIP joint moves from a flexed position of 80° to one of 40°. This tightening of the RL by extension of the PIP joint is easily demonstrated as follows (Fig. 100). If the RL is cut at b, **passive extension of P_2 is not followed by the automatic extension of P_3** and the two cut ends of RL stay apart by a distance cd or e, where d is the final position of b after rotation around a, and c is the final position of b on P_2 after rotation around O.

Conversely, with RL intact, passive flexion of the DIP joint causes automatic flexion of the PIP joint.

Contracture of RL fixes the hand in a 'buttonhole' deformity caused by rupture of the extensor expansion and leads to hyperextension of the DIP joint, as in advanced cases of Dupuytren's contracture.

In summary, it is possible to establish the effects of muscular contraction on flexion and extension of the fingers as follows:

- Simultaneous extension of $P_1 + P_2 + P_3$ (Fig. 101, A):
  - synergism of ED + IO + LX
  - passive and automatic involvement of the retinacular ligament.
- Isolated extension of P_1: ED:
  - + flexion of P_2: FDS (agonist of ED) with relaxation of the IO
  - + flexion of P_3: FDP + relaxation of IO + LX
  - + flexion of P_2: FDS + relaxation of IO + LX
  - + extension of P_3: LX and IO. (This last movement is very difficult.)
- Isolated flexion of P_1: LX (starters) and IO, the latter antagonizing ED:
  - + extension of P2 and P3 (Fig. 101, C): lumbricals, which are extensors in all portions of the MP joint, and synergistic antagonism of ED and the interossei (Fig. 101, B)
  - + flexion of P_2: FDS
  - + extension of P_3: lumbricals (a difficult movement because flexion of the PIP joint relaxes the lateral expansions)
  - + flexion of P_2: FDS
  - + flexion of P_3: FDS, whose action is made easier by the 'skidding' of the lateral expansions during flexion of the PIP joint.

The **everyday movements of the fingers** illustrate these various combinations as follows:

- During **writing** (first studied by Duchenne de Boulogne):
  - When the pencil is moved forwards (Fig. 102), the interosseus flexes P_1 and extends P_2 and P_3.
  - When the pencil is brought back (Fig. 103), ED extends P_1 and FDS flexes P_2.
- When the hand assumes the **shape of a hook** (Fig. 104) FDS and FDP both contract and the interossei relax. This movement is essential for mountain climbers as they clutch at the vertical face of a rock.
- **During tapping movements of the fingers** (Fig. 105) ED extends P_1, while FDS and FDP flex P_2 and P_3. This is the initial position of the pianist's fingers. The finger strikes the key as the **interossei and lumbricals contract** and flex the MP joint, while ED relaxes.

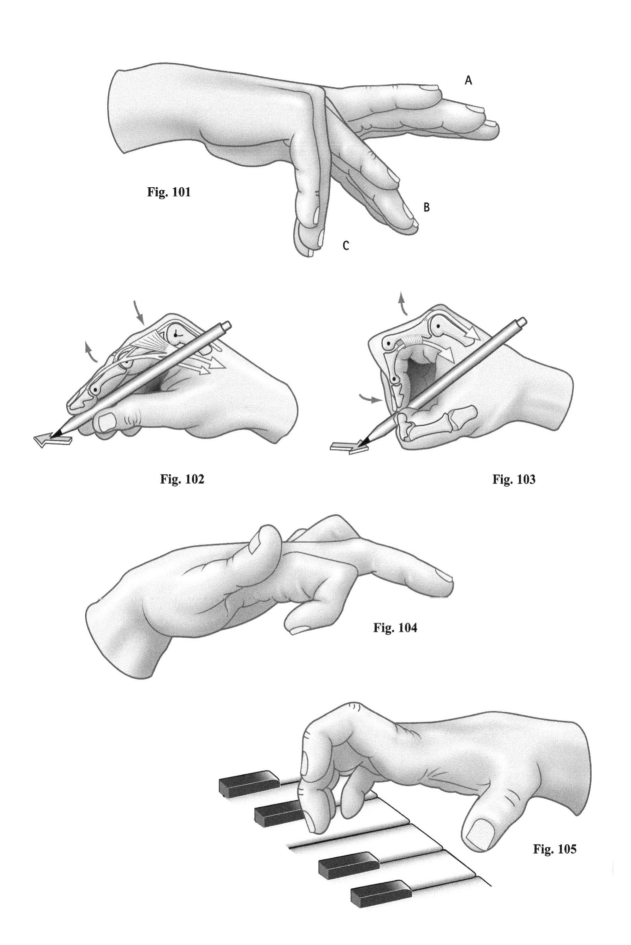

Fig. 101

Fig. 102

Fig. 103

Fig. 104

Fig. 105

Abnormal positions of the hand and fingers

These can result from either deficiency or overactivity of one of the muscles described. The following conditions produce **abnormal positions of the fingers** (Fig. 106):

- **Rupture of the extensor expansion** (a) at the level of the triangular band, which runs between the two lateral bands and whose elasticity is necessary to bring these bands back to their original dorsal position when the PIP joint moves back into extension. As a result the posterior surface of the joint herniates through the torn extensor expansion and the lateral bands remain displaced in midflexion on either side of the PIP joint while the DIP joint is hyperextended. This **'buttonhole deformity'** can also be produced by cutting ED at the PIP joint.
- **Rupture of the extensor tendon** (b) just proximal to its insertion into P_3 causes flexion of P_3, which can be reduced passively but not actively and is due to the activity of FDP, now unbalanced by ED. This leads to the **'mallet finger'** deformity.
- **Rupture of the long extensor tendon distal to the MP joint** (c) causes flexion of the joint because the action of the interossei predominates over that of ED. This is the **intrinsic plus deformity**, which arises because the interossei become more powerful than ED.
- **Rupture or deficiency of FDS** (d) leads to hyperextension of the PIP joint because of the enhanced activity of the interossei. This 'inverted position' of the joint is accompanied by a slight flexion of the DIP joint due to relative shortening of FDP following hyperextension of the PIP joint. Hence the name of **'swan-neck deformity'**.
- **Paralysis or sectioning of the FDP tendon** (e) prevents all active flexion of the distal phalanx.
- **Deficiency of the interossei** (f) is followed by **hyperextension of the MP joint** due to the contraction of ED and **hyperflexion of the two distal phalanges** caused by the combined action of FDS and FDP. This paralysis of the intrinsic muscles disrupts the longitudinal arch at the level of its keystone. This **claw-hand or intrinsic minus position** (Fig. 108) is seen mainly with **paralysis of the ulnar nerve**, which supplies the interossei, and this is why this deformity is also called the **ulnar claw**. It is associated with **atrophy of the hypothenar eminence and of the interosseous spaces**.
- The **loss of the extensors of the wrist and of the fingers**, most commonly caused by **radial nerve paralysis**, produces **'wrist drop'** (Fig. 107), i.e. increased flexion of the wrist, flexion of the MP joint and extension of the two distal phalanges owing to contraction of the interossei.
- **In advanced Dupuytren's contracture** (Fig. 109), caused by **shortening of the pretendinous fibres of the central palmar aponeurosis**, the fingers are irreducibly flexed, with flexion of the MP and PIP joints and extension of the DIP joint. The last two fingers are usually the most severely involved, the middle finger and the index finger are involved later in the progression of the disease, and the thumb is involved only exceptionally.
- **Volkman's contracture** (Fig. 110) is caused by ischaemic shortening of the flexor muscles as a result of arterial insufficiency. The fingers assume a hook-like position, which is particularly obvious during extension (a) and is attenuated when the wrist is flexed (b) and the flexors are slackened.
- The **hook-like deformity** (Fig. 111) can also be due to **suppurative synovitis of the common flexor sheath**. It becomes more marked from the lateral to the medial fingers (the fifth finger being the most afflicted). Any attempt at reversing it is extremely painful.
- Finally the hand can become fixed in a position of **massive ulnar drift** (Fig. 112, taken from the painting *The Musicians' Brawl* by Georges Latour), when all the fingers are markedly deviated medially so that the metacarpal heads become abnormally prominent. This deformity allows one to make the (retrospective) diagnosis of rheumatoid arthritis.

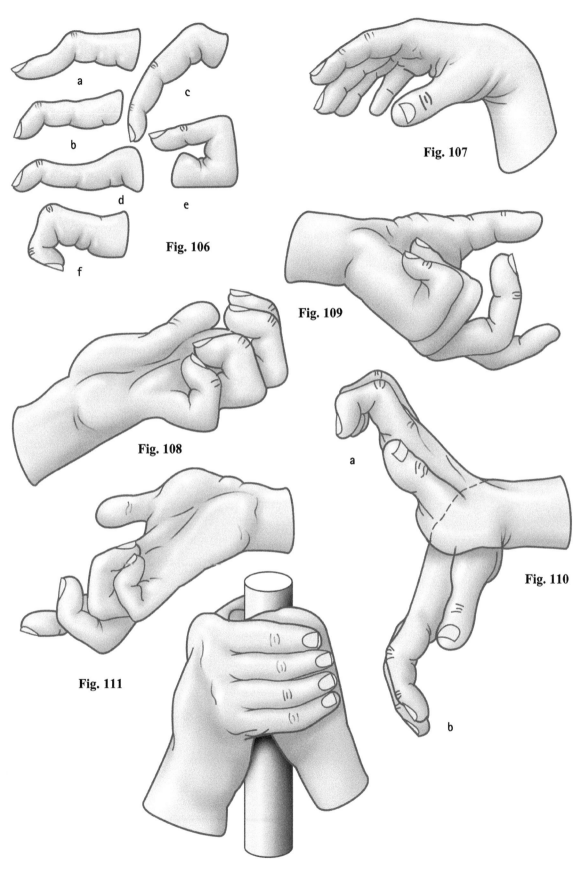

a

b

c

d

e

Fig. 106

f

Fig. 107

Fig. 109

Fig. 108

a

Fig. 110

Fig. 111

b

Fig. 112

The muscles of the hypothenar eminence

These are **three** in number (Fig. 113):

1) **Flexor digiti minimi brevis** (1), inserted into the ulnar aspect of the base of P_1, runs obliquely distally and medially from its fleshy origin located in the palmar surface of the *flexor retinaculum* and the hook of the hamate.

2) ***Adductor quinti/abductor digiti minimi** (2), which adducts the finger towards the plane of symmetry of the body, is inserted like an interosseus. Its flat tendon divides into two slips: one inserted (along with the *flexor digiti minimi brevis*) into the ulnar aspect of P_1 by a dorsal expansion shared with the fourth anterior interosseus; and the other into the ulnar border of the dorsal digital expansion of the ED. It arises from the anterior surface of the *flexor retinaculum* and from the pisiform.

3) **Opponens digiti minimi** (3) runs distally and medially from its origin at the distal border of the *flexor retinaculum* and the hook of the hamate, skirts round the anterior border of the fifth metacarpal (Fig. 113) and is inserted into its ulnar margin.

Physiological actions

The physiological actions of these muscles are as follows:

- **Opponens digiti minimi** (Fig. 114) flexes the fifth carpo-metacarpal joint about the axis XX′ and pulls the metacarpal anteriorly (arrow 1) and laterally (arrow 2) along an oblique path collinear with the axis of the fleshy belly of the muscle (pink and white arrow). But at the same time, it rotates the metacarpal around its long axis (marked by a cross) into supination (arrow 3) so that the anterior aspect of the metacarpal now faces laterally towards the thumb. Hence its name of *opponens* is justified, since it **brings the little finger into opposition with the thumb**.

- **Flexor digiti minimi brevis** (1) and ***adductor quinti/abductor digiti minimi** (2) together have roughly similar actions (Fig. 115):

  - **Flexor digiti minimi brevis** (blue arrow) flexes the MP joint and abducts the little finger from the axis of the hand.

  - ***Adductor quinti/abductor digiti minimi** (red arrow) also abducts the finger relative to the axis of the hand and so can be viewed as similar to a posterior interosseus. Like the interossei, it flexes P_1 via the digital interosseous expansion and extends the two distal phalanges via its lateral extensor expansion.

  -

---

* The author uses *adductor quinti* in French for the English *abductor digiti minimi*. This discrepancy in terminology is due to the fact that the author uses the plane of symmetry of the body rather than the axis of the hand as his point of reference for the lateral movements of the little, finger in the coronal plane.

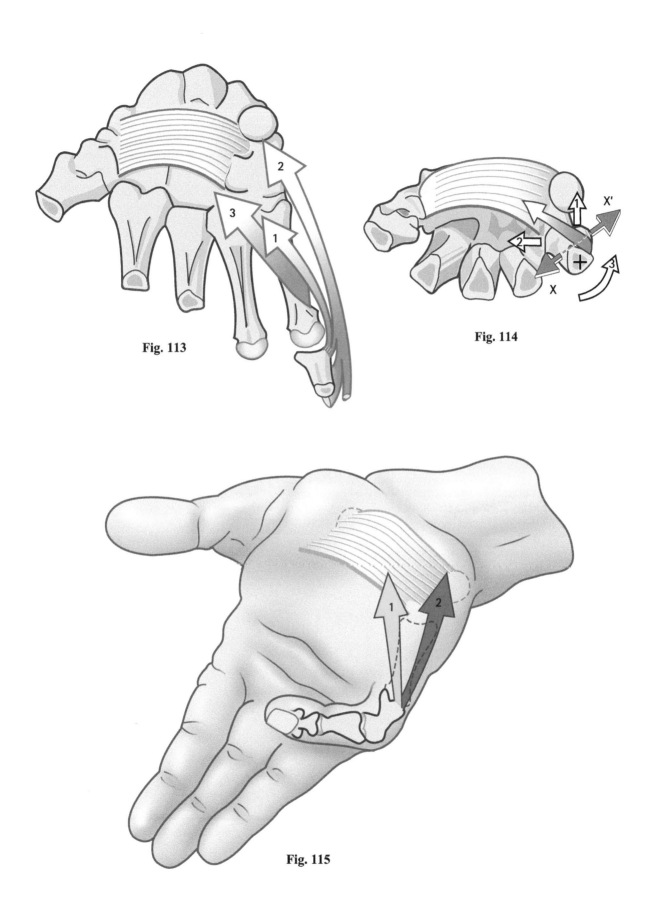

Fig. 113

Fig. 114

Fig. 115

249

The thumb

The thumb plays a unique role in the function of the hand, being essential for the formation of the pollici-digital pincers with each of the fingers and for the development of a powerful grip with the help of the other four fingers. It can also take part in actions associated with the gripping of objects by the same hand. Without the thumb the hand loses most of its prehensile capabilities.

The thumb owes its preeminent role to its location anterior to the palm and to the other fingers (Fig. 116), which allows it to move towards the fingers individually or together (the movement of opposition) or away from them (the movement of counter-opposition*) to release the grip. It also owes its role to its great functional adaptability secondary to the peculiar organization of its osteo-articular column and its motor muscles.

The osteo-articular column of the thumb (Fig. 117) consists of five bones forming the lateral ray of the hand:

1) the scaphoid (S)
2) the trapezium (TZ), which embryologically is homologous to a metacarpal
3) the first metacarpal (M_1)
4) the first phalanx (P_1)
5) the second phalanx (P_2).

Anatomically the thumb has only two phalanges, but, more important, it is attached to the hand at a point far more proximal than the other fingers. Thus its column is far shorter and its tip reaches only as far as the middle of P_1 of the index finger. This is in fact its optimal length for two reasons:

1) If it is shorter (as after partial amputation), it cannot carry out opposition because it is too short and cannot be sufficiently adducted and flexed.

2) If it is longer (as the congenitally malformed thumb with three phalanges), the delicate termino-terminal (tip-to-tip) opposition can be hampered by inadequate flexion of the DIP joint of the finger in opposition.

This illustrates Occam's principle of universal **parsimony** (also known as Occam's razor), which states that optimal function is ensured by a minimum of structural components and organization. Thus, for the thumb, five components are needed and are sufficient to ensure optimal function.

There are four joints in the column of the thumb:

1) the scapho-trapezial (ST) joint, which, as we have seen already, allows the trapezium to move anteriorly for a short distance along the distal tubercle-bearing surface of the scaphoid, i.e. a movement of flexion of small range
2) the trapezo-metacarpal (TM) joint with two degrees of freedom
3) the metacarpo-phalangeal (MP) joint with two degrees of freedom
4) the interphalangeal (IP) joint with only one degree of freedom.

Thus all five degrees of freedom are necessary and are adequate to achieve opposition.

---

* To avoid confusion the translator has elected to follow the author's terminology. *Counter-opposition*, well defined in the text, is not normally used in English, where the terms *retroposition* or *reposition* are used instead. The author also uses *retroposition* in a different sense.

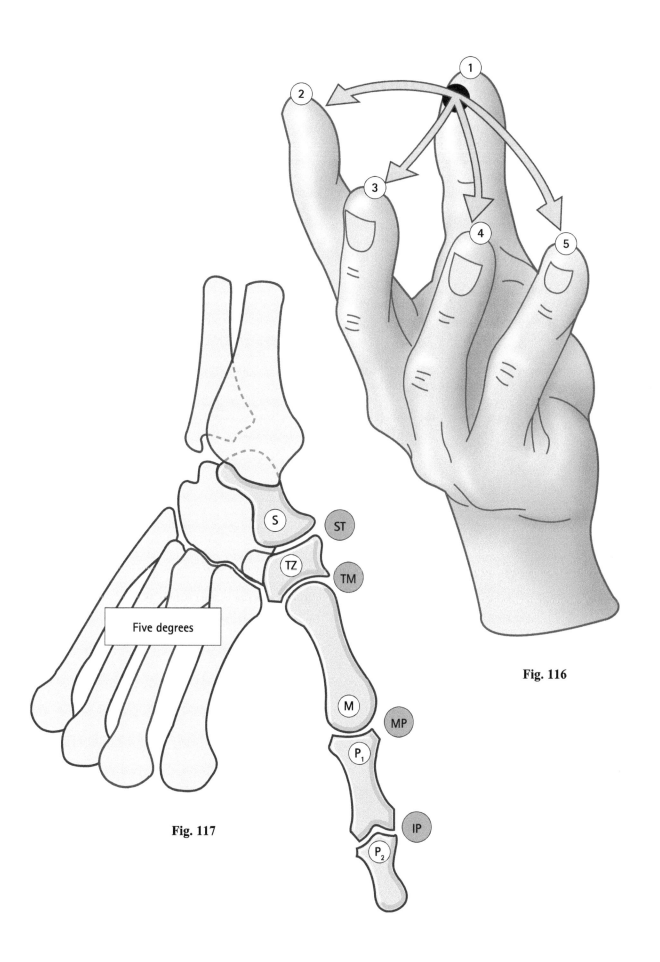

Fig. 116

Fig. 117

Five degrees

Opposition of the thumb

This is the movement bringing into contact the pulp of the thumb with that of any other finger to form a **pollici-digital pincer**, and it is the basis of the functional capability of the hand. When it is lost, the hand is almost useless, and complex surgical procedures are carried out to restore these pincers from the residual structures subserving this movement. These operations rely on the **replacement of the thumb by another finger** (the **pollicization of a finger**).

During opposition the thumb moves to meet another finger (see Figs. 200-201, p. 285), most often the index finger. This movement is the **sum of the elementary movements**:

1) **Antepulsion of M_1** and secondarily of P_1.
2) **Adduction of M_1** and ulnar flexion of P_1 towards the radial border of M_1. The range of movements increases as the thumb opposes the more medial fingers and is maximal when the thumb opposes the little finger.
3) **Axial rotation of M_1 and P_1 in the direction of pronation.**

The first two movements depend on the combined action of the *abductor pollicis longus* and of the lateral muscles of the thenar group.

Axial rotation deserves more detailed analysis.

It can be illustrated by **Sterling Bunnell's experiment** (Figs 118-120), which can easily be performed on oneself as follows. First, place markers on the bones concerned (one matchstick transversely across the nail, one perpendicular to each phalanx and a fourth one perpendicular to the metacarpal). Now bring the hand into the starting position (Fig. 118) with the palm wide open, the thenar eminence flattened and the thumb in maximal extension and abduction. Then move the thumb to oppose the index finger, i.e. in the intermediate position (Fig. 119), and finally move the thumb farther to oppose the little finger, in the extreme position (Fig. 120). When the hand is viewed head-on in a mirror, one can observe that the plane of the nail has undergone an axial rotation of 90-120°.

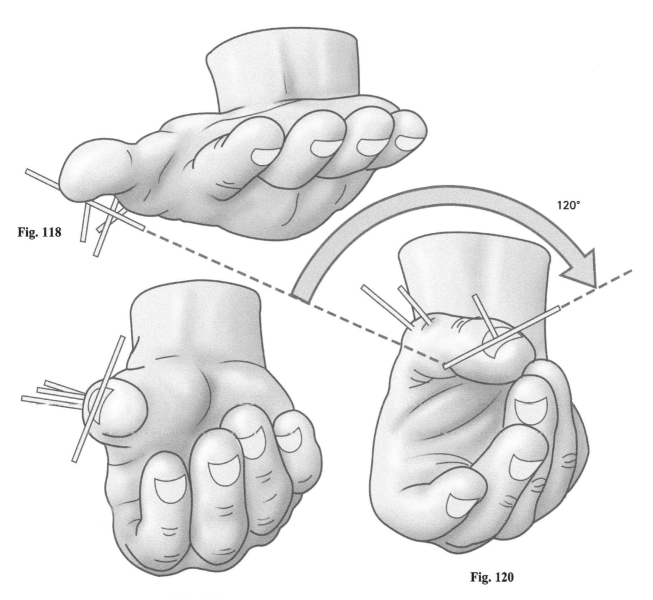

Fig. 118

Fig. 119

Fig. 120

120°

It is incorrect to assume that this axial rotation has occurred entirely in the TM and MP joints.

To test this (Fig. 121), let us use a mechanical model of the thumb (developed by the author). The strip of cardboard representing the thumb articulates with the palm around an axis O for movements of abduction-adduction and is folded along three lines perpendicular to the long axis of the strip representing the three distal joints of the thumb.

When one successively performs the following two movements on the model, i.e. **120° abduction** around O and **180° flexion** along the three folds, one completes the movement of opposition. Arrow 3 moves directly towards the fourth and fifth fingers, although the strip has not been axially rotated. The axial rotation is the geometric resultant of the combined movements of abduction and flexion. In real life, however, owing to mechanical factors at the joints, abduction cannot exceed 60°. Under these conditions (Fig. 122), the axial rotation is no longer enough to move P_2 (arrow 3) towards the last finger, and P_2 then moves anteriorly and proximally.

To perform opposition despite this limited degree of abduction (Fig. 123), a torsion of the strip must occur, i.e. a certain degree of axial rotation associated with flexion of the different segments.

On the model this is easily achieved by making the axes of flexion oblique (dotted lines), so that flexion is inevitably associated with an axial rotation. In real life, however, this axial rotation is not due to the obliquity of the axes of flexion but is the result of **a combination of many factors**:

- An **automatic axial rotation** resulting from the composite movement taking place around the two axes of the TM joint (see later) as the lateral thenar muscles contract. This active and automatic rotation is mainly responsible for opposition of the thumb.
- An **active axial rotation** due to a movement of pronation in the MP joint produced by the *flexor pollicis brevis* and the *abductor pollicis brevis* (see above).
- An **automatic axial rotation** into pronation at the IP joint (see later).

The '**play**' in the TM and MP joints, which is due to the laxity of the ligaments when the lateral thenar muscles contract, is yet another factor but is not essential.

By passively rotating the second phalanx of the thumb held between the thumb and the index finger, the range of this movement can be measured empirically; it lies between 60° and 80° but it is not a natural movement.

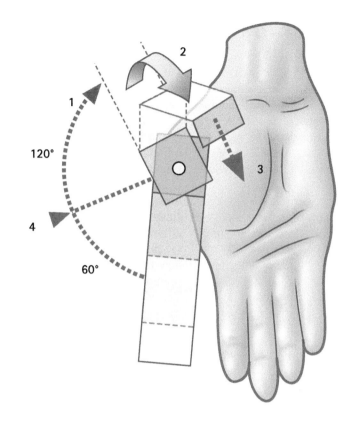

Fig. 121

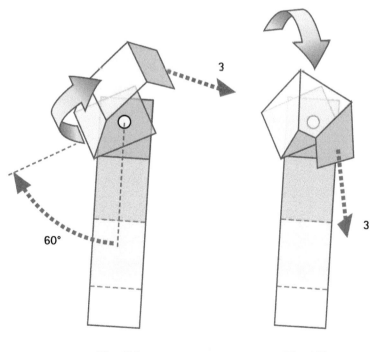

Fig. 122   **Fig. 123**

The geometry of thumb opposition

Geometrically speaking (Fig. 124), opposition of the thumb consists of moving the thumb in such a way that a point A′ on its pulp or pad becomes tangential to a corresponding point A on the pulp of another finger, e.g. the index, and that the tangential planes of A and A′ merge in space into a single point (A + A′).

For two points to coincide in space (Fig. 125), three degrees of freedom are necessary in keeping with the three space coordinates X, Y and Z. Two additional degrees of freedom are necessary for the planes of the pulps to coincide perfectly by rotation around axes t and u. Since the pulps cannot rotate into a back-to-back position, a third degree of freedom around an axis perpendicular to the preceding ones is not needed.

In sum, to achieve the coincidence of these pulpar planes **five degrees of freedom** are required:

- three for coincidence of the points of contact
- two for more or less extensive coincidence of the pulpar planes.

It can easily be demonstrated that each axis of a joint represents a degree of freedom and that these degrees of freedom can be added numerically. Thus the **five degrees of freedom of the column of the thumb are both necessary and adequate to achieve opposition of the thumb**.

Let us consider in one plane only (Fig. 126) the movements of the three mobile segments (M_1, P_1 and P_2) of the column of the thumb about the three axes of flexion YY′ for the TM joint, f_1 for the MP joint and f_2 for the IP joint. It is clear (Fig. 126)

that two degrees of freedom are needed to position the tip of P_2 at a point H in the plane. If no movement is allowed about f_1 and f_2, then there is only one way of reaching H, but the introduction of a third degree of freedom allows H to be reached from many angles. The diagram contains two pulpar orientations, O and O′, at an angle of α and β respectively. It is clear that three degrees of freedom are needed.

In space (Fig. 127), the addition of a fourth degree of freedom around the second axis $Y_2Y_2′$ of the TM joint increases by one the range of orientations for the pulp of the thumb, which can now face in yet another direction and can choose any position to oppose another finger.

The addition of a fifth degree of freedom (Fig. 128), introduced by the second axis of the MP joint, improves the degree of coincidence of the two pulpar planes by allowing them to rotate slightly with respect to each other around their point of contact. In fact, we can see that the axis of flexion f_1 of the MP joint is strictly transverse only during direct flexion but is mostly oblique in one direction or another:

- Oblique in f_2: flexion is associated with ulnar deviation and supination.
- Oblique in f_3: flexion is associated with radial deviation and pronation.

Therefore, thanks to the five degrees of freedom available in the mechanical system of the column of the thumb, **the pulp of the thumb can be brought into contact with that of any other finger in multiple ways**.

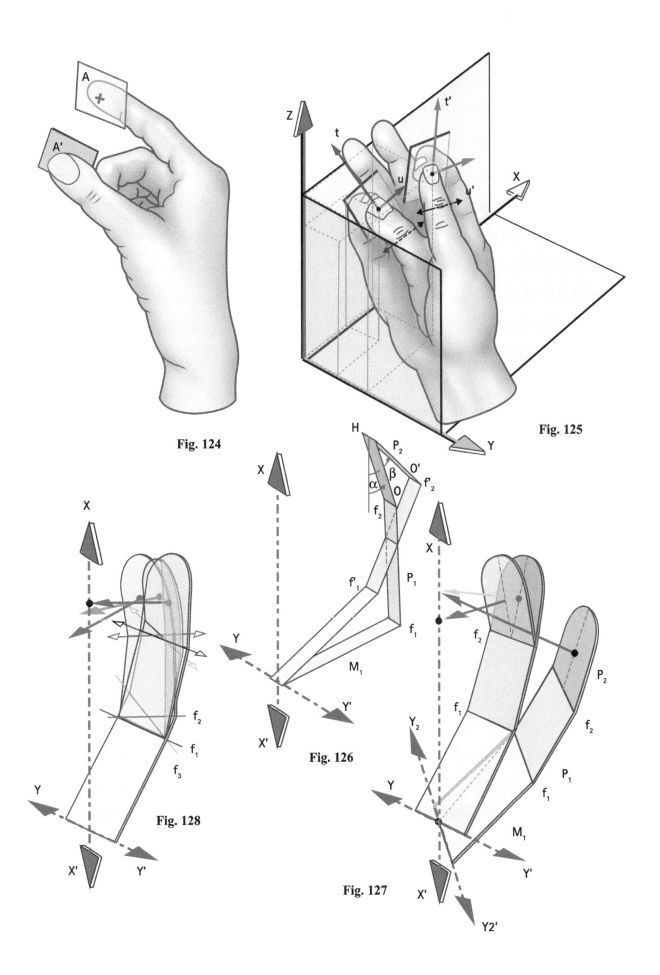

Fig. 124

Fig. 125

Fig. 126

Fig. 128

Fig. 127

257

The trapezo-metacarpal (TM) joint

Topographic features of the articular surfaces

The TM joint, lying at the base of the mobile column of the thumb, **plays a vital role in the movements of the thumb, especially in opposition,** by allowing the thumb **to take up any position in space.** Anatomists have labelled the TM joint as the '**joint of mutual interlocking**', which is not very meaningful, or as the **saddle joint** (Fig. 129), which is better, since it draws attention to its saddle shape, concave in one direction and convex in the other. In reality it consists of two saddle-shaped surfaces, i.e. one on the distal surface of the TZ and the other on the base of M_1; these surfaces are congruent only after a 90° rotation, when the convexity of one surface fits into the concavity of the other and vice versa.

A very accurate topographic study, carried out by an Italian investigator (A. Caroli) using serial sections and mounting procedures, demonstrates (Fig. 130) that the trapezial (a) and the metacarpal (b) surfaces do actually have a double inverse curvature in the shape of a saddle, but their congruence (c) is not perfect.

The exact contours of these articular surfaces have been studied extensively but still remain controversial. The first accurate account comes from a Scottish investigator (K. Kuczynski, 1974).

When the TM joint is opened and the base of M_1 is tilted laterally (Fig. 131), the articular surfaces of the trapezium (TZ) and of the first metacarpal (M_1) show the following features:

- The **trapezial surface** (TZ) bears a median ridge (CD), which is slightly bent so that its concavity faces medially and anteriorly. The dorsal part of this ridge (C) is clearly more pointed than that of its palmar part (D), which is almost flat. This ridge is indented transversely in its middle portion by a furrow (AB) running antero-laterally from its postero-lateral border A to its antero-medial border B. More important, this furrow is curved, with its convexity pointing antero-laterally. The postero-lateral part (E) is almost flat.

- The **metacarpal surface** (M_1) is inversely shaped, with a ridge A′B′ corresponding to the furrow AB of TZ, and a furrow C′D′ corresponding to the ridge CD on TZ.

When applied to TZ (Fig. 132), M_1 overhangs the borders of TZ at the ends a and b of the furrow. Also, on the section (Fig. 133), it is clear that the congruence of these surfaces is far from perfect, since their radii of curvature are slightly different. When they are firmly pressed together, however, the interlocking of the surfaces prevents any axial rotation of M_1 (Kuczynski). Because the saddle is curved along its long axis, Kuczynski compares it to a soft saddle placed on the back of a scoliotic horse (Fig. 134). It can also be likened to a **pass curving between two mountains** (Fig. 135). Thus the path (blue arrow) of a truck going uphill forms an angle R with that (pink arrow) of the same truck going downhill on the other side of the pass. According to Kuczynski, this angle, which is equal to 90° between points A and B of the furrow on TZ, accounts for the axial rotation of M_1 during opposition of the thumb. This could only be true if the base of M_1 swept the entire length of the trapezial furrow (like the truck on the mountain pass) and caused total dislocation of the joint in one or both directions. Since the displacement of M_1 is only partial in real life, we believe that **another mechanism** (to be discussed later) **underlies this rotation**.

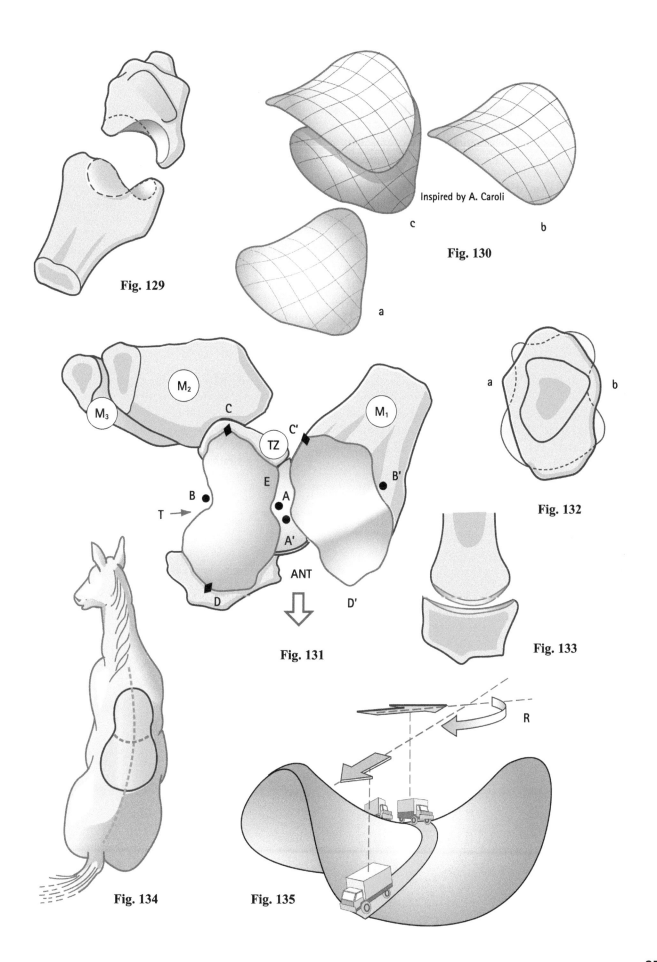

Inspired by A. Caroli

Fig. 129

Fig. 130

c

b

a

Fig. 131

M₃

M₂

C

C'

TZ

M₁

E

B'

B

A

A'

T

ANT

D

D'

Fig. 132

a

b

Fig. 133

R

Fig. 134

Fig. 135

259

Coaptation of the articular surfaces

The capsule of the TM joint is considered to be lax with considerable play, which, according to classical authors and even some modern authors, is responsible for the axial rotation of M_1. This is incorrect, as we shall see later.

In fact, the laxity of the capsule allows only the articular surface of M_1 to move over that of TZ, but the joint works by **axial compression like a pivot** (Fig. 136). Thus M_1 can assume any position in space, just like a pylon, whose direction can be altered by varying the degree of stretch of any one of its stays, which correspond here to the thenar muscles. These muscles therefore keep the articular surfaces together in all positions. In reality this pivot P is not spherical but has the shape of an O-ring (see page 265) and, as such, shares two perpendicular axes XX′ and YY′, which form a **universal joint**.

Likewise the ligaments of the TM joint direct the movements at the joint and keep the articular surfaces together by changing their degree of stretch. Their anatomy and their functions have recently been described by J.-Y. de la Caffinière (1970). There are many other accounts of their ligaments but de la Caffinière's remains valid because of its coherence and simplicity. Four ligaments are recognized (Fig. 137, anterior view; Fig. 138, posterior view):

1) The **intermetacarpal ligament** (IML) (4), which is a short thick band of fibres bridging the bases of M_1 and M_2 in the most proximal region of the first interdigital cleft.
2) The **oblique postero-medial ligament** (OPML) (3), long recognized as a wide but thin band applied to the joint posteriorly and coursing anteriorly round the medial aspect of the base of M_1.
3) The **oblique antero-medial ligament** (OAML) (2), running from the distal tip of the ridge on TZ to the base of M_1. It crosses the anterior aspect of the joint after wrapping itself round the lateral aspect of the base of M_1.
4) The **straight antero-lateral ligament** (SALL) (1), stretching directly from TZ to the base of M_1 antero-laterally to the joint. Its medial border, well defined and sharp, bounds a small gap in the capsule, through which runs a synovial sheath for the tendon of the *abductor pollicis longus* (APL).

According to de la Caffinière, **these ligaments can be paired** as follows:
- **IML and SALL**: the widening and the narrowing of the first interdigital cleft in the plane of the palm are checked by IML and SALL respectively.
- **OPML and OAML**: these are stretched essentially during rotation of M_1, with OPML limiting pronation and OAML limiting supination.

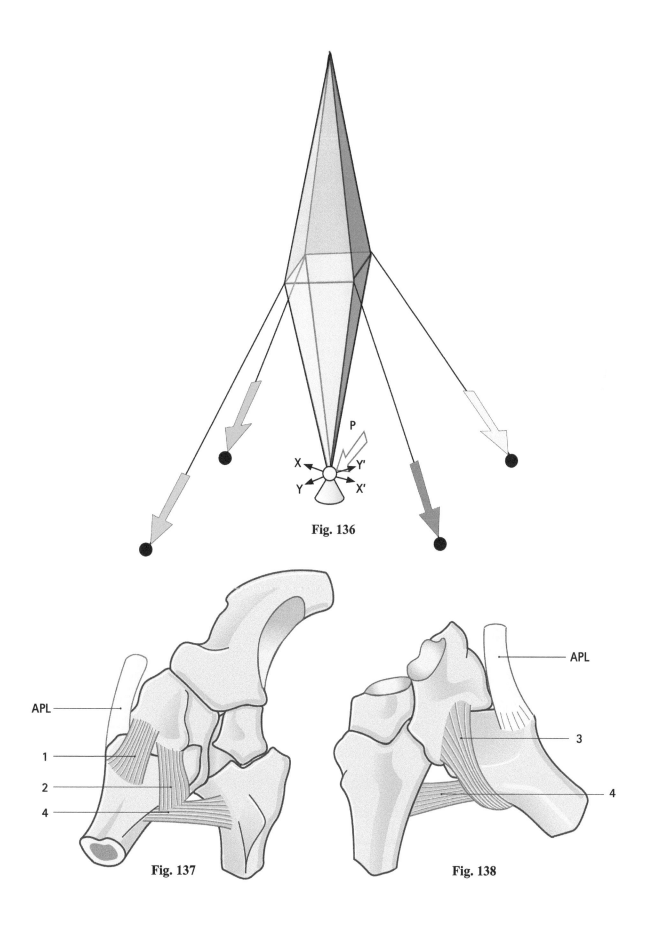

Fig. 136

APL

1

2

4

Fig. 137

APL

3

4

Fig. 138

261

The role of the ligaments

In reality we feel that the situation is more complex, since one must also describe the action of the ligaments **relative to the movements of antepulsion/retropulsion and of flexion-extension** of M_1 (which we will further define later).

During movements of antepulsion and retropulsion we observe the following:

- Figure 139 (**anterior view, taken in anteposition** (A)) shows that OAML is stretched, SALL is slackened and OPML is stretched posteriorly (Fig. 140).
- Figure 141 (**anterior view taken in retroposition** (R)) shows that SALL is stretched, OAML is slackened and OPML is also slackened posteriorly (Fig. 142).
- IML (Fig. 143, **anterior view**) is tightened in anteposition, when it pulls the base of M_1 towards M_2, and in retroposition, when it pulls back M_1, which is already displaced on TZ. It is relaxed only in the intermediate position, which bisects the angle formed by its extreme positions.

During movements of flexion-extension:

- **During extension** (E) (Fig. 144), the anterior ligaments SALL and OAML are stretched and OPML is slackened.
- **During flexion** (F) (Fig. 145), the opposite takes place, with slackening of SALL and OAML and stretching of OPML.

Being wrapped around the base of M_1 in opposite directions (Fig. 146, axial view of M_1 lying on TZ and M_2 and M_3), OPML and OAML maintain the stability of M_1 during its axial rotation as follows:

- OAML is stretched during pronation (P) and so would produce supination, if it were pathologically shortened.
- OPML is stretched during supination (S), so that, if it were to act alone, it would pronate M_1.

During opposition, which combines anteposition and flexion, all the ligaments are stretched except SALL, which runs parallel to the contracting muscles (*abductor pollicis brevis, opponens pollicis* and *flexor pollicis longus*). It is worth noting that the most stretched of these ligaments is OPML, which maintains the posterior stability of the joint. Opposition thus corresponds to the **close-packed position** of the TM joint, as already noted by MacConaill. It is the position in which the articular surfaces are the most closely apposed, thus preventing, with the help of the two concurrently stretched oblique ligaments, any axial rotation of M_1 and so any degree of play within the joint.

In the intermediate position, which will be defined later, all the ligaments are relaxed and 'play' is at a maximum within the TM joint, without any advantage during axial rotation of M_1. It is in this position that one can passively demonstrate the 'play' in the TM joint, which is thus not involved during opposition.

In counter-opposition, only the OAML is stretched, thus favouring some degree of axial rotation of M_1 into supination.

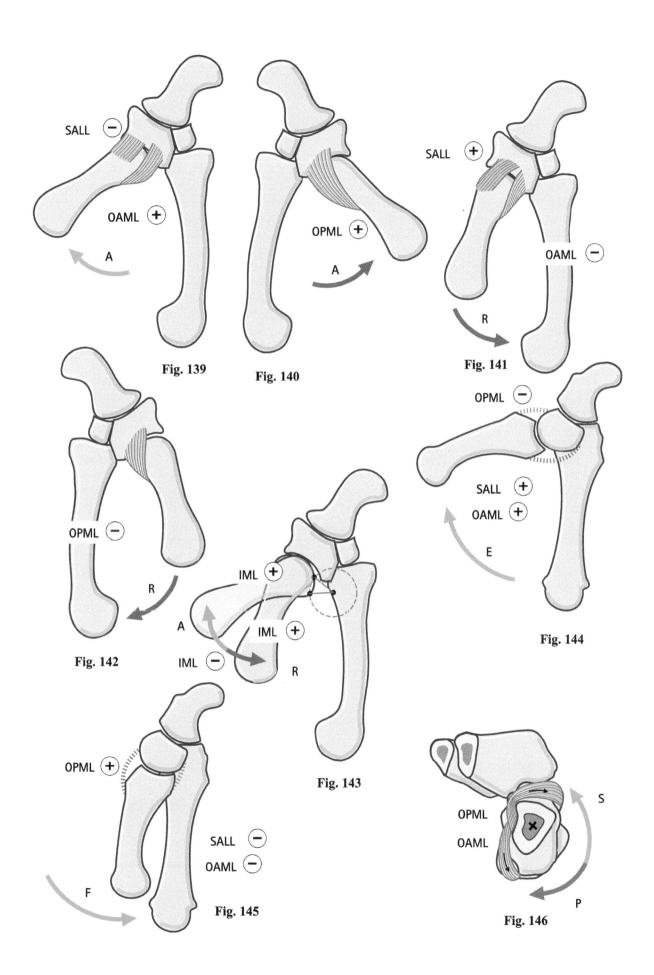

Fig. 139

Fig. 140

Fig. 141

Fig. 142

Fig. 143

Fig. 144

Fig. 145

Fig. 146

Geometrical analysis of the articular surfaces

If the axial rotation of M_1 cannot be explained by the play in the joint or by the action of the ligaments, the explanation must rest with the structure of the articular surfaces. It is worth stressing that such an explanation is accepted for the hip joint. Mathematically speaking, **saddle-shaped surfaces** have **negative curvature**, i.e. they are convex in one direction and concave in the other, so that they cannot be closed on themselves, like a sphere, which is the perfect example of positive curvature. The **non-Euclidean properties** of these surfaces have become better known since Gauss and Riemann.

These saddle-shaped surfaces have been likened to the following:

- **A segment of a circular hyperboloid** according to Bausenhart and Littler (Fig. 147): the surface of revolution (deep green) is generated by the hyperbola (HH) revolving around its conjugate axis along a circular path (CC).
- **A segment of a parabolic hyperboloid** (Fig. 148): the surface (pink) is generated by a hyperbola (HH) revolving along a parabolic path (PP).
- **A segment of a hyperbolic hyperboloid** (Fig. 149): the surface (blue) is generated by the hyperbola (HH) revolving along a hyperbolic path (H′H′).

We feel that it is more instructive to liken these saddle-shaped surfaces to an **axial segment of a torus** (Fig. 150; C = circle generating the toroidal surface). The inner border of a tyre, which provides a good representation of a **torus**, has a **concave surface** whose centre lies on the axis of the wheel XX′, and a **convex** surface whose centre lies on the axis of the tyre. In reality there is a series of axes p, q, s etc., with q corresponding to the centre of the saddle. **This toroidal surface with negative curvature**, cut out on the axial surface of the torus, therefore has **two main orthogonal axes** and consequently **two degrees of freedom** corresponding to its two curvatures.

If we take into account Kuczynski's description, which stresses the lateral curvature of the ridge of the saddle (the 'scoliotic horse', Fig. 134, p. 259), then this axial segment must be demarcated asymmetrically (Fig. 151) on the surface of the torus, as if the saddle **had slipped to one side** on the back of a normal horse. The long axis, the ridge of the saddle (nm), is bent to one side so that the radii u, v, w, passing through every point of the ridge, converge at a point O′, which lies on the axis XX′ of the torus outside its plane of symmetry and thus fails to coincide with the centre O of the torus. This saddle-shaped surface still corresponds to an **asymmetrical toroidal surface with negative curvature**, which has two main orthogonal axes and two degrees of freedom.

Under these conditions, it is logical and permissible to **construct a theoretical model of the TM joint**, just as the hip joint is biomechanically modelled as a ball-and-socket structure, although it is well known that the femoral head is not perfectly spherical. **The mechanical model of a biaxial joint is the universal joint*** (Fig. 152), with its two orthogonal convergent axes XX′ and YY′, arranged as a crossbar and allowing movements to occur in two planes AB and CD at right angles to each other. Likewise, **two saddle-shaped surfaces (a and b) lying one on top of the other** (Fig. 153) allow movements to occur relative to each other (Fig. 154) and in planes AB and CD respectively. But a study of the mechanics of the universal joint reveals that biaxial joints have an accessory movement, i.e. **automatic rotation of the mobile part on its long axis (i.e. the first metacarpal)**. This will be further discussed later.

---

* In French this joint is called the cardan after its inventor, Gerolamo Cardano (1501-1576)

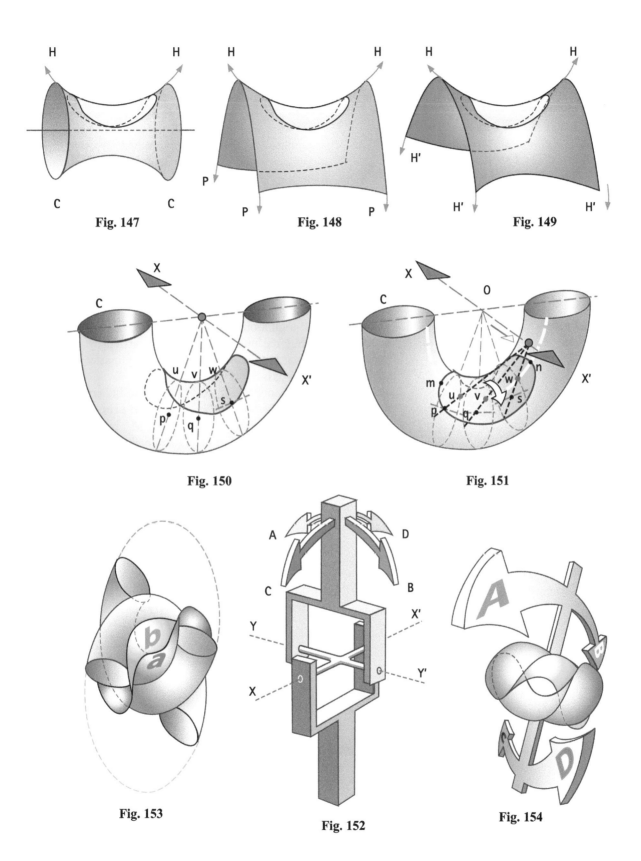

H   H

C   C

Fig. 147

H   H

P

P   P

Fig. 148

H   H

H′

H′   H′

Fig. 149

X

C

u v w

X′

p

q

s

Fig. 150

X   O

C

m

u v w

n

p

q

s

X′

Fig. 151

b
a

Fig. 153

A   D

C   B

Y   X′

X   Y′

Fig. 152

A

D

Fig. 154

Axial rotation

To understand the illustrations discussed on this page, the reader is advised to cut out pieces of cardboard and glue them together in order to construct **a mechanical model of the column of the thumb**, with a **universal joint** at its base (corresponding to the TM joint) and **two hinge joints** (corresponding to the MP and the IP joints), which **link** its three bony segments (Fig. 155). Start by cutting out three pieces from a strip of cardboard 1 mm thick. The first piece T (blue) represents the trapezium (TZ), and it has a fold (shown as a solid line) corresponding to a hinge. The second piece (yellow) has three parallel folds, which run in the same direction and separate the first metacarpal M_1, the first phalanx P_1 and the second phalanx P_2. In order to obtain neat folds, use a sharp blade to make a superficial cut into the back of the cardboard, and thus facilitate folding towards its front. The third piece (in blue and yellow) is a circle with a diameter equal to the width of the strip of cardboard. On each of its two surfaces draw a diameter; these two diameters should be perpendicular to each other.

When these pieces are ready they are glued together as follows. The blue piece is glued to one face of the circle so that the fold coincides with the diameter; the yellow piece is glued to the other face of the circle after being rotated 90° so that its fold coincides with the diameter. These two folds form the universal joint. The model is now ready and will allow us to demonstrate in space the automatic axial rotation of the mobile segment thanks to the mechanical properties of the universal joint.

Begin by **mobilizing the universal joint on its own** (Figs 156-159):

- Fold the two hinges separately and then simultaneously (Fig. 156). At hinge 1, the yellow piece revolves while staying in its own plane. At hinge 2, the yellow piece moves in two directions perpendicular to its own plane.
- You will notice (Fig. 157) that when the yellow piece is rotated about axis 1, it always moves in the same direction (a). This is an example of a **flat rotation**, i.e. rotation in one plane.

- If, before rotating the yellow piece around axis 1 (Fig. 158), you move it upwards through an angle (a), you will notice that, as it rotates (b) around axis 1, it changes direction while heading for the same point O, which corresponds to the summit of the cone described by the mobile segment. This is an example of **conical rotation**.
- If the yellow piece is flexed further to 90° (Fig. 159), it changes direction progressively relative to its rotation R around axis 1. This is an example of **cylindrical rotation**, which foreshadows the axial rotation of the column of the thumb. You can now understand what happens during opposition of the thumb (Fig. 160). As a 90° flexion cannot occur along the second axis of the TM joint, represented in the model by axis 2 of the universal joint, **this flexion is spread over the three hinge joints**.

The first movement of flexion is of moderate range and involves M_1 at the TM joint; the second involves P_1 at the MP joint, taking place around an axis 3; the third is flexion of P_2 at the IP joint around an axis 4.

Thus the pulp of the thumb, carried by P_2, can always face towards O while undergoing a cylindrical rotation around its long axis.

In summary, this axial rotation of the column of the thumb is **basically due to the mechanical properties of the universal joint** located between TZ and M_1, in particular the automatic rotation typical of this joint, i.e. the **conjunct rotation** of MacConaill. Its value can be calculated using a simple trigonometric formula that takes into account the two rotations; this is not included here.

Of course between zero automatic conjoint rotation in the case of plane rotation and maximal conjoint rotation in the case of cylindrical rotation all intermediate values are possible in biaxial universal joints.

Thus the axial rotation of the thumb is due to the coordinated function of the TM, MP and IP joints, but the initiating movement occurs in the key joint, i.e. the TM joint.

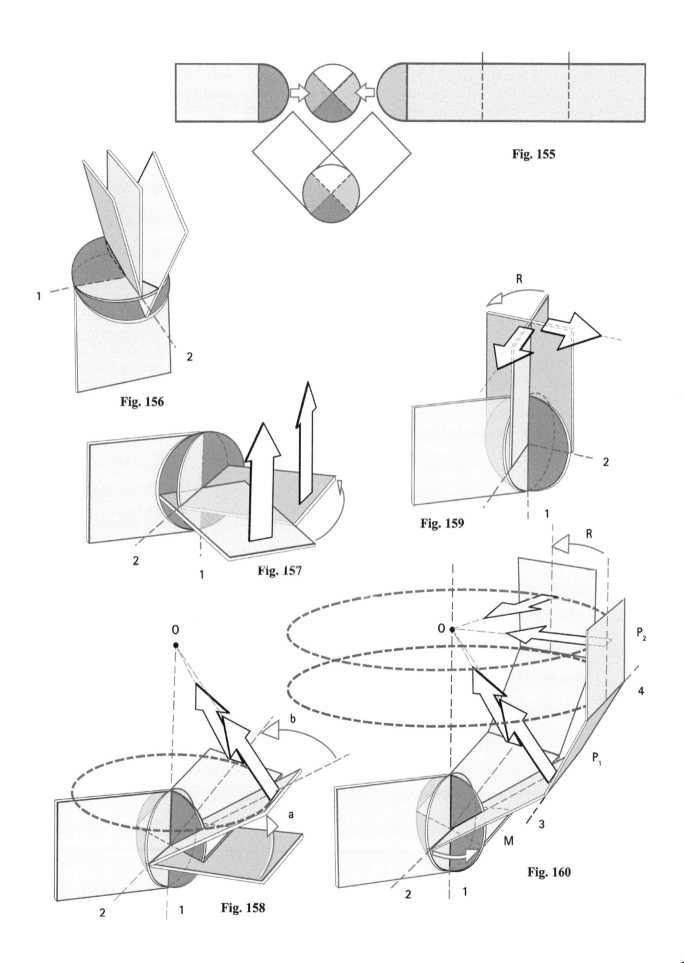

Fig. 155

Fig. 156

Fig. 157

Fig. 159

Fig. 158

Fig. 160

267

The movements of the first metacarpal (M₁)

M_1 can undergo single or combined movements about its two orthogonal axes and automatic axial rotation that **results from the movements taking place about these two axes.** We must define the **position in space of the two main axes of the TM joint,** which **do not lie in the usual three planes of reference.**

If, **on the skeleton** (Fig. 161), a metallic pin is inserted through the centre of the mean curvature of the articular surfaces of TZ and M_1, the following can be observed:

- The axis (1) corresponding to the concave curvature of TZ is seen to pass through the base of M_1.
- The axis (2) corresponding to the concave surface of the saddle-shaped M_1 passes through TZ. Of course, these axes are not fixed in reality but vary in position with the movements. (The pin represents only the mean position.) To a first approximation, however, we may consider these axes as the two axes of the TM joint, keeping in mind that this model is only a partial representation of reality meant to help in the understanding of a complex problem. These two **orthogonal axes,** which are perpendicular to each other but do not converge in space, form a universal joint. Hence it is reasonable to view the TM joint as endowed with the mechanical properties of a universal joint.

The joint has two important additional characteristics:

- Firstly, axis 1 is parallel to the axes of flexion-extension occurring at the MP joint (3) and at the IP joint (4). We will soon discuss the consequences of this arrangement.
- Secondly, axis 1 is perpendicular in space to axes 2, 3 and 4, and so lies in the plane of flexion for P_1 and P_2, i.e. **in the plane of flexion of the column of the thumb.**

Finally, an important point: the two orthogonal axes 1 and 2 of the TM joint are **oblique relative to the three planes of reference,** i.e. coronal (C), sagittal (S) and transverse (T). Hence **the pure movements of M_1** take place in a plane oblique to the three planes of reference; they therefore cannot be described in terms of classical anatomy, at least as regards abduction, which occurs in a coronal plane. Recent radiological studies have made it clear that the axis of flexion-extension of M_1 passes through TZ, that the axis of abduction-adduction lies at the base of M_1, and that these axes are close to each other. On the other hand, they do not form a right angle in space and so are not orthogonal; they actually form **an acute angle close to 42°.** This joint can still be likened to a universal joint, but it is active only in preferential sectors in accordance with its known functions.

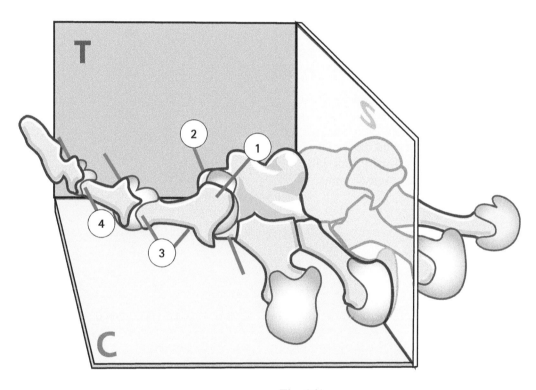

Fig. 161

The pure movements of M₁ (Fig. 162) **relative to the trapezial system of reference** can be defined as follows:

- **Around axis XX′** (axis 1 of the previous diagram), which we call the **main axis** because it allows the thumb to 'select' a particular finger during opposition, the movements of **antepulsion and retropulsion** take place. During these the column of the thumb moves in a plane AOR perpendicular to axis 1 and parallel to that of the thumbnail:
  - **During retropulsion** (R), the thumb is moved posteriorly to reach the plane of the palm while staying at an angle of 60° with M₂.
  - **During antepulsion** (A), the thumb moves anteriorly to a position almost perpendicular to the palm of the hand. This movement is confusingly called abduction by anglophone authors.
- **Around the axis YY′** (axis 2 of the previous diagram), which we call the **secondary axis**, occur the movements of flexion-extension in a plane FOE perpendicular to axis 2 of the previous diagram:
  - **During extension (E)**, M₁ moves posteriorly and laterally and the range of extension is increased by extension of P₁ and P₂, so that the column of the thumb assumes a superolateral orientation almost in the plane of the palm.
  - **During flexion** (F), P₁ moves distally, anteriorly and medially without crossing the sagittal plane, which

passes through M₂, and the range of flexion is increased by flexion of the phalanges, so that the pulp of the thumb touches the palm at the base of the little finger.

Thus the **concept of flexion and extension of M₁ is perfectly justified** by the occurrence of similar movements at the other two joints of the column of the thumb.

Aside from these pure movements of antepulsion-retropulsion and of flexion-extension, **all the other movements of M₁ are complex**, i.e. combined with varying degrees of successive or concurrent movement about the two axes and with the resultant automatic or conjunct axial rotation. The latter plays a vital role in opposition of the thumb.

The movements of flexion-extension and antepulsion-retropulsion of M₁ start from the **neutral position** or the position of rest of the thumb muscles (Fig. 163). This position is also defined as the position of **electromyographic silence** (Hamonet and Valentin), when the relaxed muscles give rise to no recordable action potentials. It (N) has also been defined radiographically as the position where M₁ and M₂ form an angle of 30° in the coronal plane (C), an angle of 40° in the sagittal plane (S) and an angle of 40° in the transverse plane (T).

This position (N) also corresponds to the position of relaxation of the ligaments and maximal congruence of the articular surfaces, which overlie each other almost perfectly.

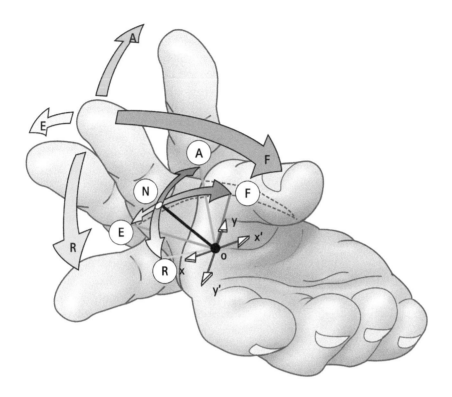

Fig. 162

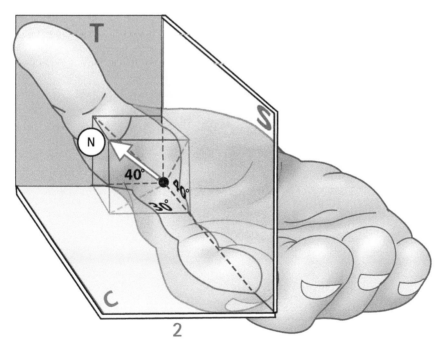

Fig. 163

Measurement of the movements of M₁

Now that we have described the real movements of M_1, how do we measure these movements in practice? The problem is complicated by the current use of three methods.

In the **first method**, which could be called the **classical** method (Fig. 164), M_1 is made to move in a rectangular solid of reference, formed by the three perpendicular planes, i.e. transverse (T), coronal (C) and sagittal (S). The latter two planes intersect along the long axis of M_2 and the plane of intersection of the three planes passes through the TM joint according to the classical method of evaluation. The reference position is achieved when **M₁ touches M₂ in the plane of the palm**, which is roughly the same plane as C.

Two comments deserve attention:

1) This position is not natural.

2) M_1 cannot strictly be made to lie parallel to M_2.

Abduction (arrow 1) occurs when M_1 moves away from M_2 in plane F, and the converse applies to adduction.

Flexion (arrow 2) or anterior (palmar) displacement occurs when M_1 moves anteriorly, and **extension** or posterior (dorsal) displacement occurs when M_1 moves posteriorly.

The position of M_1 is thus defined by two angles (Fig. 165): the angle (a) for abduction (Ab) and adduction (Add), and the angle (b) for flexion or anterior displacement (A) and extension or posterior displacement (P).

This method has two disadvantages:

1) The movements are measured as projections on abstract planes and not as real angles.

2) Axial rotation is not measured.

The **second method**, which could be called the **modern** method as proposed by Duparc, de la Caffinière and Pineau (Fig. 166), determines not movement but rather positions of M_1 according to a system of polar coordinates. The position of M_1 is defined by its position on a cone whose **axis** coincides with the long axis of M_2 and whose **apex** lies at the TM joint. The half-angle at the apex of the cone (arrow 1) is its **angle of separation**, which is valid only when M_1 moves along the surface of the cone. The position of M_1 is established precisely by the angle (arrow 2) between the plane passing through M_1 and M_2 and the coronal plane (C).

With respect to the rectangular solid of reference (Fig. 167), this angle (b) is called by these authors the **angle of rotation in space**, which is tautological, since rotation must take place in space. It would be more appropriate to call it the **angle of circumduction**, since the movement of M_1 on the surface of the cone is analogous to circumduction.

The value of this second method, relative to the first, rests on the ease with which these two angles can be measured with a protractor.

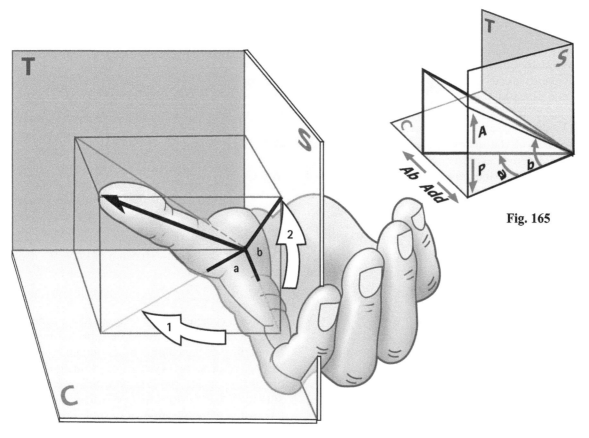

Fig. 164

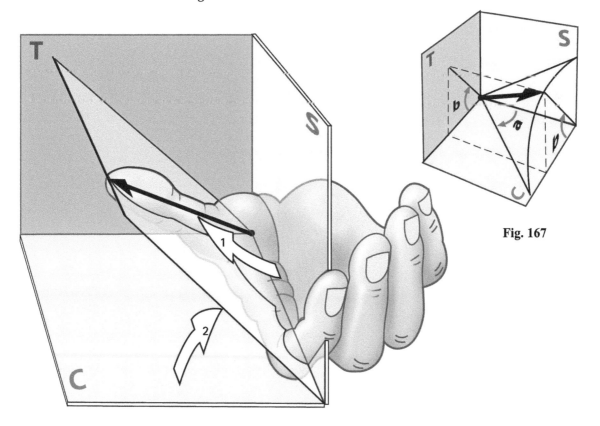

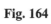

Fig. 165

Fig. 167

Radiographic features of the TM joint and of the trapezial system

The following discussion is based on **radiographic studies**, including radiographs taken head-on and from the side **at specific angles**, as defined by the author in 1980. The principle involved is to orient the main X-ray beam so as to take into account the obliquity of the axes of the joint and to demonstrate the **true curvatures of the articular surfaces without any distortions** in perspective, as observed in radiographs of the hand being taken head-on and from the side at the so-called classical angles. In this way one accurately measures both the range of the pure movements of the TM joint and its structural characteristics, which are very important in its physiology and pathology.

On the basis of radiographs taken of the hand from the front and from the side at specific angles, we propose a **third method of measurement of the ranges of movement** of the TM joint, i.e. the **trapezial system of reference**.

On an **anterior radiograph of the column of the thumb** (Fig. 168), the curvature of TZ and the convex curvature of M_1 are seen strictly in profile without the benefit of any perspective. A radiograph is then taken in retroposition R and another in anteposition A. The ranges of movement are measured between the long axes of M_1 and M_2. By subtracting the value obtained in retroposition from that obtained in anteposition one obtains the **range of antepulsion-retropulsion**:

- Retropulsion causes the axis of M_1 to come to lie almost parallel to that of M_2.

- Antepulsion widens the angle between M_1 and M_2 up to 50-60°.

The **range of antepulsion-retropulsion** is 22° ± 9°, varying with the sex of the subject:

- In men it is 19° ± 8°.
- In women it is 24° ± 9°.

On a **radiograph of the column of the thumb taken in profile** (Fig. 169) the convex curvature of TZ and the concave curvature of M1 are seen without any distortion. One radiograph is taken in extension (E) and another in flexion (F).

- Extension widens the distance between M1 and M2, which form an angle of 30-40°.
- Flexion brings M1 closer to M2 and causes them to become almost parallel.

The **range of flexion-extension** is 17° ± 9°, depending on the sex of the subject:

- In men it is 16° ± 8°.
- In women it is 18° ± 9°.

All things considered, the range of movements at the TM joint is much smaller than would be expected for the great degree of mobility of the column of the thumb.

Neither of these two systems of evaluation of the movements of the first metacarpal is satisfactory or easy to use. On pages 306-307 I put forward an opposition and counter-opposition test that is very revealing and extremely easy to use.

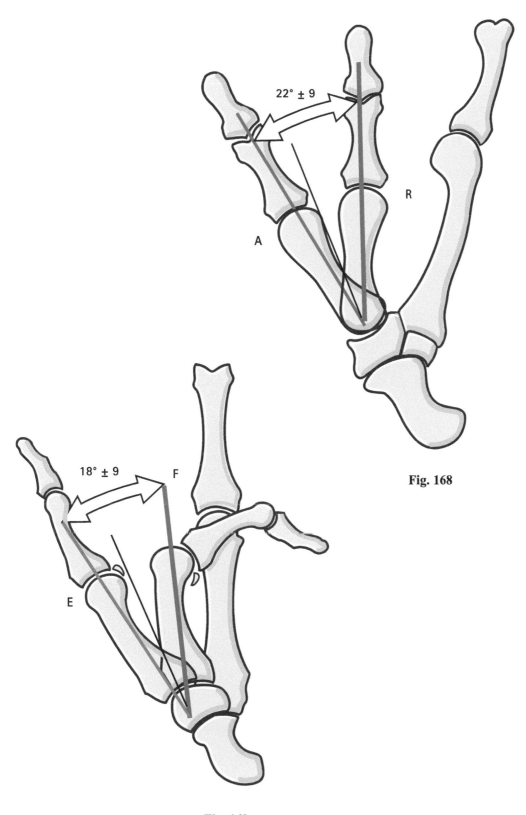

22° ± 9

A

R

Fig. 168

18° ± 9

F

E

Fig. 169

The structural and functional features of the TM joint

Structural and functional studies of 330 cases, carried out in 1993 by A.I. Kapandji and T. Kapandji, revealed the following:

- The **range of the movements of TZ** (Fig. 170) is 2.9° ± 2° between antepulsion (A) and retropulsion (R), a small range but none the less real.
- The **base of M$_1$** (Fig. 171) **in retroposition** is almost dislocated laterally on the trapezial saddle but **in anteposition** (Fig. 172) it regains its place within the concavity of the trapezial saddle.
- A head-on view (Fig. 173) shows evidence of **early rhizarthrosis**, i.e. the base of M$_1$ fails to move snugly into the trapezial saddle and stays stuck to the cantle (the raised hind part) of the saddle during antepulsion. Normally on radiographs taken from the side (Fig. 174) the 'beak' of the base of M$_1$ fits perfectly under the convex surface of TZ.
- In **early rhizarthrosis** (Fig. 175) the beak-like base of M$_1$ does not regain its normal position and remains stuck to the convex surface of TZ under the pull of the tendon of the *abductor pollicis longus* (white).
- The measurement of the angle **between the base and the ridge of the saddle** made on anterior radiographs is of vital importance in the diagnosis of **early rhizarthrosis**. Normally (Fig. 176), this angle, as measured between the axis of M$_2$ and that of the trapezial saddle (red line), has a mean value of 127° and the intermetacarpal ligament (green dotted line) is able to bring back the base of M$_1$ on to the trapezial saddle.
- **When this angle approaches 140°** (Fig. 177) one can suspect the early development of rhizarthrosis, especially if the patient feels pain occasionally over the TM joint. The congenital condition of the '**sliding saddle**', i.e. dysplasia of the trapezial saddle, predisposes to rhizarthrosis of the TM joint, since in the long run the intermetacarpal ligament loses its ability to bring back the base of M$_1$, and produces a state of chronic lateral subluxation, which wears out the trapezial surface and reduces the width of the joint space as is evident in frontal X-rays.

To end the discussion of the TM joint, it is quite clear that it corresponds mechanically to a **universal joint**, and that it is totally inappropriate to replace it with a spherical prosthesis, as favoured by some surgeons who have not yet understood that a universal joint is mechanically able to allow longitudinal rotation of the first metacarpal to occur. For this reason there is no need for the extra degree of freedom provided by a spherical joint. This is another example of the universal principle of Occam's razor.

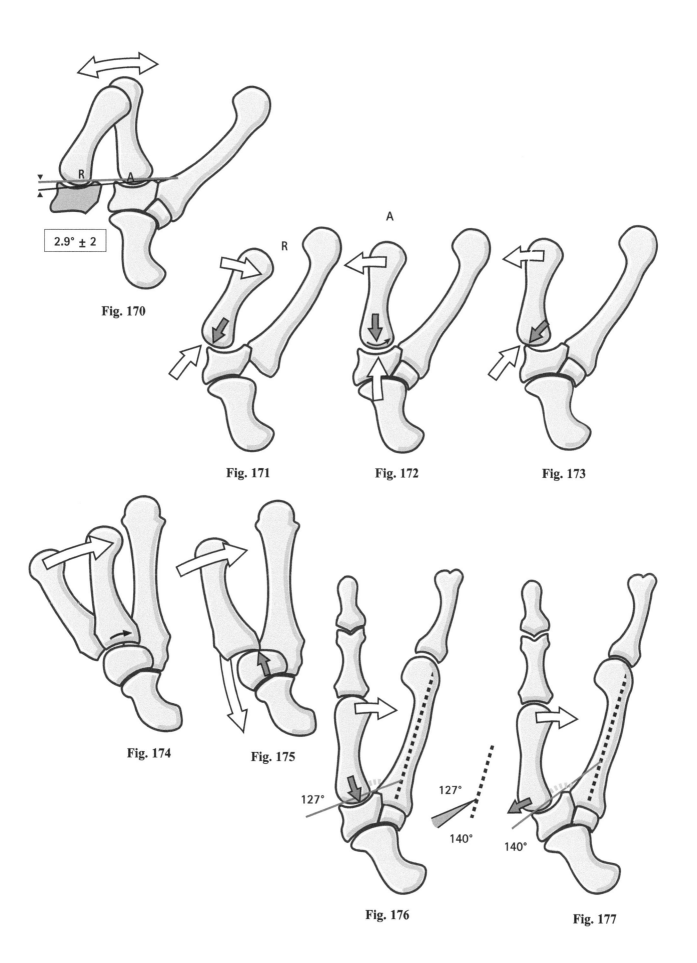

2.9° ± 2

Fig. 170

R A

Fig. 171

Fig. 172

Fig. 173

Fig. 174

Fig. 175

127°

127°

140°

140°

Fig. 176

Fig. 177

The metacarpo-phalangeal (MP) joint of the thumb

The **MP joint of the thumb** is considered by anatomists to be of the **condyloid** variety, though anglophone authors think of it as an ellipsoid joint. Like every condyloid joint, it has two degrees of freedom, allowing flexion-extension and lateral inclinations. In reality, as a result of its complex biomechanical structure, it has also a **third degree of freedom** allowing **axial rotation of P**$_1$ (pronation and supination), which is both passive and active and essential for thumb opposition.

In Figure 178 (the joint is opened anteriorly and P$_1$ is displaced posteriorly and proximally) the **head of M**$_1$ (1) appears biconvex, being longer than it is wide and expanded anteriorly by two asymmetrical swellings, with the medial swelling (a) being more prominent than the lateral one (b). To the cartilage-coated biconcave **base of P**$_1$ (2) and its anterior border is attached the **fibro-cartilaginous palmar plate** (3), which bears **two sesamoid bones** near its distal edge. The medial (4) and the external (5) sesamoid bones have a cartilaginous surface continuous with that of the palmar plate. The **medial (6) and the lateral (7) sesamoid muscles** are attached to these sesamoid bones. The capsule, seen sliced in the diagram (8), is thickened on either side by the **medial (9) and the lateral (10) collateral ligaments** attaching M$_1$ to the palmar plate. Also seen are **the anterior (11) and the posterior (12) recesses of the capsule** and the collateral ligaments, the medial ligament (13) being shorter than the lateral (14). The arrows XX′ and YY′ represent respectively the **axis of flexion-extension** and the **axis of lateral inclinations**.

Figure 179 (**anterior view**) shows the same structures, i.e. M$_1$ (15) below and P$_1$ (16) above, and provides a more detailed view of the palmar plate (3) and the medial (4) and the lateral (5) sesamoid bones. These bones are linked by the **intersesa-moid ligament** (not shown), are attached to the head of M$_1$ by the medial (18) and lateral (19) collateral ligaments of the MP joint, and are bound to the base of P$_1$ by the **straight** (20) and **crossed** (21) fibres of the phalango-sesamoid ligament. The medial sesamoid muscles (6) are inserted into the medial sesamoid bone and send an expansion to the base of P$_1$ (22), which partially masks the medial ligament (13). The **phalangeal expansion** (23) of the lateral sesamoid muscles (7) has been cut to display the lateral collateral ligament (14).

In Figures 180 (**medial view**) and 181 (**lateral view**) can also be seen the **posterior (24) and the anterior (25) recesses of the capsule**, the insertion of the tendon of the **extensor pollicis brevis** (26) and the clearly off-centre metacarpal attachment of the medial (13) and lateral (14) collateral ligaments and of the ligaments attaching the metacarpal to the palmar plate (18 and 19). One can see that the medial collateral ligament is shorter and more readily tightened than the lateral so that the movements of the base of P$_1$ are less marked on the medial than on the lateral aspect of the head of M$_1$. A transparent diagram of the head of M$_1$ (Fig. 186, p. 281) explains how the differential displacement of M$_1$ medially (SM) and laterally (SL) produces an axial rotation into pronation of the base of P$_1$, when the lateral sesamoid muscles (7) contract more vigorously than the medial sesamoid muscles (6).

This differential displacement is further enhanced by the **asymmetry of the head of M**$_1$ (Fig. 182, seen head-on) with its **more prominent medial swelling** (a) extending less distally than its **lateral swelling** (b). Thus laterally the base of P$_1$ moves farther anteriorly and distally, giving rise to a combined movement of flexion, pronation and radial deviation of P$_1$.

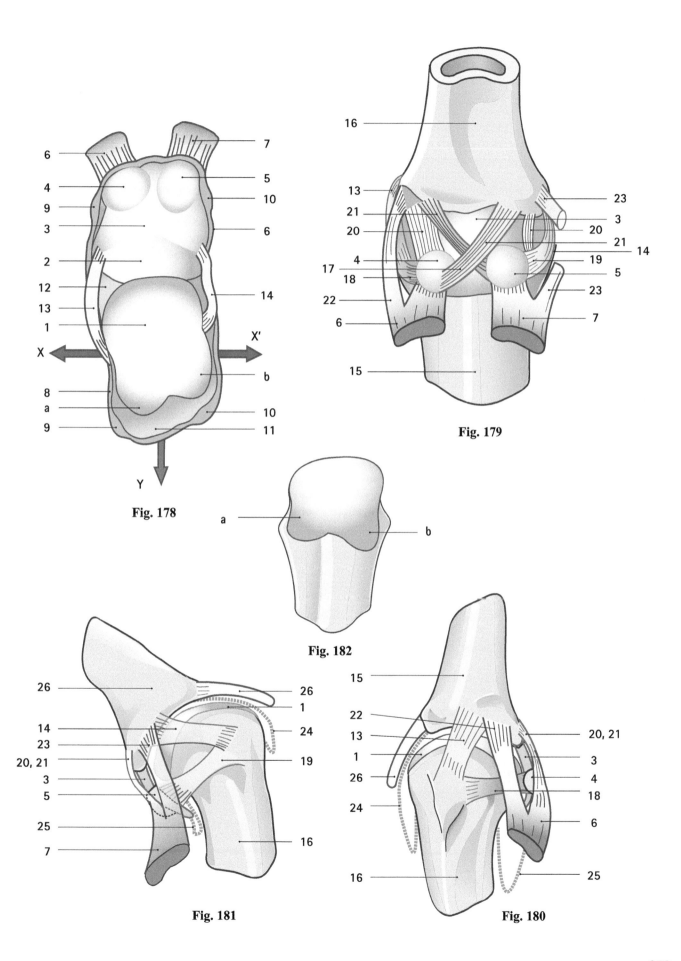

Fig. 178

Fig. 179

Fig. 182

Fig. 181

Fig. 180

The extent of the lateral inclinations and axial rotation of P_1 depend on its degree of flexion.

In the neutral position or in extension (Fig. 183), the **collateral ligaments** (1) are slack, while the **palmar plate** (2) and **the ligaments attaching M_1 to the plate** (3) are taut, thus preventing axial rotation and lateral movements. This is therefore the first locked position and it occurs in extension, as the sesamoids (4) are firmly applied to the metacarpal head. Note that the **posterior (5) and anterior (6) synovial recesses** are relaxed in the intermediate position.

In the intermediate or mid-flexion position (Fig. 184) the collateral ligaments (1) are again slack, the lateral more than the medial one, while the palmar plate (2) and the ligaments binding it to M_1 are slackened as the **sesamoid bones** (4) slip under the anterior swellings of the head of M_1.

This is the **position of maximal mobility**, where lateral inclinations and axial rotation can be produced by the sesamoid muscles. Thus contraction of the medial sesamoid muscles leads to ulnar deviation and more limited supination, while that of the lateral sesamoid muscles produces radial deviation and pronation.

In full flexion (Fig. 185) the palmar plate and the ligament attaching it to M_1 are slackened, while the **collateral ligaments are maximally stretched**, so that the base of P_1 undergoes **radial deviation and pronation**. The joint is literally locked by the interaction of the collateral ligaments and the posterior synovial recess (5), when the thumb is in the **extreme position of thumb-to-little finger opposition** produced by the predominant, if not exclusive, action of the **lateral thenar muscles**.

This corresponds to the close-packed position of MacConaill. It is the second locked position and occurs in flexion.

Figure 186 (**superior view**, with the base of P_1 transparent) shows how $\mathbf{P_1}$ **is pronated** mostly by the lateral sesamoid muscles (SL).

On the whole the MP joint of the thumb can undergo **three types of movement** (Kapandji, 1980), starting from the neutral position (Fig. 187, posterior view of the head of M_1, showing the axes of the various movements):

- **Pure flexion** (blue arrow 1) around a transverse axis f_1, produced by the balanced action of the medial and lateral sesamoid muscles up to the position of mid-flexion.
- Two types of complex movements combining flexion, lateral deviation and axial rotation:
  - **Combined flexion, ulnar deviation and supination** (green arrow 2) around a mobile oblique axis f_2, giving rise to a conical rotation; this is produced largely by the medial sesamoid muscles.
  - **Combined flexion, radial deviation and pronation** (orange arrow 3) around a mobile axis f_3, which is more oblique than f_2 and points in the other direction. Again there is conical rotation produced largely by the lateral sesamoid muscles.

Thus full flexion is always combined with radial deviation and pronation because of the asymmetrical shape of the head of M_1 and the unequal degree of stretching of the collateral ligaments, **both of which promote the overall opposition of the column of the thumb**.

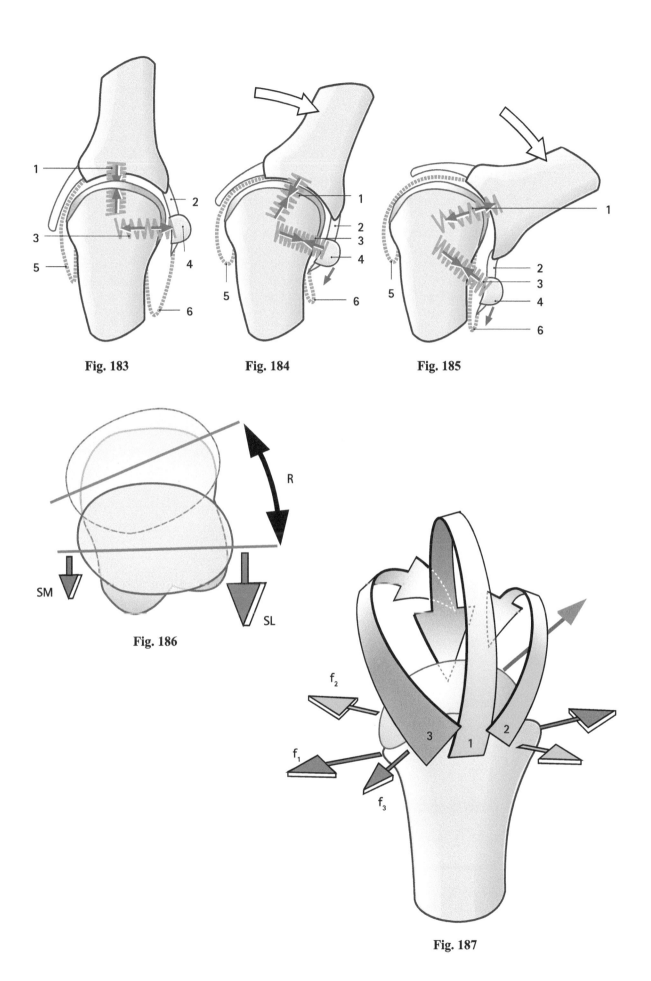

Fig. 183

Fig. 184

Fig. 185

Fig. 186

Fig. 187

Movements of the MP joint of the thumb

The **position of reference for this joint** is achieved when the **thumb is straight** and the axes of P_1 and M_1 are collinear (Fig. 188). To understand the elementary movements of the joints of the fingers, it is a good idea to construct **two trihedral structures** with three matchsticks arranged orthogonally and to glue each of these structures on either side of the joint.

Starting from this position, **no active or passive extension is possible in a normal person**.

Active flexion (Fig. 189) is 60-70°, while **passive flexion** can attain 80° or even 90°. The elementary components of this movement are well brought out with the use of the trihedral structures.

In the position of reference (Fig. 190, dorsal view) the trihedral structures are glued so that the matchsticks are parallel or collinear. In this way the components of rotation and lateral deviation can be observed during movements.

In the position of mid-flexion one can voluntarily contract either the medial or the lateral sesamoid muscles.

When the medial sesamoid muscles contract (Fig. 191, distal view with the thumb lying slightly anterior to the plane of the palm; Fig 192, proximal view with the thumb lying in the plane of the palm), with the help of the matchsticks one can observe ulnar deviation of a few degrees and supination of 5-7°.

When the lateral sesamoid muscles contract (Fig. 193, distal view; Fig. 194, proximal view), one can observe radial deviation (well shown in Fig. 194), which is greater than the previous ulnar deviation, and pronation of 20°.

We shall discuss later the full significance of this combined movement of flexion, radial deviation and pronation during opposition of the thumb.

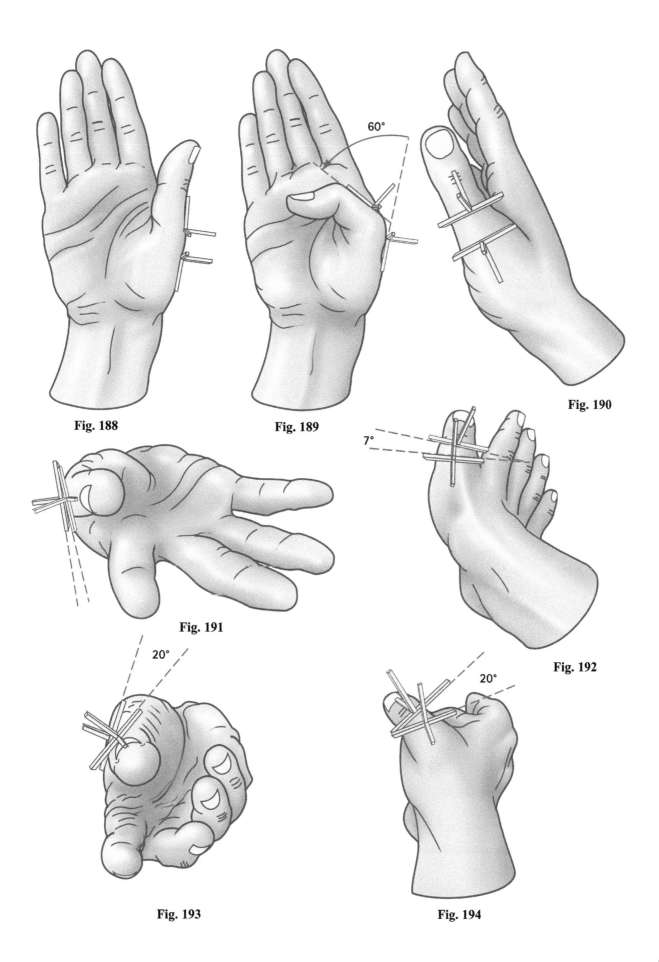

Fig. 188

Fig. 189

60°

Fig. 190

Fig. 191

7°

Fig. 192

20°

Fig. 193

20°

Fig. 194

Combined lateral and rotational movements of the MP joint of the thumb

In full palmar cylindrical grips, the grip is firmly locked by the **action of the lateral sesamoid muscles** at the MP joint. When the thumb is inactive (Fig. 195) and stays parallel to the axis of the cylinder, the grip is incompletely locked and the object can easily slip through the gap between the fingertips and the thenar eminence.

If, on the other hand, **the thumb moves towards the fingers** (Fig. 196), the object cannot escape. The **radial deviation of P_1**, seen clearly with the help of the trihedral structures, brings M_1 into full anteposition. Thus the thumb takes the shortest, i.e. circular, path (f) around the cylinder; this path would be elliptical and longer (d) without the radial deviation of P_1.

Radial deviation is therefore essential for locking the grip, the more so as the ring formed around the object by the thumb and the index finger is more completely closed and is the shortest (Fig. 197). In position **a** the thumb lies along the axis of the cylinder and the ring-like structure of the grip is absent. In positions **b-e**, the ring closes progressively, and finally in position **f** the thumb is perpendicular to the long axis of the cylinder. The ring is now completely closed and the grip is locked. Furthermore, **pronation of P_1** (Fig. 198), shown by the 12° angle formed by the two transverse matchsticks, allows the thumb to apply itself to the object with the bulk of its palmar surface instead of its medial border. Thus, by increasing the surface of contact, pronation of P_1 helps to strengthen the grip.

If **a small cylinder is being held** (Fig. 199), the thumb comes to overlie the index partially, and so the ring of grip is narrower, the locking is more complete and the grip is stronger.

Thus the functional characteristics of the MP joint of the thumb and of its motor muscles **are remarkably adapted for prehension**.

The stability of the MP joint of the thumb depends on a combination of **articular and muscular factors**. Normally, during opposition of the thumb (Fig. 200), the successive joints of the index finger and of the thumb are stabilized by the action of antagonistic muscles (small arrows). Under certain circumstances (Fig. 201, inspired by Sterling Bunnell), the MP joint goes into extension rather than flexion, i.e. inversion of movements (white arrow):

- when paralysis of the *abductor pollicis brevis* and of the *flexor pollicis brevis* allows P_1 to be tilted posteriorly into extension
- when shortening of the muscles of the first interosseous space draws M_1 closer to M_2
- when weakness of the *abductor pollicis longus* prevents abduction of M_1.

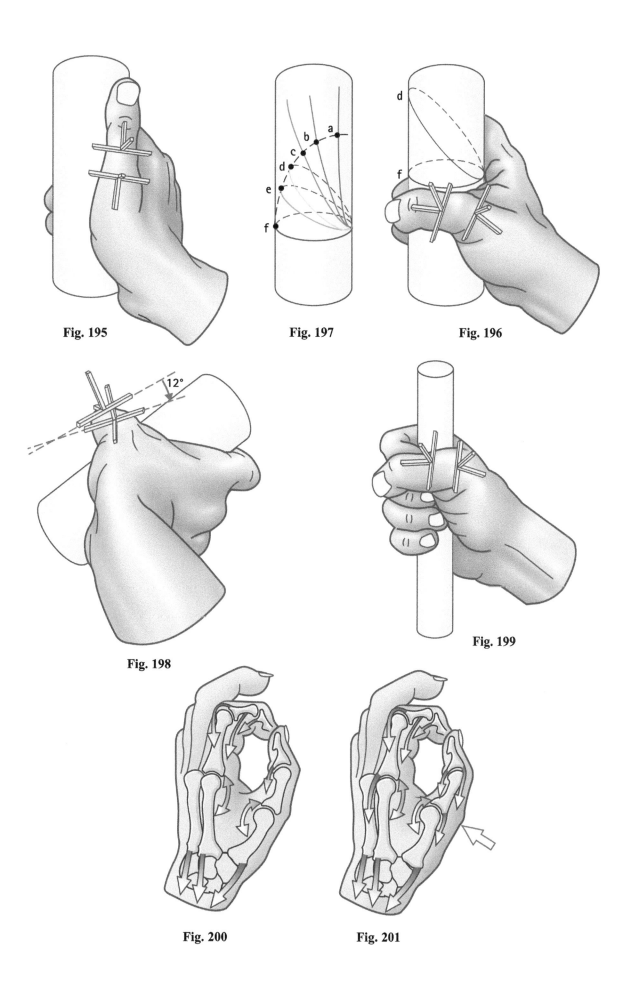

Fig. 195

Fig. 197

Fig. 196

Fig. 198

12°

Fig. 199

Fig. 200

Fig. 201

The interphalangeal (IP) joint of the thumb

At first glance the IP joint of the thumb is straightforward. It is a **hinge joint** with a fixed transverse axis, which runs through the centre of curvature of the condyles of the articular surface of P_1 and about which occur movements of flexion and extension.

Flexion (Fig. 202), when active, is 75-80° as measured by a goniometer (Fig. 203) and reaches 90° when passive.

Extension (Fig. 204) is 5-10° when active, whereas passive hyperextension (Fig. 205) can be quite marked, i.e. 30°, among certain professionals such as sculptors, who use their thumbs as spatulas to press the clay.

These movements are a little more complex in real life, since during flexion P_2 **undergoes a movement of automatic medial rotation into pronation**.

In Figure 206 (anatomical model) two parallel pins have been inserted, one (a) into the head of P_1 and the other (b) into the base of P_2 with the IP joint in full extension (A). When the IP joint is flexed (B), the pins come to lie at an angle of 5-10° open medially, i.e. in the direction of pronation.

A similar experiment done on a living subject using parallel matchsticks stuck to the posterior surfaces of P_1 and P_2 gives a similar result; **when P_2 is flexed, it is pronated 5-10°**.

This observation can be explained partly by the mechanical properties of the articular surfaces. Figure 207 (joint opened posteriorly) shows right away the differences between the two condyles; the medial condyle is more prominent and longer anteriorly and medially than the lateral condyle (Fig. 208). The radius of curvature of the lateral condyle is shorter, so that its anterior surface 'drops' more abruptly towards the surface of the palm. Therefore the medial collateral ligament is stretched sooner than the lateral counterpart during flexion and so brings the medial aspect of the base of P_2 to a halt, while its lateral aspect goes on moving.

In other words (Fig. 209), the excursion of P_2 is shorter on the medial condyle (AA') of P_1 than it is on the lateral condyle (BB'), and as a result P_2 **is medially rotated**. There is no single axis of flexion-extension but rather **a series of oblique instantaneous axes** between the initial position (i) and the final position (f). These axes trace the base circle of a cone with its apex at their point of convergence O, which lies distal to the thumb. If a model of the IP joint is made with cardboard (Fig. 210), the strip must be folded along an axis that is not perpendicular to that of the 'finger' but at an angle of 5-10° to it. The phalanx, when flexed, will then undergo conical rotation, indicating a change in its direction proportional to the degree of flexion.

This component of rotation at the IP joint contributes, as we shall see later, to the overall movement of pronation of the thumb during opposition.

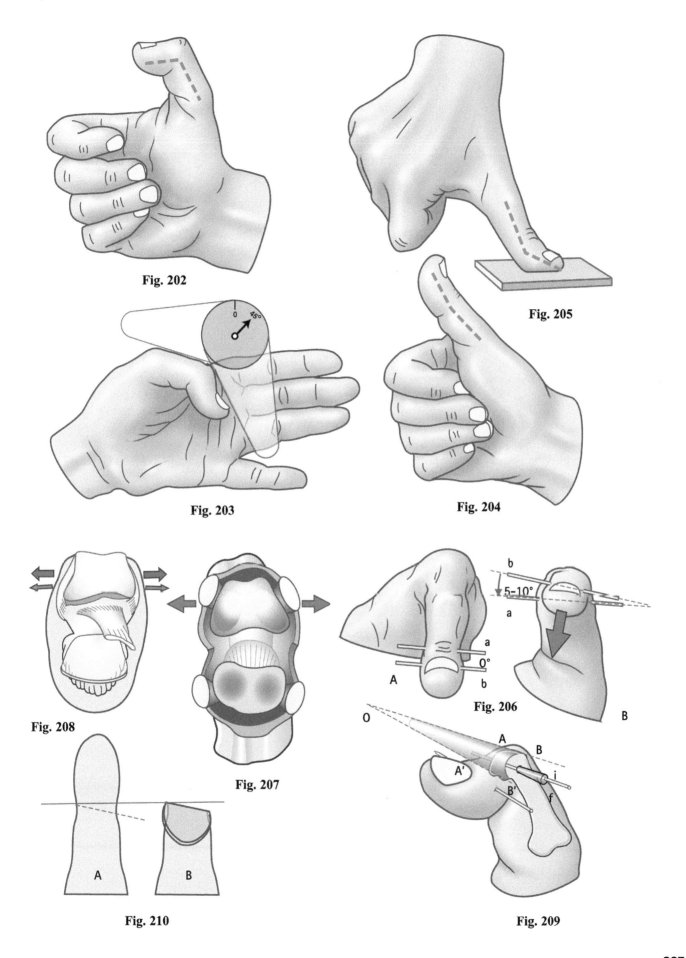

Fig. 202

Fig. 203

Fig. 204

Fig. 205

Fig. 206

Fig. 207

Fig. 208

Fig. 209

Fig. 210

The motor muscles of the thumb

The thumb has **nine motor muscles**, and this abundance of dedicated muscles, as compared with the other fingers, determines **its greater mobility and its essentiality**.

These muscles fall into two groups:

1) The **extrinsic or long muscles**, four in all and lodged mostly in the forearm. **Three of these are extensors and abductors** and are used to release the grip; **the fourth is a flexor** and is used to lock the grip.

2) The **intrinsic muscles**, lying within the thenar eminence and the first osseous space. These **five** muscles allow the hand to achieve a variety of grips and above all allow the thumb to be **opposed**. They are weak muscles and are more involved in **precise and coordinated movements**.

To understand the action of these muscles on the column of the thumb, **their paths relative to the two theoretical axes of the TM joint** must be defined. These axes (Fig. 212), i.e. the axis YY′ for flexion-extension, lying parallel to the axes of flexion of the MP joint (f_1) and of the IP joint (f_2), and the axis XX′ of antepulsion-retropulsion demarcate the following four quadrants represented by the two orthogonal pins, as follows:

1) **Quadrant X′Y′** lying dorsal to the axis YY′ of flexion-extension of the TM joint and lateral to the axis XX′ of antepulsion-retropulsion, contains one muscle, the **abductor pollicis longus** (1). As this muscle lies close to axis X′, it produces antepulsion only weakly but extends M_1 powerfully (Fig. 211, lateral and proximal view of the thumb 'running away').

2) **Quadrant X′Y**, lying medial to axis XX′ and dorsal to axis YY′, contains the tendons of the **extensor pollicis brevis** (2) and of the **extensor pollicis longus** (3).

3) **Quadrant XY** (Fig. 213), lying palmar to axis YY′ and palmar to axis XX′, contains two muscles, which lie in the first interosseous space and produce retropulsion combined with slight flexion of the TM joint:
   - the adductor pollicis with its two bundles (8)
   - the first palmar interosseus (9), if present.

These two muscles adduct M_1 and narrow the first interdigital cleft or web space by bringing M_1 closer to M_2.

4) **Quadrant XY′** (Fig. 213), lying palmar to axis YY′ and lateral to axis XX′, contains the muscles of opposition, which produce combined flexion and antepulsion of M_1:
   - the opponens pollicis (6)
   - the abductor pollicis brevis (7).

The last two muscles lie on axis XX′ and thus are flexors of the TM joint:

1) the **flexor pollicis longus** (4)
2) the **flexor pollicis brevis** (5).

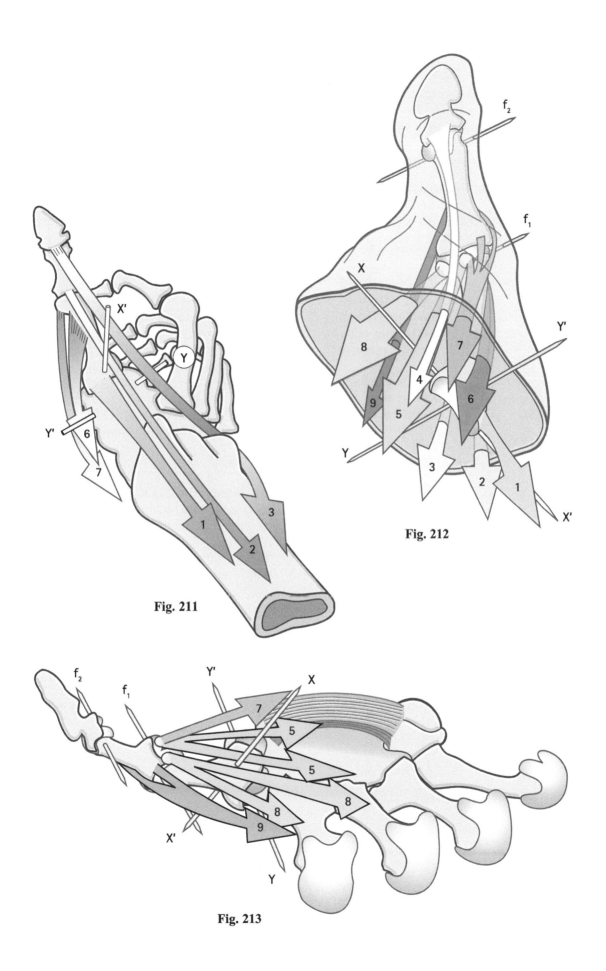

Fig. 211

Fig. 212

Fig. 213

A **brief review of the anatomy** of these motor muscles of the thumb will shed considerable light on their physiology. They fall into two groups: the extrinsic and the intrinsic muscles.

The extrinsic muscles
- The **abductor pollicis longus** (1) (Fig. 214, anterior view), inserted into the antero-lateral aspect of the base of M_1
- The **extensor pollicis brevis** (2) (Fig. 215, lateral view) running parallel to the previous muscle and inserted into the base of P_1
- The **extensor pollicis longus** (3), inserted posteriorly into the dorsal aspect of the base of P_2.

Two points must be made regarding these three muscles:
1) **Anatomically speaking**, their three tendons, present on the dorsal and lateral aspects of the thumb, bound a triangular space with its apex located distally, i.e. the **anatomical snuff-box**. In the floor of this space run the parallel tendons of the **extensor carpi radialis longus** (10) and of the **extensor carpi radialis brevis** (11).
2) **Functionally speaking**, each of these three muscles acts on a particular segment of the thumb and all three are extensors, whereas the **flexor pollicis longus** (4) is a palmar muscle (Fig. 214). It traverses the carpal tunnel, runs between the two heads of the **flexor pollicis brevis** and slips between the two sesamoid bones of the MP joint of the thumb (Fig. 214), to be inserted into the palmar aspect of the base of P_2.

The intrinsic muscles
These (Figs 214 and 215) fall into two groups: the lateral group and the medial group.

The lateral group

The **lateral group** consists of three muscles supplied by the median nerve. They are as follows, from deep to superficial:
1) The **flexor pollicis brevis** (5), which arises by two heads, one from the deep carpal surface of the carpal tunnel and the other from the lower border of the *flexor retinaculum* and the tubercle of TZ. Its single tendon is inserted into the outer sesamoid bone and the lateral tubercle of the base of P_1. Its general direction is oblique distally and laterally.
2) The **opponens pollicis** (6), arising from the *flexor retinaculum* (lateral palmar surface) runs distally, laterally and posteriorly to be inserted into the anterior aspect of M_1.
3) The **abductor pollicis brevis** (7) arises from the *flexor retinaculum* proximal to the origin of the *opponens* and the crest of the scaphoid and lies superficial to the *opponens*, forming the superficial plane of the thenar eminence. It is inserted into the lateral tubercle of the base of P_1 but some of its lateral fibres join the dorsal digital expansion of the thumb along with the **first anterior interosseus** (9). The abductor does not lie on the radial side of the metacarpal but anteriorly and medially and runs in the same direction as the *opponens*, i.e. distally, laterally and posteriorly. Contrary to what its name would suggest, the abductor does not move the column of the thumb laterally but moves it proximally and medially. These three muscles form the **lateral group**, since they are inserted into the lateral aspects of M_1 and P_1. The *flexor pollicis brevis* and the *abductor pollicis brevis* are called the **lateral sesamoid muscles**.

The medial group

The **medial group** consists of two muscles supplied by the ulnar nerve and inserted into the medial side of the MP joint:
1) the **first palmar interosseus** (9) inserted by tendon into the medial tubercle of the base of P_1 and into the dorsal expansion
2) the **adductor pollicis** (8) with its transverse and oblique heads converging by a common tendon upon its insertion into the medial sesamoid bone and the medial aspect of P_1.

For reasons of symmetry these two muscles are called the **medial sesamoid muscles** and are **synergists-antagonists** of the lateral sesamoid muscles.

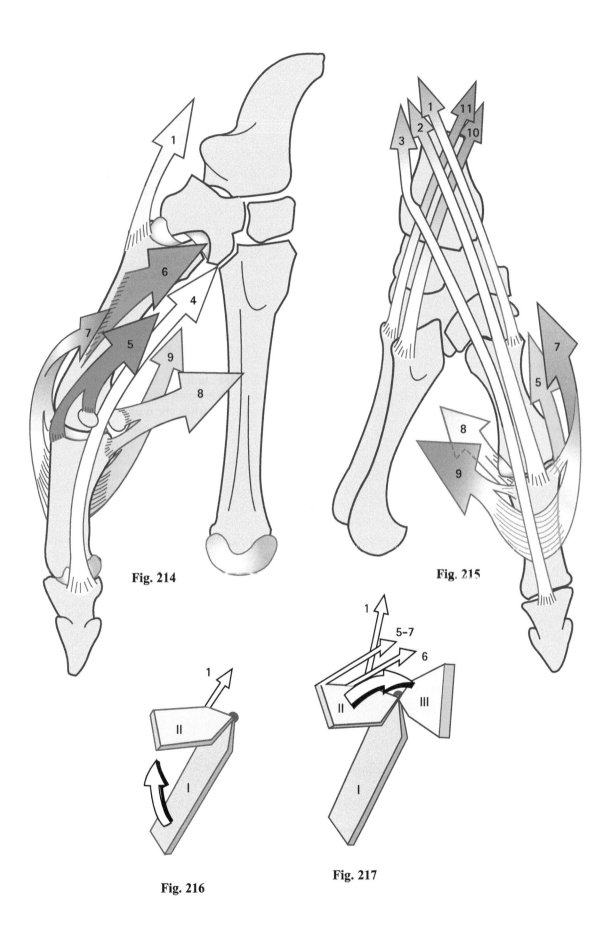

Fig. 214

Fig. 215

Fig. 216

Fig. 217

The actions of the extrinsic muscles of the thumb

The abductor pollicis longus (Fig. 218) moves M_1 laterally and anteriorly. Therefore it produces both **abduction** and **antepulsion** of M_1, especially when the wrist is slightly flexed. This antepulsion is due to the fact that the abductor tendon runs anterior to the tendons of the muscles of the anatomical snuffbox (Fig. 215, p. 291). When the wrist is not stabilized by the radial extensors, especially the *brevis*, the *abductor pollicis longus* also **flexes the wrist**; when the wrist is extended, it produces retropulsion of M_1.

Functionally speaking, the **force couple formed by the abductor pollicis longus** and the **lateral group of intrinsic muscles** plays a very important role in opposition. For opposition to start, M_1 must be raised directly above the plane of the palm so that the thenar eminence forms a conical mass at the edge of the palm. This action is produced by this functional couple of muscles (p. 291) in the following two stages:

1) **In the first stage** (Fig. 216, M_1 is stylized), the **abductor pollicis longus** (1) extends M_1 anteriorly and laterally from position I to position II.

2) **In the second stage** (Fig. 217), from position II the lateral group of muscles, i.e. *flexor brevis* (5), *abductor brevis* (7) and *opponens* (6), tilt M_1 anteriorly and medially into position III while rotating it slightly on its long axis.

This movement has been divided into two successive stages for descriptive purposes, but in reality these stages occur simultaneously and the final position III of M_1 is the resultant of the simultaneous forces exerted by these two sets of muscles.

The **extensor poflicis brevis** (Fig. 219) has two actions:

1) It **extends P_1 over M_1.**

2) It moves M_1 and the thumb directly laterally, and therefore is a **true abductor of the thumb** by producing extension-retropulsion at the TM joint. For pure abduction to occur, the wrist joint must be stabilized by the synergistic contraction of the *flexor carpi ulnaris* and especially of the *extensor carpi ulnaris*; otherwise the *extensor pollicis brevis* also produces abduction at the wrist.

The **extensor pollicis longus** has three actions (Fig. 220):

1) It **extends P_2 over P_1.**

2) It **extends P_1 over M_1.**

3) It **moves M_1 medially and posteriorly.** Medially it 'closes' the first interosseous space and thus adducts M_1; posteriorly it causes retropulsion of M_1 because it is bent at the distal tubercle of the radius (Lister's tubercle, Fig. 211). It is therefore an antagonist of the muscles of opposition, since it helps to flatten the palm and makes the pulp of the thumb face anteriorly.

The **extensor pollicis longus** forms a functional set of antagonistic-synergistic muscles with the lateral group of thenar muscles. In fact, when one wants to extend P_2 without extending the thumb, these external thenar muscles must act to stabilize M_1 and P_1 and prevent their extension. They therefore act as brakes on the *extensor pollicis longus*, and if the thenar muscles are paralysed the thumb is irresistibly moved medially and posteriorly. An accessory action of the *extensor pollicis longus* is **extension of the wrist**, unless cancelled by the action of the *flexor carpi radialis*.

The **flexor pollicis longus** (Fig. 221) **flexes P_2 over P_1** and **secondarily flexes P_1 over M_1** For flexion of P_2 to occur alone, the *extensor pollicis brevis* must contract and prevent flexion of P_1 (synergistic action). We shall see later the indispensable role of the *flexor pollicis longus* in terminal prehension.

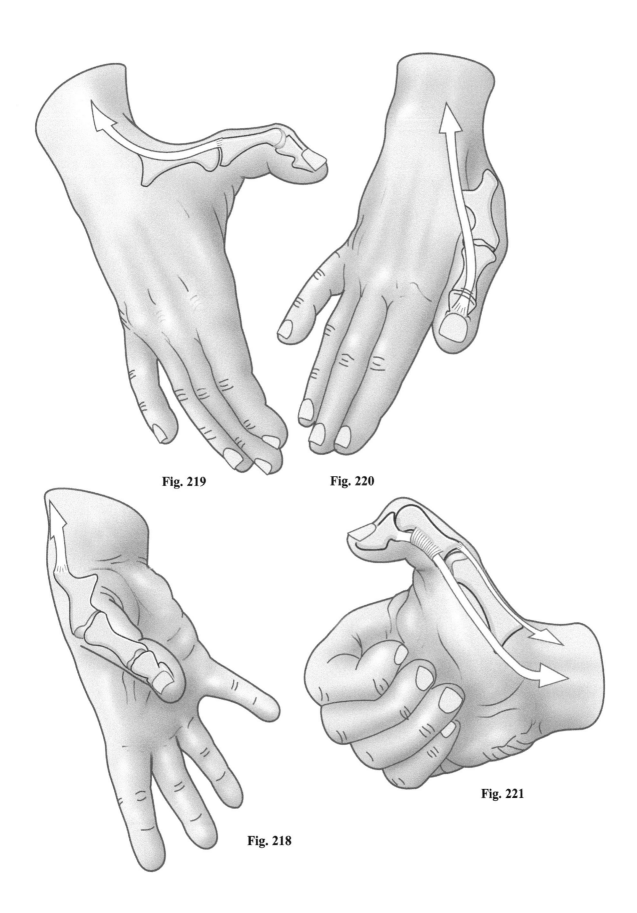

Fig. 219

Fig. 220

Fig. 218

Fig. 221

The actions of the medial group of thenar muscles (the medial sesamoid muscles)

The adductor pollicis (Fig. 222, 8), with its oblique (upper white arrow) and its transverse (lower white arrow) heads, acts on the three bones of the thumb:

1) Contraction of the adductor (Fig. 223, diagrammatic section) moves M_1 to a position of equilibrium (A) slightly lateral and anterior to M_2. The direction of the movement produced by the muscle depends on the starting-point of M_1 (Duchenne de Boulogne), as follows:
   - The adductor is effectively an adductor if M_1 starts from a position of full abduction (1).
   - The adductor becomes an abductor if M_1 starts from a position of full adduction (2).
   - If M_1 is initially in a position of full retroposition under the pull of the *extensor pollicis longus* (3), the adductor brings M_1 back into anteposition.
   - It brings M_1 back into retroposition if M_1 is already in anteposition as a result of contraction of the *abductor pollicis brevis* (4).
   - The position of rest of M_1 corresponds to R halfway between 1 and 3.

Electromyographic studies have shown that the *adductor pollicis* is active not only during adduction but also during retropulsion of the thumb, during full palmar prehension, during subterminal or pulpar (pulp-to-pulp) prehension, and especially during subtermino-lateral or pulpo-lateral (pulp-to-side) prehension. When the thumb opposes the other fingers, the *adductor pollicis* becomes progressively more active as the thumb opposes the medial fingers. Hence it is **maximally active when the thumb opposes the little finger**. The adductor is inactive during abduction, antepulsion and termino-terminal (tip-to-tip) prehension.

Later **electromyographic studies** (Hamonet, de la Caffinière and Opsomer) have confirmed that it is particularly active when the thumb and M_2 are brought closer together during all phases of opposition. It is less active in the long path of opposition than in the short path (Fig. 224, diagram showing the action of the adductor, according to Hamonet, de la Caffinière and Opsomer).

2) **On P_1** (Fig. 222) it has a triple action: slight flexion, ulnar deviation and lateral axial rotation or supination (curved white arrow).

3) **On P_2** it acts as an extensor insofar as its insertion blends with that of the first interosseus.

The **first palmar interosseus** has very similar actions:
- adduction, i.e. M_1 is drawn towards the axis of the hand
- flexion of P_1 via the dorsal extensor expansion
- extension of P_2 via the lateral extensor expansion.

The **global contraction of the medial thenar muscles** brings the pulp of the thumb into contact with the radial aspect of P_1 of the index (Fig. 222) and also produces supination of the column of the thumb. These muscles, supplied by the ulnar nerve, are essential for holding an object firmly between the thumb and the index finger.

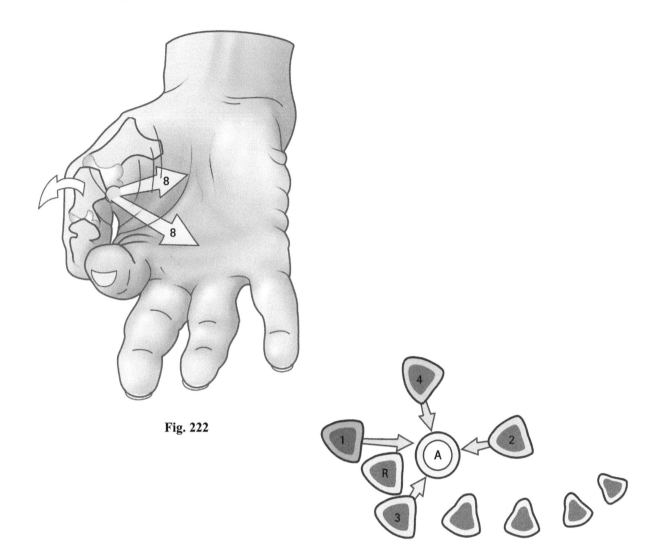

Fig. 222

Fig. 223

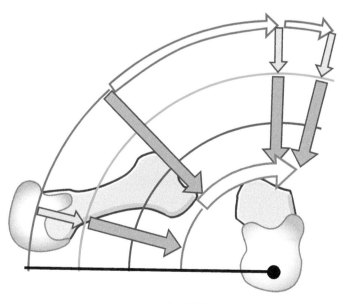

Fig. 224

The actions of the lateral group of thenar muscles

The **opponens pollicis** (6) has three actions corresponding to those of the *opponens digiti minimi*.

The **electromyographic diagram** (Fig. 226, inspired by Hamonet et al.) brings out its components:

- **antepulsion** of M_1 with respect to the carpus, especially in the long path of opposition
- **adduction** bringing M_1 and M_2 closer together during maximal movements of opposition
- **axial rotation in the direction of pronation.**

As these three simultaneous movements are essential for opposition, this muscle deserves its name. The *opponens* therefore is active in every type of grip involving the thumb. In addition, electromyographic studies have shown that it is paradoxically recruited during abduction when it stabilizes the column of the thumb.

The **abductor pollicis brevis** (7 and 7′) pulls apart M_1 and M_2 at the end of opposition (Fig. 227, electromyographic diagram, after Hamonet et al.):

- It **moves M_1 anteriorly and medially** during the long path of opposition, i.e. when M_1 and M_2 are farthest apart (Fig. 225).
- It **produces flexion** of P_1 on M_1 with some **radial deviation** on its lateral border.
- It causes axial rotation of P_1 into **pronation (medial rotation).**
- Finally, it **extends P_2 on P_1** via an expansion, which joins the *extensor pollicis longus.*

When it contracts on its own as a result of electrical stimulation, it brings the pulp of the thumb into contact with the index and the middle finger (Fig. 225). It is thus an essential muscle for opposition. As shown previously, it forms with the *abductor pollicis longus* a force couple essential for opposition.

The **flexor pollicis brevis** (Fig. 228, 5 and 5′) takes part in the overall movements produced by the lateral group of thenar muscles. Nevertheless, when it is made to contract on its own by electrical stimulation (Duchenne de Boulogne), it is primarily an **adductor**, as it brings the pulp of the thumb into opposition with the last two digits. On the other hand, its ability to move M_1 into anteposition is more restricted because its deep head (5′) antagonizes its superficial head (5) during this movement. It produces a marked degree of medial rotation into pronation. Action potentials recorded from the superficial head (Fig. 229, diagram inspired by Hamonet et al.) demonstrate that it has a similar action to that of the *opponens* and is maximally active during the long path of opposition.

It also flexes P_1 on M_1 with the help of the *abductor pollicis brevis*, another medial sesamoid muscle, and of the first palmar interosseus, both of which form the dorsal expansion of P_1.

The combined action of the lateral thenar muscles produces opposition of the thumb with the help of the *abductor pollicis longus.*

Extension of P_2 can be produced (Duchenne de Boulogne) by **three sets of muscles**, which act differentially as follows:

1) **By the extensor pollicis longus** in combination with extension of P_1 and flattening of the thenar eminence. These movements occur when one opens and flattens the hand.

2) **By the medial group of thenar muscles** (first anterior interosseus) in combination with adduction of the thumb. These movements take place when the pulp of the thumb is opposed to the lateral aspect of P_1 of the index (Fig. 249, p. 309).

3) **By the lateral group of thenar muscles**, especially the *abductor pollicis brevis*, when the pulp of the thumb opposes the other fingers.

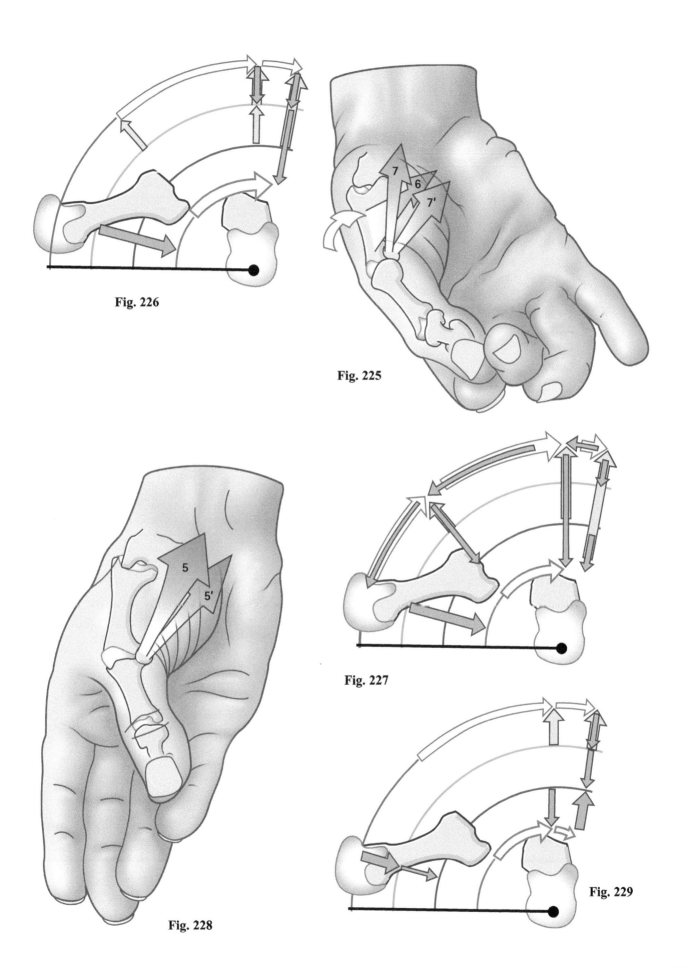

Fig. 226

Fig. 225

Fig. 227

Fig. 228

Fig. 229

Opposition of the thumb

Opposition is the essential movement of the thumb, because it allows the pulp of the thumb to come into contact with that of any other finger to form the **pollici-digital pincer**. There is thus not one movement of opposition but a series of movements, which underlie **a wide variety of static and dynamic grips,** depending on the number of fingers involved and the ways they are called into action. Thus the thumb only assumes its full functional significance when it is recruited in conjunction with the other fingers and vice versa. **Without the thumb the hand is virtually useless,** and complicated surgical procedures have been developed to reconstitute the thumb from the other structures of the hand, e.g. **pollicization of a finger** or, more recently, **transplantation**.

The full spectrum of the movements of opposition lies within a **conical sector of space**, whose apex lies at the TM joint, i.e. the **cone of opposition**. This cone is markedly distorted because its base is restricted by 'the short and long paths of opposition' (J. Duparc and J.-Y. de la Caffinière).

The **long path of opposition** (Fig. 230) has been well illustrated by Sterling Bunnell's classical match-stick experiment (Fig. 234, p. 301). This movement is described in detail on page 300.

The **short path of opposition** (Fig. 231) is defined as 'an almost linear movement of M_1 in one plane so that its head comes progressively to lie anterior to M_2'. **This crawling movement of the thumb across the palm** is seldom used and of little functional value. It should not be classified as a movement of opposition, since it is not associated with a **rotational component**, which, as we shall see later, is of fundamental importance in opposition. Furthermore, this crawling movement of the thumb is still present when opposition is impaired by **dysfunction of the median nerve**.

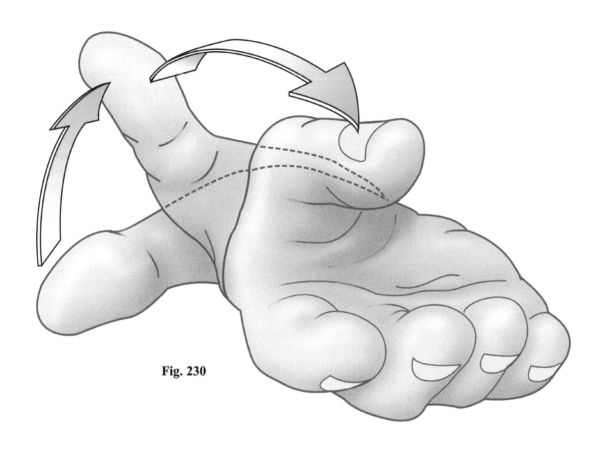

Fig. 230

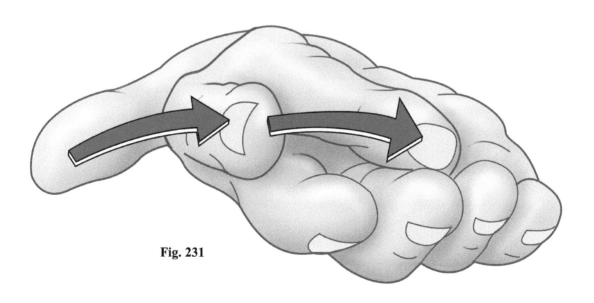

Fig. 231

Mechanically speaking, thumb opposition is a **complex movement** variably made up of **three components: antepulsion, flexion** and **pronation** of the osteoarticular column of the thumb.

Antepulsion

Antepulsion (Fig. 232) is the movement that brings the thumb to **lie anterior to the plane of the palm**, so that the thenar eminence looks like a cone at the proximal lateral angle of the hand. It occurs essentially at the **TM joint** and to a lesser degree at the MP joint, where radial deviation makes the thumb look more erect. This movement of M_1 away from M_2 is called abduction in anglophone literature, which contradicts the presence of a second component of adduction in the movement of the thumb medially. Thus it is better to use abduction only when M_1 moves away from M_2 strictly in the coronal plane.

Flexion

Flexion (Fig. 233) moves the entire column of the thumb medially and so is classically called adduction. But we have already shown that it is a movement of flexion involving all the joints of the column, as follows:
- It involves mostly the **TM joint**, but movement in this joint cannot bring M_1 past the sagittal plane running through the axis of M_2. It is thus truly a movement of flexion, as it is continuous with flexion at the MP joint.
- The **MP joint** promotes flexion to a variable degree depending on the finger 'targeted' for opposition.
- The **IP joint** allows flexion to reach completion by prolonging the movement of flexion at the MP joint.

Pronation

Pronation is an essential component of the opposition of the thumb in that it allows the pulps of the thumb and the fingers to achieve full contact. It can be defined as the change in the spatial orientation of P_2 so that it faces in different directions depending on the degree of rotation on its long axis. The term pronation is used by analogy with the movement of the forearm and has the same meaning. This medial rotation of P_2 is produced by the **summation of movements, which occur to a variable degree and by various mechanisms in the column of the thumb**. This is well demonstrated by **Sterling Bunnell's matchstick experiment** (Fig. 234). A matchstick is glued across the base of the nail of the thumb and the hand is viewed head-on. (You can perform this experiment on yourself while looking in a mirror.) The angle between its initial position (I) (with the hand flat) and its final position (II) in full opposition (with the thumb touching the little finger) is 90-120°. It was first thought that this rotation of the column of the thumb was the result of the laxity of the capsule of the TM joint. Recent studies, however, have shown that it is precisely in full opposition that the TM joint is in the close-packed position with a minimal degree of play, because of the direction of all the thenar muscles, whose contraction strongly presses the base of the metacarpal against the trapezial saddle and ensures that the degree of play in the joint is at a minimum, so that it is not mechanically responsible for the longitudinal rotation of the first metacarpal. It is now recognized that the rotation occurring at the TM joint is **due to the mechanical properties of this biaxial joint**. Moreover, a **biaxial prosthesis** of the TM joint allows opposition to occur normally.

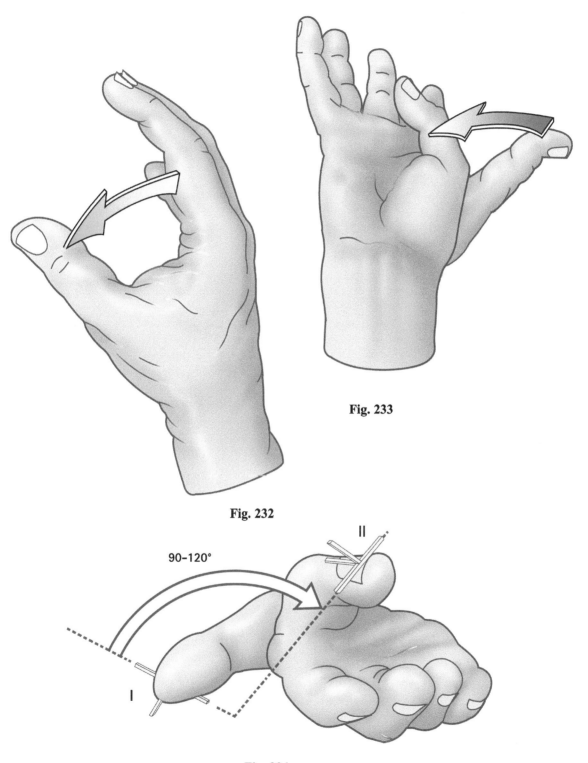

Fig. 232

Fig. 233

90–120°

I

II

Fig. 234

The component of pronation

Pronation of the column of the thumb results from two types of rotation: automatic 'conjunct' rotation and voluntary or 'adjunct' rotation.

Automatic 'conjunct' rotation

Automatic 'conjunct' rotation is due to the movement at the TM joint, as shown previously. The MP and IP joints contribute to this rotation by adding their movement of flexion to that of the TM joint. As a result the long axis of P_2 comes to lie almost parallel to the axis XX' of antepulsion-retropulsion, and P_2 undergoes a cylindrical rotation so that any rotation in the TM joint about that axis causes the pulp of the thumb to rotate and alter its orientation.

From the initial position (Fig. 235, antero-superior view of the model) to the final position (Fig. 236) the changes in the spatial orientation of P_2 during its opposition to P_2 of the little finger have occurred about four axes XX', YY', f_1 and f_2 without any twisting of the cardboard, which would signify free 'play' at one of the joints.

For a detailed study of this movement (Fig. 237 A, B, C), simply perform successively (or simultaneously) the following four operations on the universal joint model of the TM joint as shown on page 267:

A. The **universal joint model** with its fixed part (T) (the trapezium) and the first metacarpal (M), which articulates with (T) by the intermediate circular piece. This figure corresponds to the position of retroposition of the thumb, which is 'stuck' against the base of the Index in the plane of the palm.

B. **Rotation of the circular intermediate piece** of the universal joint model of the TM joint around the axis XX' in the direction of **anteposition** (red arrow) associated with an initial anteposition (green arrow) of the first metacarpal (M1).

C. **Flexion of the first metacarpal** (blue arrow) about the second axis (YY') of the universal joint to reach position M2. It is then possible to observe that it has undergone an automatic rotation on its long axis (R), which can be measured on the small diagram (above C).

This movement of flexion is followed by flexion of the first phalanx about the axis f1 in the metacarpophalangeal joint (Fig. 236) and by flexion of the second phalanx about the axis f2 in the inter-phalangeal joint. This movement of flexion is extended by **flexion of the first phalanx** about the axis f1 in the metacarpophalangeal joint (Fig. 236) and by **flexion of the second phalanx** about the axis f2 in the interphalangeal joint. Thus we have demonstrated, not by theoretical arguments but by practical experiments, that the universal TM joint plays an essential role in the axial rotation of the thumb.

Voluntary or 'adjunct' rotation

Voluntary or 'adjunct' rotation (Fig. 238) is well brought out by fixing matchsticks transversely to the three mobile segments of the thumb and moving the thumb into full opposition. One can see that axial rotation into pronation of nearly 30° takes place at two joints:

- **at the MP joint**, where a 24° pronation is produced by the *abductor pollicis brevis* and the *flexor pollicis brevis*. (This is **active rotation**.)
- **at the IP joint**, where a 7° pronation, **purely automatic**, occurs as a result of conical rotation (Fig. 206).

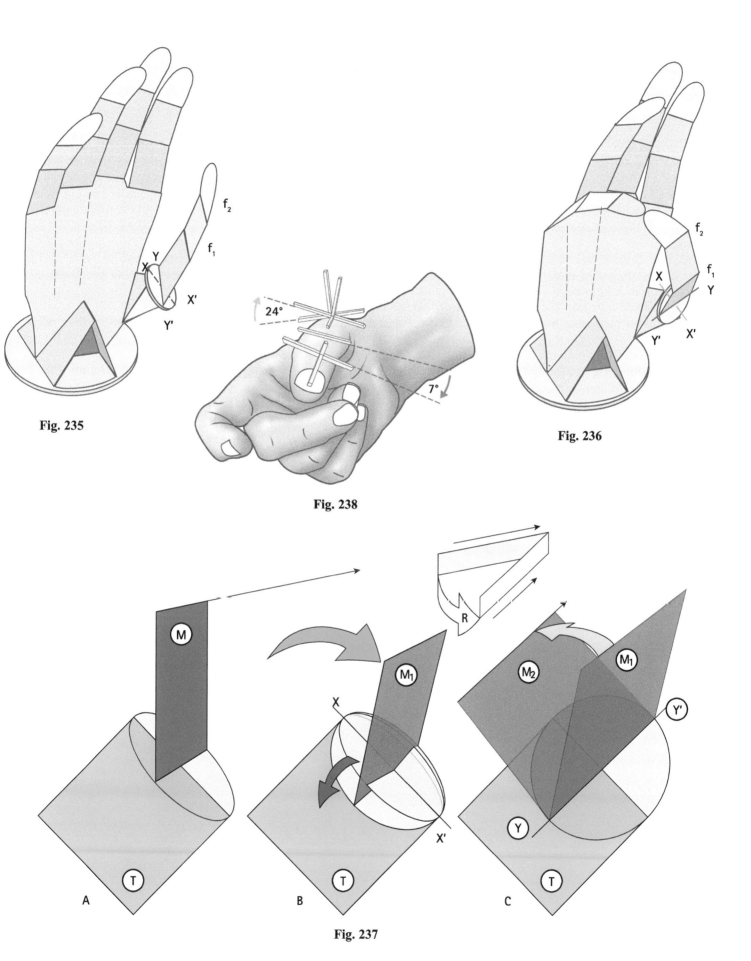

Fig. 235

Fig. 238

24°

7°

Fig. 236

M

T

A

X

M₁

T

B

X'

R

M₂

M₁

Y'

Y

T

C

Fig. 237

Opposition and counter-opposition

We have seen the crucial role played by the TM joint during opposition of the thumb, but the **MP and IP joints are critical in determining** which of the four fingers the thumb will select for opposition. In fact it is the **presence of variable degrees of flexion at these joints** that allows the thumb to pick a finger for opposition.

When the thumb and index are opposed pulp to pulp (Fig. 239), there is very little flexion at the MP joint, with no pronation or radial deviation of P_1, which is prevented by the medial collateral ligament. The IP joint is **extended**. There are other modes of opposition between the thumb and the index finger, e.g. termino-terminal (tip-to-tip), when the MP joint is in full extension and the IP joint is flexed.

When the thumb is opposed to the little finger tip to tip (Fig. 240), the MP joint is flexed with concurrent radial deviation and pronation of P_1, while the IP joint is flexed. Note that the thumbnail is seen almost head-on, which suggests that it has undergone rotation. During pulp-to-pulp opposition the IP joint is extended.

Opposition with the ring finger and the middle finger occurs as a result of an intermediate degree of flexion at the MP joint, with concurrent radial deviation and pronation of P_1.

Thus one can say that, during opposition, once the base of M_1 has started to move from any initial position, **it is the MP joint that allows the thumb to choose a finger for opposition.**

Opposition, essential as it is for gripping an object, would be useless without **counter-opposition**, which allows the hand to release its grip or to get ready to grip very large objects. This movement (Fig. 241), which brings the thumb into the plane of the palm, consists of three components starting from the position of opposition:

- extension
- retropulsion
- supination of the column of the thumb.

The motor muscles of counter-opposition are these:
- the *abductor pollicis longus*
- the *extensor pollicis brevis*
- especially the *extensor pollicis longus*, which is the only one able to bring the thumb into full retroposition in the plane of the palm.

The motor nerves of the muscles of the thumb (Fig. 242) **are these:**
- the **radial nerve** (R) for counter-opposition
- the **median nerve** (M) for opposition
- the **ulnar nerve** (U) to firm up a grip.

The movements used to test the integrity of the nerve supply are these:
- for the radial nerve: **extension of the wrist and of the MP joints** of the four fingers and extension and radial abduction of the thumb
- for the ulnar nerve: **extension of the distal phalanges of the fingers** and **their approximation or separation**
- for the median nerve: **making a fist** and **opposition of the thumb**.

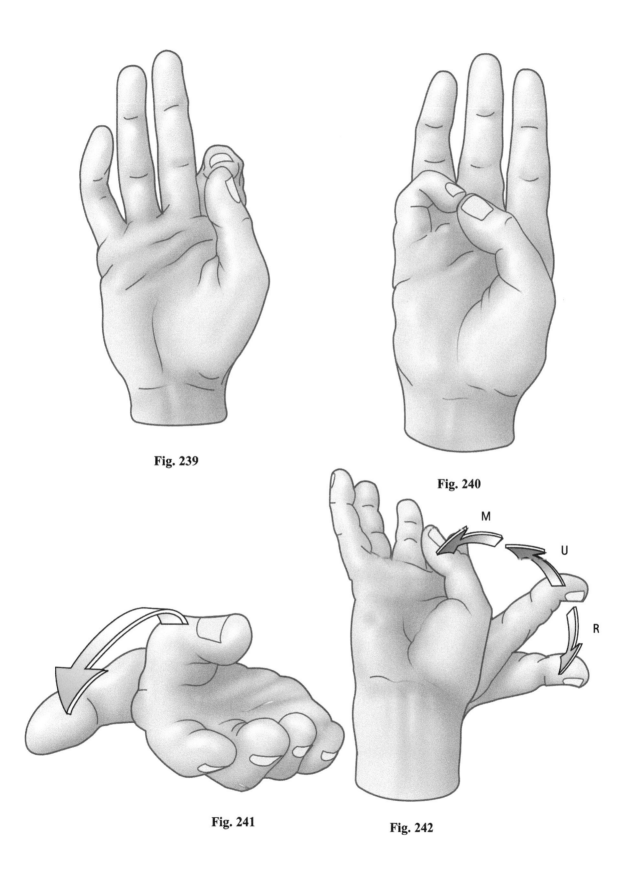

Fig. 239

Fig. 240

Fig. 241

Fig. 242

It is difficult to measure the complex movement of opposition accurately, since the methods in use (p. 254) do not take into account the axial rotation of the column of the thumb. In 1986 the author proposed a method of quantitation that has been adopted more or less universally, i.e. the **opposition and counter-opposition tests**. It avoids the use of any measuring device and uses the patient's body as the reference system; it can be applied in any setting and follows the Hippocratic method. The result is recorded as a **single number**, which can easily be included in **statistical tables**.

During the **total opposition test** (TOT) (Fig. 243), now included in the international classification, the patient's hand itself serves as the reference system, as follows. From its starting-point, i.e. the position of maximal abduction, the thumb will follow the long path of opposition as it makes contact sequentially with the pulps of the other fingers, until it reaches the palmar surface of the little finger and the palm itself.

The **method of measurement** comprises **ten stages** from opposition zero to maximal opposition:

- **Stage 0**: the pulp of the thumb touches the outer border of P_1 of the index finger; the hand is flat and there is no opposition of the thumb.
- **Stage 1**: the pulp of the thumb touches the external border of P_2 of the index finger following a slight degree of anteposition of the thumb and a slight flexion of the index finger.
- **Stage 2**: the pulp of the thumb reaches the lateral border of P_3 of the index, which has undergone some flexion, while the column of the thumb moves farther into anteposition.
- **Stage 3**: the tip of the thumb touches the tip of P_3 of the index finger, which is flexed, while the column of the thumb is slightly adducted.
- **Stage 4**: the tip of the thumb reaches the tip of P_3 of the middle finger as the thumb is adducted further, the MP joint is slightly flexed and the IP joint stays extended.
- **Stage 5**: the thumb reaches the tip of P_3 of the ring finger as the thumb moves farther into adduction and anteposition, the MP joint is flexed some more and the IP joint is slightly flexed.

- **Stage 6**: the thumb reaches the tip of P_3 of the little finger, while the thumb and the MP joint lie in maximal anteposition and the right IP joint stays extended.
- **Stage 7**: the thumb touches the slightly flexed little finger at the level of the distal interphalangeal crease, while the IP joint is more flexed and flexion of the MP joint is maximal.
- **Stage 8**: the thumb reaches the slightly flexed little finger at the level of the proximal inter-phalangeal crease, while the IP joint is more flexed and the TM and MP joints are maximally flexed.
- **Stage 9**: the thumb touches the base of the little finger at the level of the digito-palmar crease, while the IP joint becomes fully flexed.
- **Stage 10**: the thumb reaches the palm at the level of the distal palmar crease, while the IP, TM and MP joints are fully flexed. This point represents the maximal range of opposition.

If the test gives a result of 10, then opposition is normal. However, for this test to retain its full value, the thumb must follow the long path of opposition, i.e. **there must always be a space between the thumb and the palm** (Fig. 244), especially in stages 6-10. It is true that a value of 10 can be obtained by allowing the thumb to follow the short path, but then the test is useless.

The **test of counter-opposition** is carried out on a horizontal plane such as a table (Fig. 245). The hand to be examined is placed flat on the table, while the other is placed on its ulnar border in front of the thumb to serve as control. Counter-opposition is then measured in four stages:

- **Stage 0**: the thumb cannot actively leave the surface of the table.
- **Stage 1**: the distal end of the thumb is raised actively up to the level of MPJ5.
- **Stage 2**: the thumb is actively raised up to the level of MPJ4.
- **Stage 3**: the thumb is only rarely raised actively up to the level of MPJ3.

If stage 2 or stage 3 is reached, the **efficiency of the *extensor pollicis longus*** is intact.

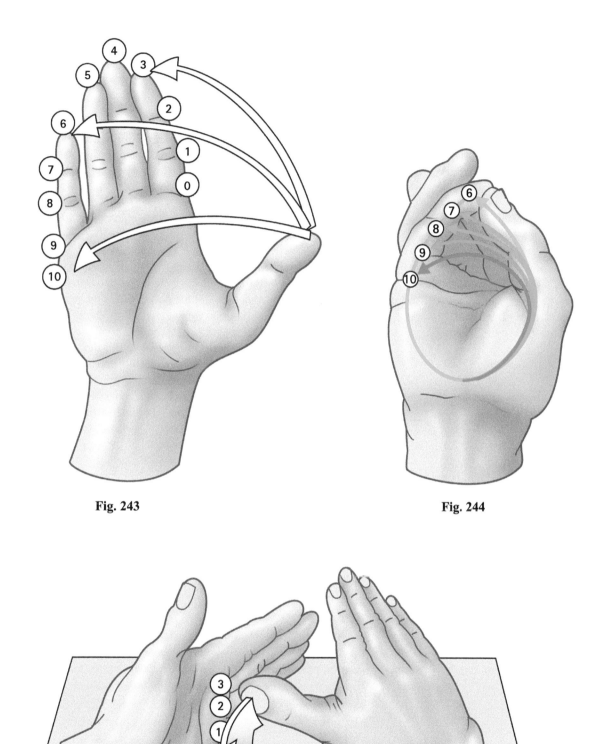

Fig. 243

Fig. 244

Fig. 245

The modes of prehension

The complex anatomical and functional organization of the hand contributes to prehension. The numerous modes of prehension fall into three broad categories: **static grips**, which can be likened to pincers, **grips associated with gravity** and **dynamic grips associated with actions**. In addition to prehension the hand can act as an instrument of percussion, as a means of contact and in the performance of gestures. These will be discussed sequentially.

Static grips

These pincer-like grips can be classified into **three groups: digital, palmar and symmetrical**. They do not require the help of gravity and are therefore effective in space capsules.

Digital grips

The **pincer-like digital grips** can be further subdivided into **bidigital** and **pluridigital**.

A. Bidigital grips give rise to the classic pollici-digital pincer, usually between the thumb and the index finger, and they also fall into three types, depending on whether opposition occurs by terminal, subterminal or subtermino-lateral contact.

1) **Prehension by terminal (tip-to-tip) opposition** (Figs 246 and 247) is the finest and most precise. It allows one to hold a thin object (Fig. 246) or to pick up a very fine object like a match or a pin (Fig. 247). The thumb and the index finger (or the middle finger) are opposed at the tips of their pulps or even at the edge of their nails when very fine objects (e.g. a hair) are being gripped. This requires that the pulp be elastic and properly supported by the nail, which plays an all-important role in this mode of so-called **pulpo-ungual** (pulp-to-nail) prehension. It is the mode of prehension that is the first to be disturbed by any disease of the hand, as it requires the entire range of movements of the joints with full flexion and especially the intactness of the muscles and tendons, the following in particular:
   - for the index, the **flexor digitorum profundus** tendon, which stabilizes the flexed P_3 and must be repaired surgically at all costs when the flexor tendons have been cut

   - the **flexor pollicis longus**, which has a similar action on the thumb and therefore needs to be repaired. Note also the associated automatic flexion of the middle finger and of the ring finger

2) **Prehension by sub-terminal or pulpar (pulp-to-pulp) opposition** (Fig. 248) is the most common. It allows one to hold relatively larger objects like a pencil or a sheet of paper. The efficiency of this mode of prehension can be tested by attempting to pull a sheet of paper out from between the thumb and the index finger. If prehension is efficient, the sheet cannot be pulled out. This test, known as **Froment's sign**, assesses the strength of the **adductor pollicis** and thus the integrity of its motor nerve, the ulnar nerve. In this mode of prehension the thumb and the index finger (or any other finger) are in contact on the palmar surfaces of their pulps. The state of the pulp is of course important, but not the DIP joint, which can be frozen by arthrodesis either in extension or in mid-flexion. The muscles needed for this mode of prehension are these:
   - the index tendon of the *flexor digitorum superficialis* tendon, which stabilizes the flexed P_2
   - the thenar muscles, which flex P_1 of the thumb: the *flexor pollicis brevis*, the first anterior interosseus, the *abductor pollicis brevis* and especially the *adductor pollicis*.

3) **Prehension by subtermino-lateral or pulpo-lateral (pulp-to-side) contact** (Fig. 249), e.g. holding a coin. It can replace the first two types when the last two phalanges of the index finger have been amputated. The grip is less fine but none the less strong. The palmar aspect of the pulp of the thumb presses on the lateral surface of P_1 of the index finger. This requires the following muscles:
   - the first dorsal interosseus to stabilize the index laterally while it is supported medially by the other fingers
   - the *flexor pollicis brevis*, the first palmar interosseus and above all the *adductor pollicis*, whose involvement has been confirmed electromyographically.

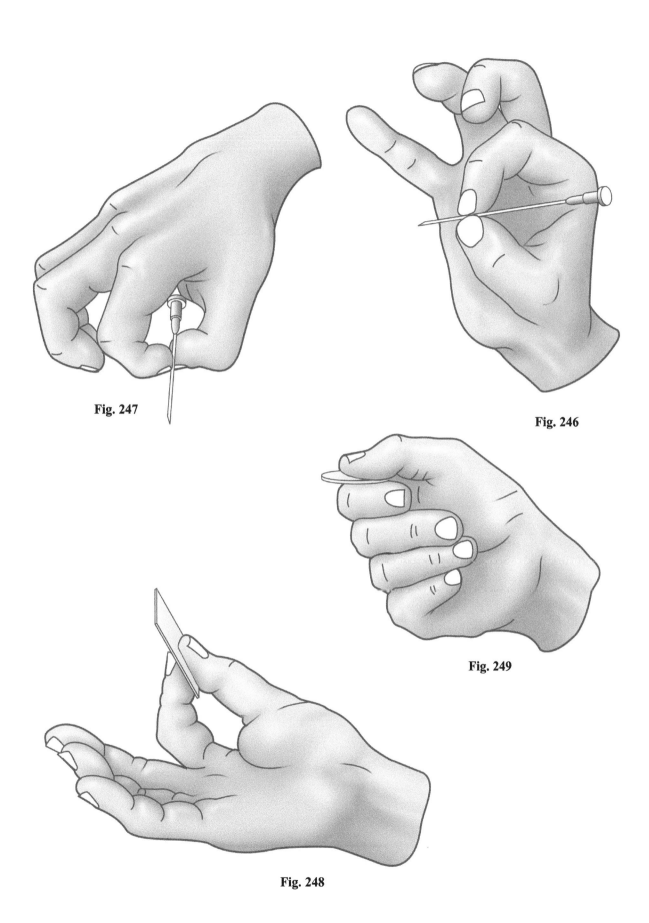

Fig. 247

Fig. 246

Fig. 249

Fig. 248

4) **Interdigital latero-lateral prehension** (Fig. 250) is the only type of bidigital grip without involvement of the thumb and is a grip of secondary importance usually involving the index and the middle fingers, as in holding a cigarette or another small object. The muscles concerned are the interossei (the second interossei, palmar and dorsal). The grip is weak with little precision, but thumb amputees can develop this grip to an astonishing degree. It is a supplementary type of grip.

B. **The pluridigital grips**, involving the thumb and more than one finger at a time, are much stronger than the bidigital grips, which are essentially concerned with precision.

The **tridigital grips (three-point palmar pinches)** are the most commonly used and involve the thumb, and the index and middle fingers. The greater part of the world population does not eat with cutlery and uses this grip to bring food to the mouth; it is the grip used for feeding. **It is a form of subterminal (pulp-to-pulp) tridigital prehension** (Fig. 251), as when a ball is held tight between the pulp of the thumb and those of the index and middle fingers. It is also used when writing with a pencil or a pen (Fig. 252), which is held between the pulps of the index finger and the thumb and the lateral aspect of the middle finger. The grip is supported by the latter and also by the first interdigital cleft.

In this sense this grip is directional and resembles symmetrical grips and dynamic grips (see later), since writing results from movements of the shoulder and of the hand, which slides on the table on its ulnar border and its little finger, and also from the movements of the first three fingers. The to-and-fro movements of the pencil are produced by the *flexor pollicis longus* and the index tendon of the *flexor digitorum superficialis*, while the lateral sesamoid muscles and the second dorsal interosseus keep the pencil in place.

When the cap of a flask is unscrewed (Fig. 253), the grip is tridigital, with the lateral aspects of the thumb and of P_2 of the middle finger holding the cap on one side and the pulp of the index finger helping to jam it on the other side. The thumb presses the cap strongly against the middle finger as a result of contraction of all the thenar muscles. The grip is locked initially by the *flexor pollicis longus* and finally by the *flexor digitorum superficialis*. After the cap is loosened, it is unscrewed without the help of the index by flexing the thumb and extending the middle finger. This is an example of a dynamic action-associated grip (see later).

If the cap is loose from the start, it can be unscrewed by a pulpar tridigital grip, as the thumb is flexed, the middle finger extended and the index finger abducted by the first dorsal interosseus. This is another dynamic movement-associated grip.

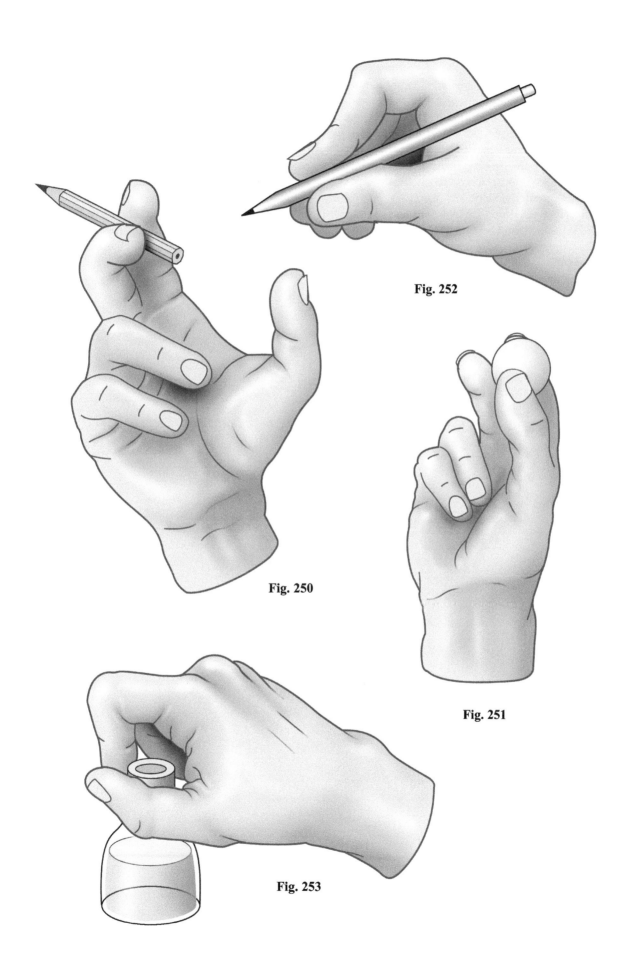

Fig. 252

Fig. 250

Fig. 251

Fig. 253

311

Tetradigital grips are used when objects are larger and must be gripped more firmly, as follows:

- **Pulpar (pulp-to-pulp) tetradigital** grip (Fig. 254), as when the hand takes hold of a spherical object like a ping-pong ball. The thumb and the index and middle fingers make pulp-to-pulp contact, while the ball is pressed against the lateral aspect of P_3 of the ring finger, whose function is to stop the ball from slipping away medially.

- **Tetradigital grip with pulpo-lateral contact** (Fig. 255), as when a lid is unscrewed. The area of contact is extensive, involving the pulps and the palmar surfaces of the first phalanges of the thumb, index finger and middle finger, and also the pulp and lateral aspect of the second phalanx of the ring finger, which stops the lid from slipping away medially. As the thumb and the fingers surround the lid, the fingers move spirally and it can be shown that the resultant of the forces is nil at the centre of the lid, which moves up towards the MP joint of the index finger.

- **Pulpar (pulp-to-pulp) tetradigital grip involving the thumb and three other fingers (the dynamic quadrupod grip)**, as when one holds a charcoal pencil, an artist's paint-brush or an ordinary pencil (Fig. 256). The pulp of the thumb presses the object firmly against the pulps of the index, middle and ring fingers, which are almost fully extended. This is also how a violinist or a cellist holds the bow.

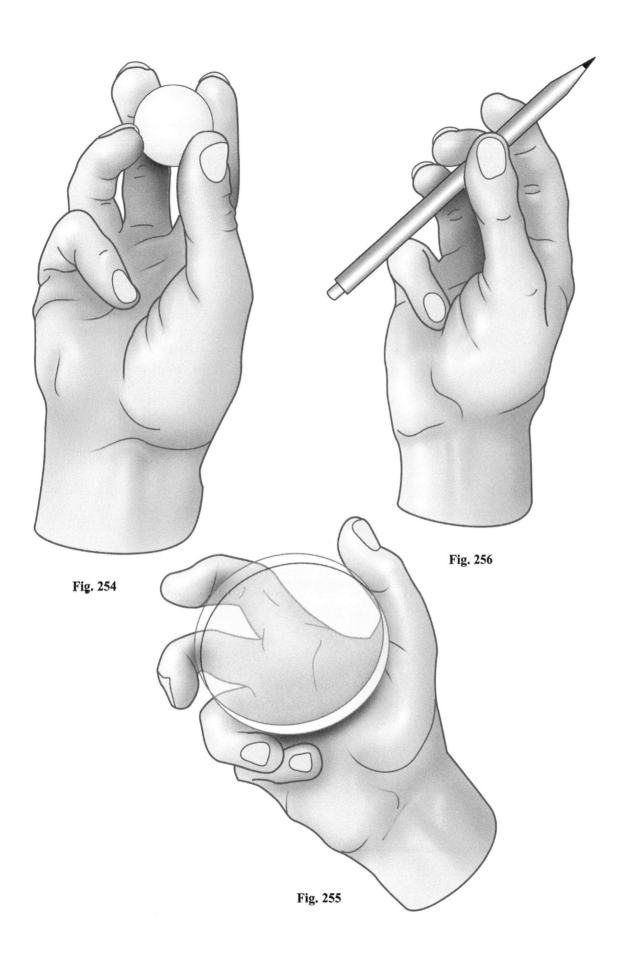

Fig. 254

Fig. 255

Fig. 256

Pentadigital grips use all the fingers (with the thumb lying in various positions of opposition), as is usual when large objects are gripped. However, even small objects can be grasped by a **pulpar pentadigital grip** (disc grip) (Fig. 257), with only the fifth finger showing lateral contact. As the object gets bigger, e.g. a tennis ball, **the pentadigital grip involves the pulps and the sides of the fingers** (Fig. 258). The palmar surfaces of the first four fingers are in contact with the ball and surround it almost completely. The thumb opposes these three fingers, while the little finger is in contact on its lateral surface and prevents the ball from slipping medially and proximally. Though not a palmar grip, since the ball is held by the fingers above the palm, it is actually very strong.

Another pentadigital grip (Fig. 259) is used to hold a large hemispherical object, e.g. a bowl, in the first interdigital cleft. The thumb and the index finger, widely extended and separated from each other, touch the object along their entire palmar surfaces. This can only occur if there is great flexibility of movement and if the first interdigital cleft can be widened

normally, which is not the case when fractures of M_1 or traumatic lesions of the cleft have caused it to retract. The bowl is also supported (Fig. 260) by the middle, ring and little fingers, which make contact with their two distal phalanges. It is thus a purely digital and not a palmar grip.

The **'panoramic' pentadigital grip** (the full disc grip) (Fig. 261) allows one to take hold of a large flat object, e.g. a saucer. It depends on the very wide separation of the fingers with the thumb in full counter-opposition, i.e. in extreme retroposition and extension. The thumb lies diametrically opposite the little finger (red arrows), and it is linked to it in space by a semicircle on which lie the index and middle fingers. The little finger lies on the major arc at an angle of 215° with the thumb. These two fingers are maximally separated, as when spanning an octave on the piano, and form a 'triangular' grip with the index finger and a **'spider-like' grip** with the others, from which the object cannot escape. Note that the efficiency of this grip depends on the integrity of the DIP joints and the action of the deep flexors.

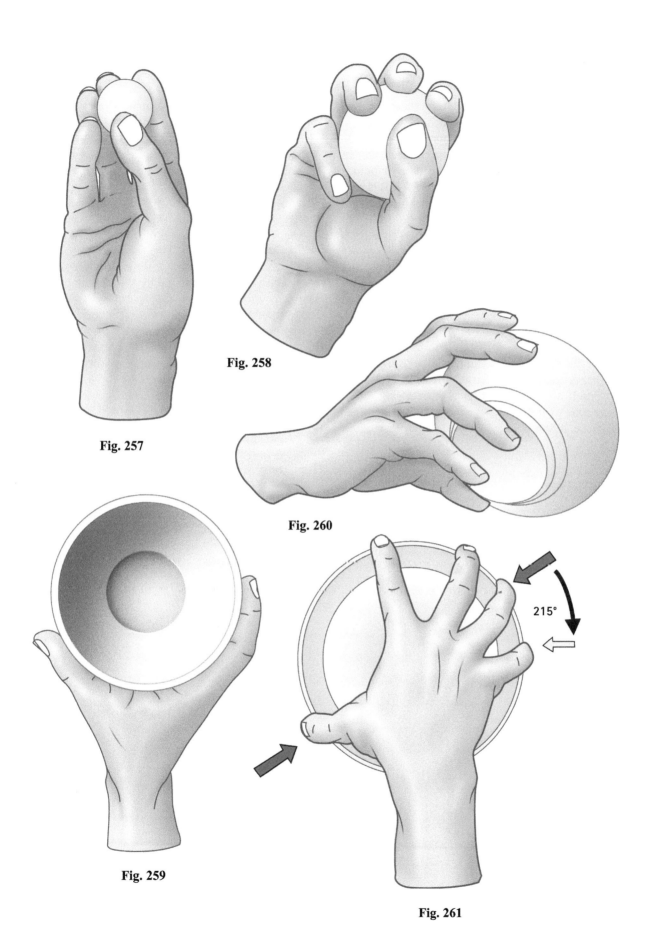

Fig. 257

Fig. 258

Fig. 259

Fig. 260

215°

Fig. 261

Palmar grips

These involve both the fingers and the palm; there are two types depending on whether the thumb is included or not.

A) **Digito-palmar prehension** draws the four fingers towards the palm (Fig. 262). It is of secondary importance but in fairly common use, e.g. to manipulate a handle or hold a steering wheel. The object of small diameter (3-4 cm) is held between the flexed fingers and the palm without involvement of the thumb. The grip is strong up to a point distally, but proximally, when the object is held close to the wrist, it can easily slip away, since the grip is not locked. The axis of the grip is set obliquely with respect to the axis of the hand and follows the oblique direction of the palmar gutter. This digito-palmar grip can also be used to hold a larger object, e.g. a glass (Fig. 263), but the greater the diameter of the object, the weaker the grip.

B) **Full palmar prehension** (Figs 264 and 265), i.e. using the whole palm or the whole hand (oblique palmar grip), allows one to grip heavy and relatively large objects strongly. The hand wraps itself around a **cylindrical object** (Fig. 264), and the long axis of the object coincides with that of the palmar gutter, i.e. it runs obliquely from the hypothenar emi-nence to the base of the index finger. The obliquity of this axis with respect to the axis of the hand and that of the forearm corresponds to the obliquity of the handle of a tool (Fig. 265), which forms an angle of 100-110° with the body of the tool. Unfortunately this also applies to a weapon. It is easy to note that one can compensate more easily for a wider (120-130°) than a narrower (90°) angle, because radial deviation of the wrist is smaller than its ulnar deviation.

The volume of the object gripped determines the strength of the grip, which is maximal when the thumb can touch or nearly touch the index finger. The thumb in fact forms the only buttress against the force generated by the other four fingers, and its efficiency is greater the more flexed it is. Hence the diameter of tool handles is determined by this observation.

The shape of the object gripped is also important, and nowadays handles are made with depressions appropriate for the fingers.

The **important muscles** for this mode of prehension are these:

- the *flexor digitorum superficialis*, the *flexor digitorum profundus* and above all the interossei, which strongly flex the first phalanx of each finger
- all the muscles of the thenar eminence, the *adductor pollicis brevis* and particularly the *flexor pollicis longus*, which lock the grip thanks to flexion of P_2.

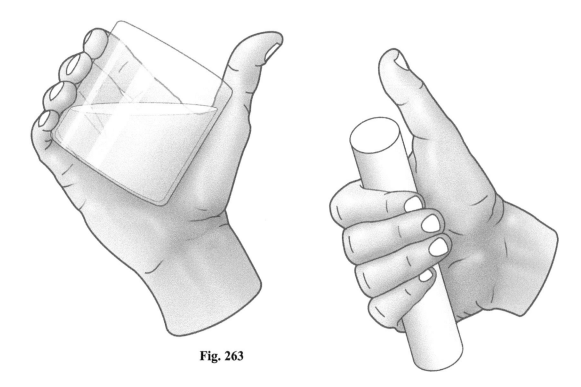

Fig. 263

Fig. 262

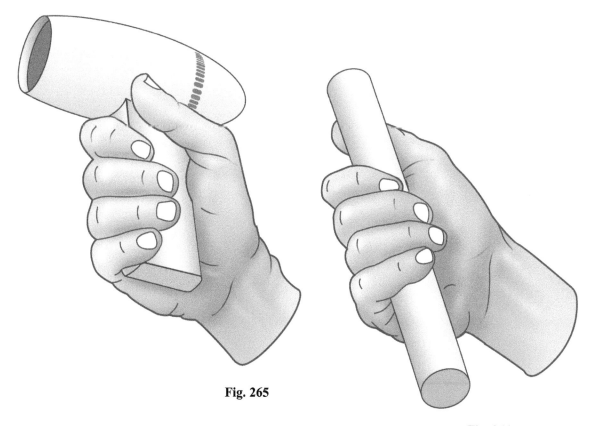

Fig. 265

Fig. 264

Cylindrical palmar grips are used to grasp large objects (Figs 266 and 267), but the grip gets weaker as the object gets bigger. The grip is locked, as we have already shown, because movements at the MP joint allow the thumb to move along the directrix of the cylinder, i.e. a circular path, which is the shortest path needed for the thumb to surround the object. Conversely, the volume of the object requires maximal widening of the first interdigital cleft.

Spherical palmar grips may involve three, four or five fingers. When three (Fig. 268) or four (Fig. 269) fingers are involved, the most medial finger, i.e. the middle finger in the tridigital grip or the ring finger in the tetradigital grip, touches the object on its lateral aspect and, with the help of the other fingers (the little finger alone or the little and ring fingers), it prevents it from escaping medially. As the object is also held by the thumb laterally, the grip is locked distally by the palmar surface of the fingers involved.

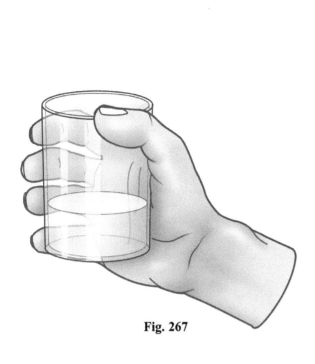

Fig. 267

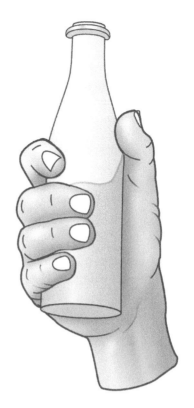

Fig. 266

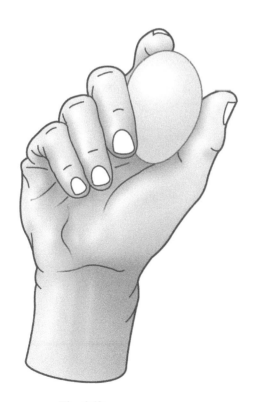

Fig. 268

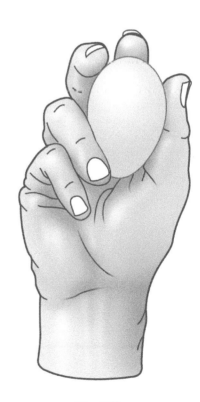

Fig. 269

During spherical pentadigital palmar grips (Fig. 270) the palmar surfaces of the fingers touch the object. The thumb lies opposite to the little finger, from which it is the most widely separated. The grip is locked distally by the index and middle fingers and proximally by the thenar eminence and the little finger, and its strength depends on the cooperation of the 'hooked' fingers and of the palm. This grip is possible only if the interdigital clefts can be widened to their limits and if the superficial and deep flexors of the fingers are working efficiently. It is much more symmetrical than the last two, and is thus much closer to the following types of grip.

Centralized grips

Centralized grips are in fact symmetrical about a longitudinal axis, which generally coincides with that of the forearm, as when the **conductor holds his baton** (Fig. 271), which is collinear with the axis of the forearm and extends the index finger in its role of indicator. This collinearity of axes is essential when one **holds a screwdriver** (Fig. 272), so that its axis coincides with the axis of pronation-supination of the forearm during the screwing or unscrewing of a nail. This is also the case when **one holds a fork** (Fig. 273) or a knife, which essentially elongates the hand distally. In every case, a long object is firmly gripped in a palmar grip using the thumb and the last three fingers, while the index plays a vital role in **determining the direction of the tool**.

Centralized or directional grips are in common use and are achieved only when the last three fingers can be flexed, the index finger completely extended with its flexors in good trim, and the thumb can be minimally opposed without the need of flexion of its IP joint.

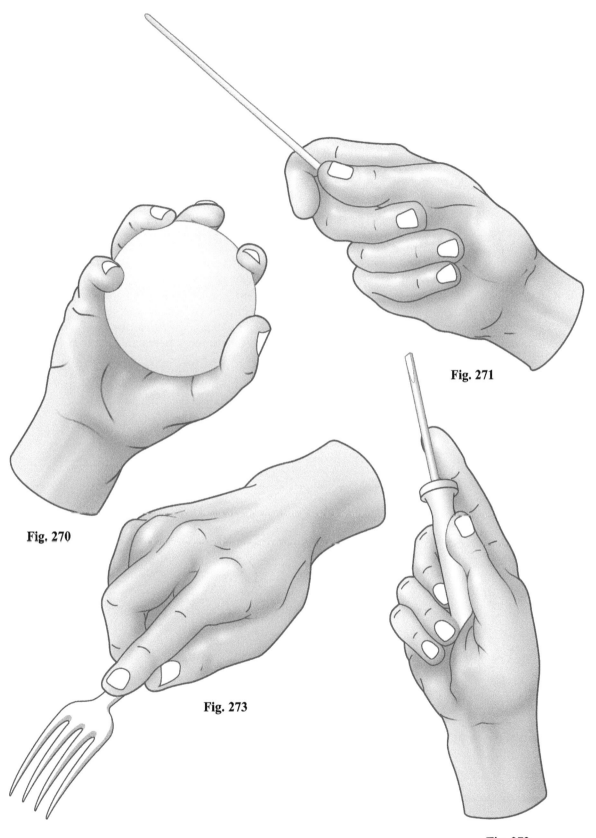

Fig. 271

Fig. 270

Fig. 273

Fig. 272

321

Gravity-assisted grips

So far only grips where gravity is not involved have been discussed, and they can occur even in a spaceship. There are others that **depend critically on the action of gravity** and are in regular use on Earth. If gravity is zero, the muscles atrophy, and if it is stronger than on Earth (as on Jupiter), the muscles must undergo hypertrophy. This is another way of 'doping' for athletes but it must be unpleasant to live in a centrifuge!

In these **gravity-assisted grips**, the hand acts as a **supporting platform**, e.g. when it supports a tray (Fig. 274), provided the hand can be flattened with the palm facing anteriorly in supination and with the fingers straight or can form a tripod under an object. The former movement is the basis of the **waiter test**. Under the force of gravity the hand can act as a **spoon**, as when it **contains seeds** (Fig. 275), flour or a liquid. The hollow of the hand is then extended by the concavity of the fingers as they are brought closer together by the palmar interossei in order to stop any leaks. The thumb is very important in that it closes the palmar gutter laterally. It is half-flexed and pulled against M_2 and P_1 of the index finger by its adductor. A **larger shell** can be formed by holding both hands together (Fig. 276) and placing both half-shells side by side along their ulnar borders **like an offering-bowl**.

All these gravity-assisted modes of prehension require the **integrity of supination**. Without it, the palm, which is the only part of the hand that can form a concave surface, cannot face anteriorly, since the shoulder is unable to offset this loss of supination.

The **tridigital grip of a bowl** (Fig. 277) needs the help of gravity, as the circumference of the bowl is held between two prongs, formed by the thumb and the middle finger, and a hook formed by the index finger. This grip depends on full stability of the thumb and of the middle finger and on the integrity of the tendon of the *flexor digitorum profundus* for the middle finger, whose third phalanx holds the sickle-shaped fold of the bowl. The *adductor pollicis brevis* is also indispensable.

Grips with one or more hooked fingers (the hook grips), as when **carrying a pail or a suitcase** or **trying to cling to a rocky surface**, also depend on gravity by opposing it and depend on the integrity of the flexors, in particular of the *flexor digitorum profundus*, which **can be ruptured accidentally when mountain climbers perform certain grips**.

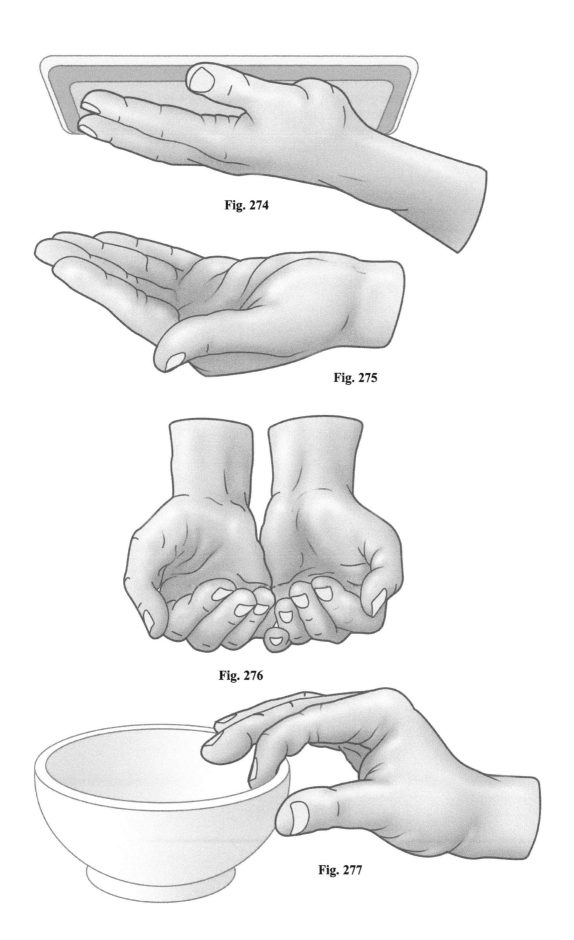

Fig. 274

Fig. 275

Fig. 276

Fig. 277

Dynamic movement-associated grips

The static grips so far described do not include all the possible grips of the hand. **The hand can also act while gripping.** We call these grips **movement-associated or dynamic grips**. Some of these actions are simple. When a **small top is twirled** (Fig. 278), it is held tangentially between the thumb and the index finger; when **a marble is shot** (Fig. 279) by a sudden flick of P_2 of the thumb produced by the contraction of the *extensor pollicis longus*, it is first held in the hollow of the index fully flexed by the *flexor digitorum profundus*. Other actions are more complex, **with the hand acting on itself, i.e. 'in-hand manipulation'.** In this case, the object held by one part of the hand is acted upon by another part of the hand. These dynamic grips where the hand acts on itself are **countless**, as for example:

- **Lighting a cigarette lighter** (Fig. 280), which is very much like flicking a marble. The lighter is held in the hollow of the index and of the other fingers, while the clawed thumb is pressed on its top with the help of the *flexor pollicis longus* and the thenar muscles.
- **Squeezing the top of a spray can** (Fig. 281): this time the can is held by a palmar grip and the flexed index is pressed on the top by contraction of the *flexor digitorum profundus*.
- **Cutting with scissors** (Fig. 282): the handles are threaded on to the thumb and the middle or ring finger. The thumb muscles provide the force needed to close the scissors (the thenar muscles) and to open them (*extensor pollicis longus*). Opening the scissors, when excessively repeated during work, can lead to rupture of the *extensor longus*. The index finger imparts direction to the scissors, turning this grip into a **directional dynamic grip**.

- **Eating with chopsticks** (Fig. 283): one stick is jammed in the first interdigital cleft by the ring finger and stays put while the other stick, held in a tridigital grip with the thumb, index finger and middle finger, forms a pincer with its partner. This is certainly a good test of manual dexterity for Europeans, while Asians use chopsticks almost unconsciously from a very young age.
- **Tying knots with one hand** (Fig. 284): this is also a test of manual dexterity that not everyone can perform. It relies on the independent but coordinated action of two bidigital pincers, i.e. the one formed by the index finger and the middle finger in lateral apposition and the other formed by the thumb and the ring finger. This is a rarely used form of pollici-digital grip. **Surgeons** use a closely related grip to tie knots with one hand. Such complex actions involving only one hand are very commonly used by **jugglers and conjurers**, whose clearly above-average manual dexterity needs to be maintained by daily exercises.
- **The left hand of the violinist** (Fig. 285) **or of the guitarist** achieves a very flexible dynamic grip. The thumb supports the neck of the violin and by moving up and down balances the force applied by the other four fingers as they play the notes. This pressure on the strings must be at once precise, firm and modulated **to produce the vibrato**. These complex actions can be performed only after many years of training and daily practice.

Readers can find for themselves the infinite variety of dynamic grips that constitute the most elaborate form of activity of the hand when it is endowed with its full functional capacity and can form the basis of **functional tests**.

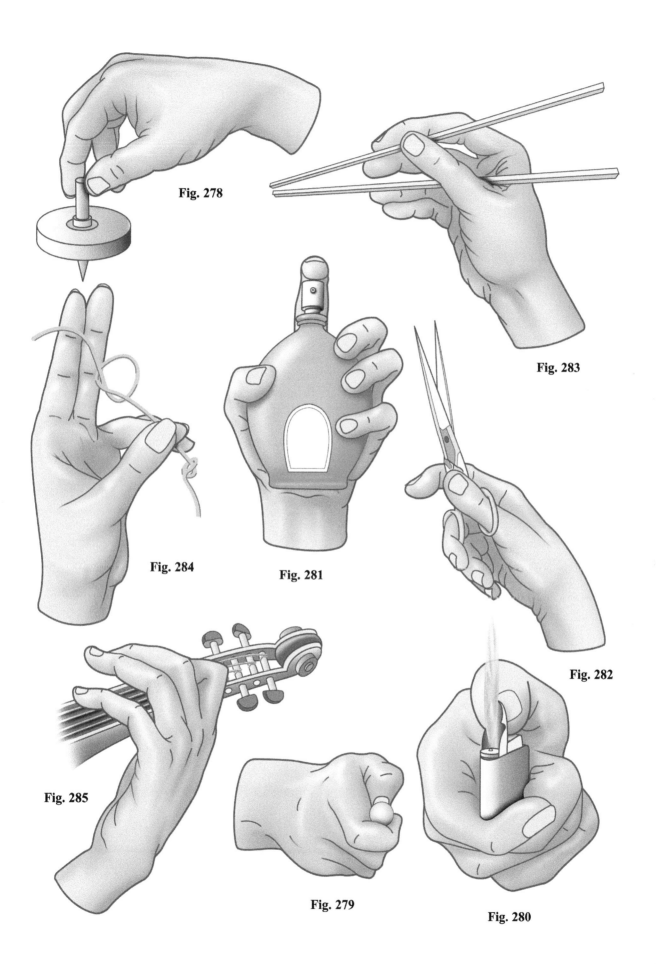

Fig. 278

Fig. 283

Fig. 284

Fig. 281

Fig. 282

Fig. 285

Fig. 279

Fig. 280

Percussion – Contact – Gestures

The human hand is used not only for prehension but also **as an instrument of percussion**:

- When one uses a **calculator**, a **typewriter** or a **computer** at work (Fig. 286) or **when one plays the piano**, each finger behaving like a little hammer, hitting the keyboard as a result of the coordinated action of the interossei and digital flexors, in particular the *profundus*. The difficulty lies in acquiring functional independence of the fingers and of the hands, and this requires special training of the brain and muscles and constant practice.
- When **blows are dealt by the fist in boxing** (Fig. 287), or by the ulnar border or distal extremity of the fingers in karate or by the outspread hand when a simple slap is given.
- When snapping one's fingers by making the middle finger shoot forcibly from the tip to the base of the thumb.

The touch of the hand is softer when it **caresses** (Fig. 288), an action of fundamental importance in social and particularly affective interaction. Note that an intact cutaneous sensitivity is essential for both the hand that caresses and the hand caressed. In some cases, contact with two hands may cause healing, as in the laying on of hands, which may be effective even at a distance. Finally, the most banal gesture of everyday life in the West, the handshake (Fig. 289), represents a social contact charged with symbolic meaning.

The **performance of gestures** is an irreplaceable function of the hand. In fact, gestures are performed by **close cooperation between the face and the hand** and are under subcortical control, since they disappear in Parkinsonism.

This **language of face and hand** is codified in the language of deaf-mutes, but the **gamut of instinctive gestures constitutes a second language**, which, unlike the spoken language, is universally understood. This mode of expression is made up of countless instinctive gestures that may show geographical differences but are generally understood all over the world, as, for example, the fist raised in threat (Fig. 287), the peace greeting with the hand wide open, the **finger pointing accusingly** (Fig. 290, representing the finger of St Thomas in the *Retable of Issenheim* of Matthias Grünewald), and finally **applause** expressing approval. This gamut of gestures is further developed professionally by actors, but it is an integral part of every human being's behaviour. Its goal is to underline and stress particular facial expressions, but often it dispenses with words and suffices by itself to express feelings and situations. Hence the **extensive use of the 'posturing hand' in painting and sculpture**. This role of the hand is as important as its role in gripping and feeling. In certain crafts, as in **pottery**, the hand is multifunctional (Fig. 291); it is the effector organ modelling the object, the sensory organ that recognizes and modifies its shape continuously, and finally the organ of symbolic expression when it offers the object of its creation to mankind. **It is the completeness of the creative gesture that makes it so valuable.**

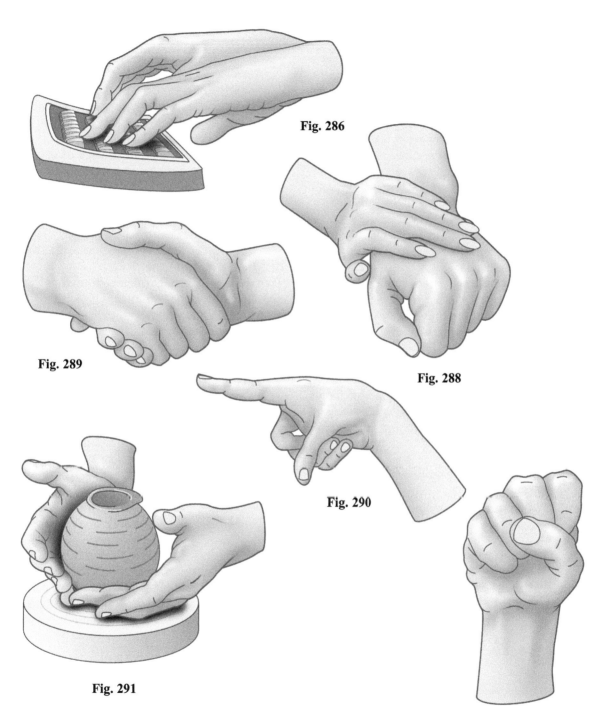

Fig. 286

Fig. 289

Fig. 288

Fig. 290

Fig. 291

Fig. 287

The positions of function and of immobilization

The **functional position of the hand**, first described by S. Bunnell as the resting position of the hand, is quite different from that observed during sleep (Fig. 292, the *Hand of Adam*, according to Michelangelo). The latter position, called the **position of relaxation**, is also maintained by the wounded hand so as to reduce pain and consists of the following: forearm pronated, wrist flexed, thumb in adduction-retroposition, the first interdigital cleft closed and the fingers relatively extended, particularly at the level of the MP joints.

The **functional position** (Figs 293 and 294) was redefined by Littler (1951) as follows: forearm in semi-pronation; wrist in 30° extension and adduction; the thumb (particularly M_1) collinear with the radius and forming an angle of 45° with M_2; the MP and IP joints of the thumb almost straight; the fingers slightly flexed and their MP joints flexed, with the degree of flexion increasing towards the little finger. As a whole, this position of function **corresponds to that in which prehension could take place in the presence of minimal articular mobility**, i.e. if one or more of the joints of the fingers and thumb were ankylosed, or to that in which recovery of useful movements would be relatively easy, since opposition is already almost maximal and could be completed by a few degrees of flexion in any of the still active joints.

There are in practice, however, **three positions of immobilization**, as defined by R. Tubiana (1973).

The temporary or 'protective' position of immobilization

The temporary or 'protective' position of immobilization (Fig. 295), which aims at preserving the mobility of the hand in the long run:

- forearm in mid-flexion and pronation with the elbow flexed at 100°
- wrist in extension at 20° and in slight adduction
- the fingers flexed, the more so as they are more medial, as follows:

- the MP joints flexed between 50° and 80°, the more so, the less flexed the PIP joints
- the IP joints moderately flexed, the less so to reduce tension and the risk of ischaemia from arterial insufficiency
- the PIP joints flexed between 10° and 40° and the DIP joints between 10° and 20°
- the thumb in the initial stage of opposition: in slight adduction but also in anteposition, keeping the interdigital cleft open; the MP and IP joints in very slight extension, so that the pulp of the thumb faces those of the index and middle fingers.

The positions of definitive immobilization or functional fixation

The positions of definitive immobilization or functional fixation depend on the individual case:

- As regards the wrist:
  - When the fingers are still able to grip, the wrist should be arthrodesed in 25° extension so as to place the hand in a gripping position.
  - When the fingers are unable to grip, it is better to fix the wrist in moderate flexion.
  - If both wrists are fused for life, then it is imperative to fix one in flexion to facilitate perineal hygiene. If a cane is to be used, it is necessary to fix the wrist in a straight position; if two canes are to be used, the wrist of the dominant hand should be fixed in 10° extension and the other hand in 10° flexion.
- The forearm is immobilized in more or less full pronation.
- The MP joints are fixed in flexion ranging from 35° for the index to 50° for the little finger.
- The IP joints are fixed in flexion from 40° to 60°.
- The TM joint is arthrodesed in a position that suits each case but, every time one of the elements of the pollici-digital pincer is permanently put out of action, the functional capabilities of the other still mobile elements must be considered.

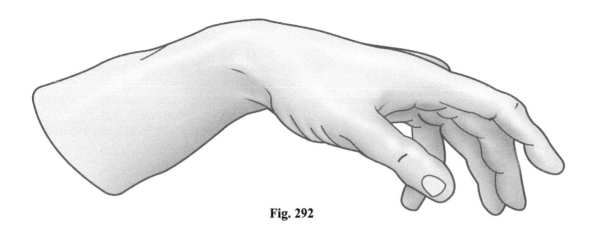

Fig. 292

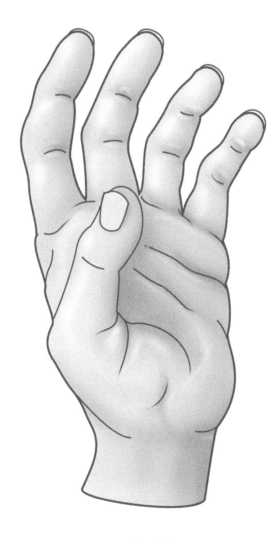

Fig. 293

The non-functional positions of 'temporary immobilization' or 'partial relaxation'

These should be used for the shortest possible time in order to stabilize a fracture or to slacken tissue tension around a sutured tendon or nerve. As a result of venous or lymphatic stasis, there is a serious risk of developing stiffness, which can be considerably reduced if the joints are actively exercised:

- **After the median nerve, the ulnar nerve or the flexor tendons have been sutured**, the wrist can be safely kept in flexion at 40° for 3 weeks, but it is crucial to immobilize the MP joints in approximately 80° flexion while keeping the IP joints in their natural state of extension, since recovery of extension is difficult to obtain after forced flexion.
- **After the dorsal structures have been repaired**, the joints must be immobilized in hyperextension but the MP joints must be kept in at least 10° flexion. The IP joints should be flexed at 20°, if the damage occurred proximal to the MP joints, but they should be fixed in the neutral position if the damage was done at the level of P_1.
- **When 'buttonhole' lesions are repaired**, the PIP joint is immobilized in extension and the DIP joint in flexion so as to pull the extensor tendons distally.
- Conversely, **if the DIP joint is close to the site of the lesion**, it should be immobilized in extension and the PIP joint in flexion so as to relax the lateral expansions of the extensors.

Whatever the position adopted, one must remember that any prolonged period of immobilization always causes some functional loss, and so immobilization must be as brief as possible.

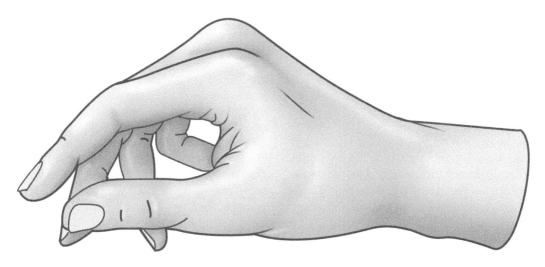

Fig. 294

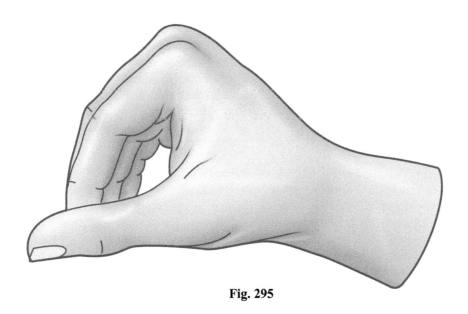

Fig. 295

Partially amputated hands and fictional hands

The study of **fictional hands** is not simply a thought experiment; it also provides a better understanding of the structural rationale behind the human hand. The types of hand that can be imagined fall into two categories: asymmetrical and symmetrical.

Asymmetrical hands are derived from the normal hand by reducing or increasing the number of fingers or by inverting its symmetry.

1) **An increase in the number of fingers**, i.e. a sixth or seventh finger added to the ulnar border of the little finger, would certainly in theory strengthen the full palmar grip, but it also gives rise to unacceptable functional complications. These supernumerary fingers are due to a congenital malformation and should be amputated.

2) **A decrease in the number of fingers to four or three** would reduce the functional capability of the hand. In some monkeys of Central America (the spider monkeys) the upper limb has a hand with four fingers and no thumb; this hand is only able to cling to branches, whereas the lower limb has a hand with five fingers, including a thumb capable of opposition. The **hand with three fingers** (Fig. 296), as seen after certain forms of amputation, retains the tridigital and bidigital grips, which are the most commonly used and the most precise, but has lost the full palmar grip needed to grip the handle of a tool or the butt of a rifle. In the **hand with two fingers** (Fig. 297), the thumb and the index finger can still form a hook and a bidigital pincer in order to grip small objects, but tridigital and full palmar grips are impossible. Yet unexpected success can be obtained when such a hand is retained or reconstructed in some patients.

3) Following amputation of the little finger for definitive treatment of Dupuytren's contracture or following avulsion of the ring finger after the ring is 'caught', hand surgeons may consider the reconstruction of a **hand with four fingers.** Whether this involves the **complete resection of the fifth ray of the hand** (Fig. 298) or **intermetacarpal resection of the fourth ray of the hand** (Fig. 299), the aesthetic and functional results can be very satisfactory, and this deformity may go unnoticed by the casual observer. Who has noticed that Mickey Mouse's hand (Fig. 300) has only four fingers?

Let us imagine a **symmetrically inverted** hand, i.e. **a hand with five fingers and an ulnar thumb located medially**. Such a hand would have a palmar gutter that ran obliquely in the opposite direction. Thus in the neutral position of pronation-supination the head of the hammer, instead of lying obliquely proximally, would lie obliquely distally. This change of orientation would prevent one from hitting a nail on the head unless the neutral position of pronation-supination were reversed by +180°, i.e. with the palm pointing laterally! The ulna would override the radius and the insertion of the biceps on the radius would reduce its efficiency. In sum, the entire architecture of the upper limb would have to be changed without any obvious functional advantage. This demonstration *ab absurdo* therefore fully justifies the normal location of the thumb on the radial side of the hand.

Let us finally imagine **symmetrical hands**, with two thumbs, one medial and one lateral, flanking two or three fingers. In the **symmetrical hand with three fingers**, the simplest form (Fig. 301), the following grips would be possible: two pollicidigital, bipollical (between the two thumbs) and tridigital (Fig. 302) with the two thumbs opposing the index. Thus four precision grips would be possible. A full palmar grip would also be possible between the two thumbs and the palm and the index. Though fairly strong, this grip would have a serious disadvantage; because of its symmetry, the handle of any tool would lie perpendicular to the long axis of the forearm. We have already seen that, for a tool to be properly oriented, the obliquity of the handle must be combined with movements of pronation-supination of the hand. The same would apply to **symmetrical hands with two or three intermediate fingers** (Fig. 303), i.e. a hand with five fingers, including two thumbs. Parrots have two posteriorly located fingers and these form a symmetrical claw, which allows them to stand firmly on a branch, but this is not a solution to our problem! Another consequence of the symmetrical hand with two thumbs would be the need for a symmetrical arrangement of the structures of the forearm, which would exclude pronation-supination.

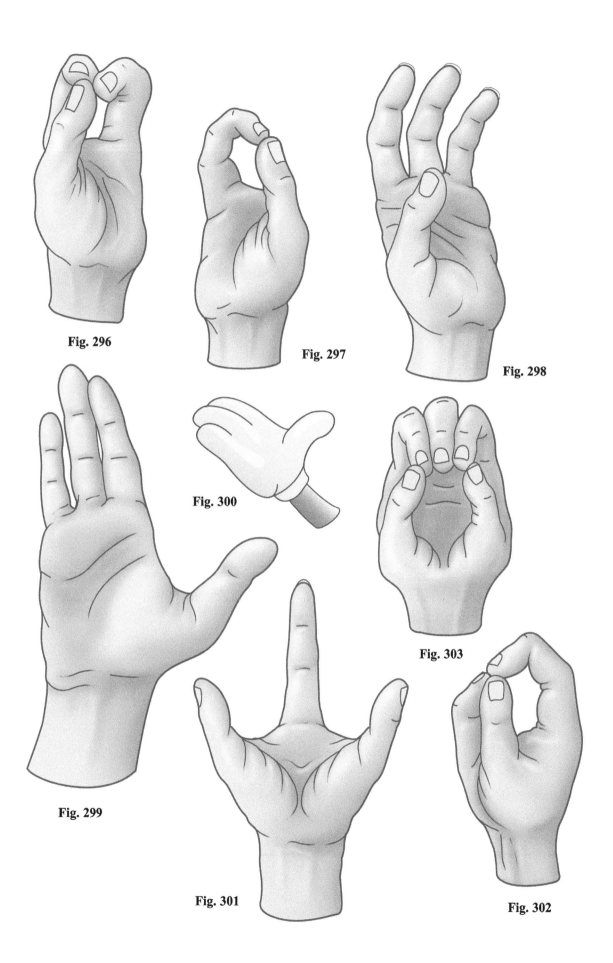

Fig. 296

Fig. 297

Fig. 298

Fig. 299

Fig. 300

Fig. 301

Fig. 303

Fig. 302

The motor and sensory function of the upper limb

This page is meant to be a memory aid for the motor and sensory supply to the hand.

A **synoptic table of the motor nerves of the upper limb** (Fig. 304) lists the nerve(s) that supply each of the muscles identified by their names using the International Classification. There is no need to itemize this list in detail. One should study it carefully and absorb it with emphasis on the overlapping of nerve supply, double innervation and also the interconnections between the nerve trunks, which can explain some paradoxical findings in cases of neurological deficit or aberrant results from some electrical investigations. This exchange among nerve fibres must be envisaged like a motorway interchange where cars leave one motorway to enter another via exit ramps. The point of arrival is not actually that of the original nerve trunk but that of the adjacent trunk. One must also bear in mind that a large nerve trunk comes from a variable number of cervical roots and that nerve fibres coming from nerve roots that do not belong to the trunk under investigation can end up in unexpected places. There are countless and unpredictable variations from the average pattern, which fortunately turns out to be the correct one most of the time.

The axillary nerve (old name: circumflex)
- Arises from the cervical roots C5 and C6.
- Receives sensory information from the deltoid region.
- Is the motor nerve to the deltoid and thus responsible for abduction.

The musculo-cutaneous nerve
- Arises from C5 to C7.
- Receives sensory information from the anterior surface of the arm and part of the forearm.
- Is the motor nerve for the *biceps* and the *brachialis* and thus responsible for elbow flexion.

The median nerve
- Arises from C5 to T1.
- Receives sensory information from the palmar surface of the hand down to the fingers (see later) and partly from the forearm.
- Is the motor nerve for the flexors of the fingers and the wrist.
- Is also responsible for opposition of the thumb.

The ulnar nerve
- Arises from C7 to T1.
- Receives sensory information from the palmar and dorsal surfaces of the hand and of the fingers (see later) and partly from the forearm.
- Is the motor nerve of the interossei and the medial thenar muscles.

The radial nerve
- Arises from C5 to T1.
- Receives sensory information from the posterior surface of the arm and of the forearm.
- Is responsible for extension of the elbow, the wrist and the fingers and for abduction of the thumb.

Fig. 304

OVERVIEW OF THE MOTOR NERVES OF THE UPPER LIMB

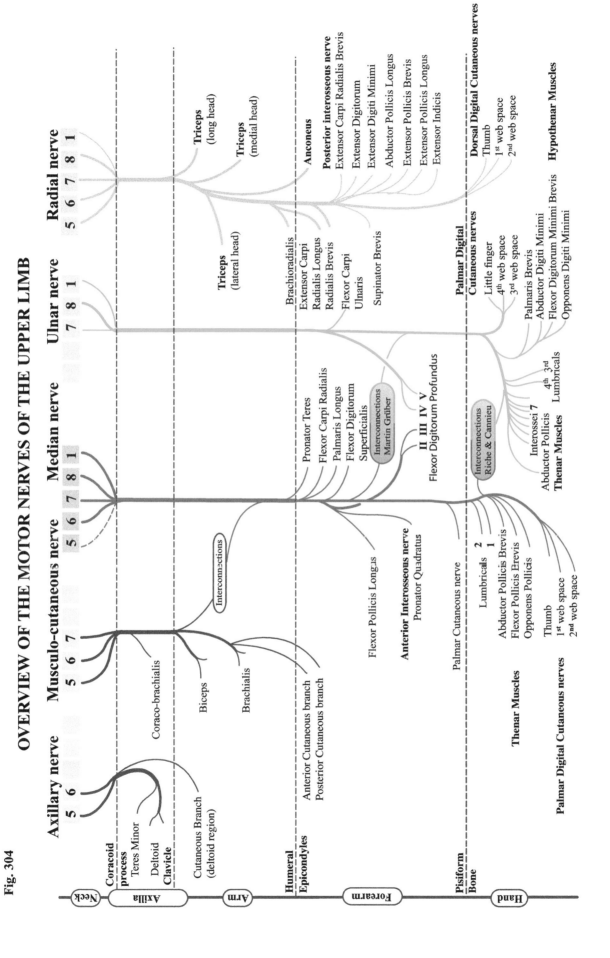

335

Motor and sensory tests of the upper limb

The pulps of the fingers

The **dynamic tests of the main motor nerves** allow one to establish whether a nerve trunk is interrupted or paralysed, as follows:

- The **test for the median nerve** (Fig. 305): making a fist.
- The **test for the ulnar nerve**: spreading the fingers (Fig. 306) and bringing the extended fingers together (Fig. 307).
- The **test for the radial nerve** (Fig. 308): active extension of the wrist, extension and radial abduction of the thumb. Note that only the MP joints of the fingers are extended. The IP joints stay flexed and are partially extended only when the wrist is flexed.
- The **combined test for the radial and ulnar nerves**: (Fig. 309) differs from the previous test only in that the IP joints are extended at the same time.

The **sensory areas of the hand** must be fully understood in order to make accurate diagnoses of nerve damage:

- It is easy for the **palmar surface** of the hand (Fig. 310); the median nerve (pink) supplies the lateral half and the ulnar nerve (green) supplies the medial half. The dividing line passes exactly through the fourth ray.
- The picture is more complicated for the **dorsal surface** (Fig. 311), which is supplied by **three nerves**:
  - Laterally, the radial nerve (in yellow).
  - Medially, the ulnar nerve (in green).
  - The dividing line between these two territories runs through the axis of the hand, i.e. the third ray.
  - Only the dorsal surfaces of the proximal phalanges and of the metacarpals are supplied by these nerves.
  - The dorsal surfaces of the two distal phalanges are supplied by the two palmar nerves. The median nerve (pink) supplies the dorsal surfaces of the lateral half of the ring finger and of the other three lateral fingers; the ulnar nerve supplies the dorsal surfaces of the medial half of the ring finger and of the little finger.

In summary, the last two phalanges are supplied by sensory nerves derived from the following:

- the median nerve for the thumb, the index finger and the middle finger
- the ulnar nerve for the little finger
- the median nerve for the lateral half of the ring finger and the ulnar nerve for its medial half.

The hand, and particularly the pulps of the fingers, have a rich nerve and blood supply, since the hand is the **main receptor for one of our five senses: touch**. As a result it has very extensive projections in the motor and sensory areas of the cerebral cortex.

The **blood supply to the pulps of the fingers** (Fig. 312) comes from the **palmar and dorsal digital arteries** (only one is shown in red), which anastomose freely in the pulps and across each of the IP joints.

The **nerve supply** (Fig. 312) comes from the rich network of fibres derived from the palmar digital nerves (only one is shown in green).

The **pulp itself** (Fig. 313) is made up of highly specialized tissue, i.e. loose areolar connective tissue with its fibres attached to the periosteum of the phalanx and to the deep dermis of the finger. As a result it has flexibility, elasticity and mechanical strength, features essential for its sensory and motor function. Distally the pulp is buttressed by the **nail bed**, which also makes an important functional contribution.

The pulps of the fingers are invaluable to craftsmen, artists, pianists and violinists. A simple whitlow can damage them and destroy their usefulness.

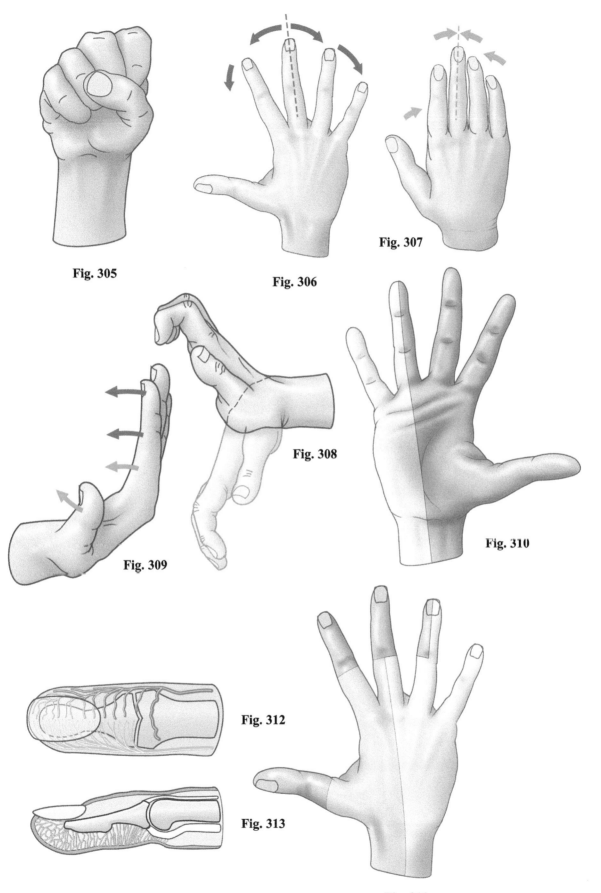

Fig. 305

Fig. 306

Fig. 307

Fig. 308

Fig. 309

Fig. 310

Fig. 312

Fig. 313

Fig. 311

Three motor tests for the hand

In addition to the motor tests described in the preceding pages, there are three tests for the ulnar nerve that deserve special attention. Two of them are standard tests and the third is a new one.

1) **Wartenberg's sign** (Fig. 314) is observed when the ulnar nerve is completely paralysed but is particularly useful in recognizing distal lesions of the nerve, i.e. at the level of Guyon's canal or the carpal ulnar neurovascular space. The little finger stays permanently separated from the ring finger (black arrow) and cannot be drawn actively towards the ring finger (shown in the background).

2) **Froment's sign** (Fig. 315) is observed when the subject is asked to pinch a sheet of paper between thumb and index finger. These two digits normally form a ring (seen in the background). When the ulnar nerve is paralysed, the pincer is loose because the *adductor pollicis*, innervated by the deep palmar branch of the ulnar nerve, is paralysed. The proximal phalanx of the thumb tilts into extension and the paper can easily be pulled away, which is not the case when the nerve is normal.

3) The **sign of the weak ulnar hook** has recently been described by the author. Normally, when the last two fingers are strongly flexed towards the palm of the hand, the examiner cannot 'unhook' the little finger by passively extending its distal phalanx. This test is carried out as follows on the patient's right hand (Fig. 316):

   – The examiner, using both hands, offers his right index to the patient and asks him to grip it tightly between his strongly flexed last two fingers.
   – The examiner then tries with his left index to extend forcibly the distal phalanx of the patient's little finger.

– Normally he fails to do so as the two hooked fingers resist successfully.
– If the ulnar nerve is paralysed, the hook of the patient's little finger gives way, and his distal phalanx is tilted into extension (black arrow).

The same manœuvre can be applied to the ring finger with similar results.

The underlying mechanism for the test

One must remember that the *flexor digitorum profundus* has a composite innervation (Fig. 317). The two lateral tendons (deep pink) for the index and middle fingers are innervated by a branch (2) of the median nerve (M), while its two medial tendons for the ring finger (light pink) and the little finger are innervated by a branch (1) of the ulnar nerve (U), which arises distal to the wrist.

This explains why flexion of the ring finger and of the little finger can be selectively compromised when the ulnar nerve is damaged and, more important, why the test is positive or negative depending on the site of damage to the nerve:

• If the damage has occurred proximal to point **a**, the test is **positive**.
• If the damage has occurred at point **b** or distal to it, i.e. at the level of Guyon's canal, the test is **negative**, whereas Froment's test is positive.

Therefore this test, very easy to carry out and very selective in its results, should be part of every complete neurological examination of the upper limb. It could also be dubbed the **nail-file test**, since it was discovered in a patient who complained that she could no longer file down the nail of her ring finger because it kept extending under the pressure exerted by the nail file.

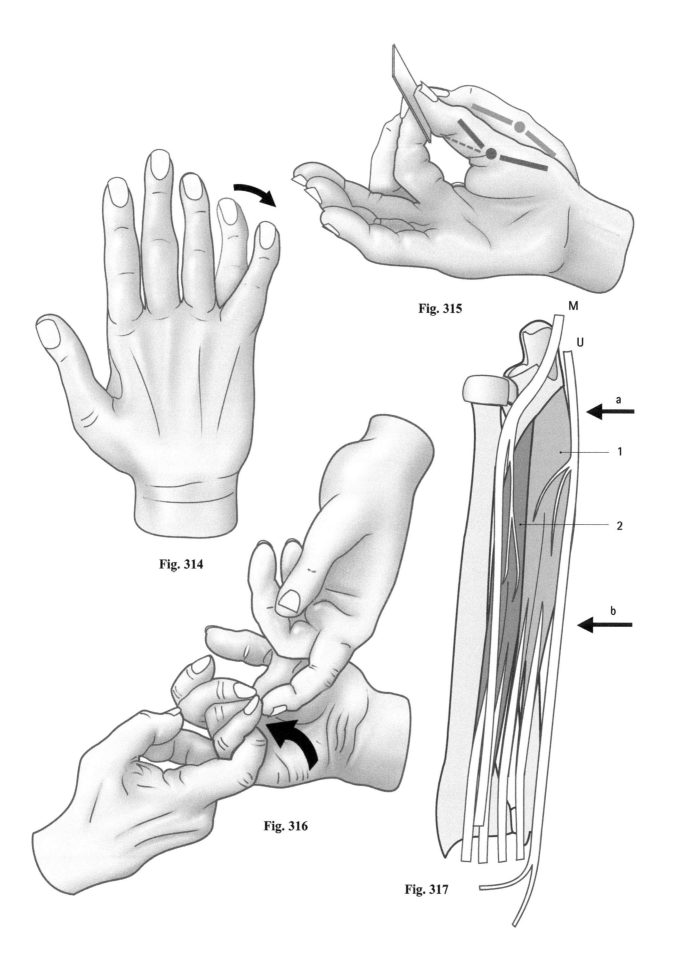

Fig. 315

Fig. 314

Fig. 316

Fig. 317

M

U

a

1

2

b

The upper limbs after the transition to bipedalism

Our first ancestor on land was the **tetrapod Icthyosega** (Fig. 318), whose four limbs are derived from the two pairs of pectoral and caudal fins of fish. All terrestrial quadrupeds have inherited its skeletal structure, consisting of a **trunk**, which is supported by a flexible **spinal column** crowned by the **head**, which is linked to the neck and contains the brain, the central computer. The trunk articulates with two pairs of limbs with the help of two girdles: **the pelvic girdle and the shoulder girdle**, the latter appearing later in evolution. This prototype was maintained and diversified over millions of years into numerous species to culminate in the primates, which split into two branches: the apes and the Homo species, the latter becoming the definitive bipeds, while the apes remain quadrupeds for the most part.

When the species Homo became **exclusively bipedal** this transition led to significant changes in the structure and function of these two pairs of limbs.

1) The posterior limb (Fig. 319) became the lower limb and retained their role as carriers and movers while supporting the entire body weight. As the anterior limbs became the upper limbs they no longer carried or moved the body but acquired a higher function by becoming **effector organs** solely devoted to **prehension**.

2) As regards the stability and range of movements:

- the lower limb is **very stably** linked to the trunk, and its range of movement is limited
- in contrast, the lower limb is 'attached' at the level of the shoulder girdle (Fig. 320), which is much more mobile because its bony connections with the thorax are mediated by the clavicle and the scapula, which articulates with the humerus and 'slides' over the postero-lateral wall of the thorax via two "false joints" consisting of gliding planes of

fibrocellular tissue (see page 140). To use a 'mechanical' analogy, the front-wheel axle unit of a car (Fig. 321), which consists of two deformable parallelograms, is much more 'flexible' than the rear-wheel axle unit.

3) The upper limb, now transformed into an effector organ totally devoted to prehension, thus becomes the 'logistical support' of the hand. This term is used to reflect its military equivalent, i.e., a specialised unit aimed at supplying the combatants with food, petrol, ammunition, weapons and spare parts. Without logistical support an army is doomed to failure, as illustrated by two historical examples: Napoleon's army in Moscow, and that of Von Paulus in Stalingrad. Their supply routes had extended beyond the reach of their logistical support.

To be effective the hand must be able to approach its target in the best possible way thanks to the seven degrees of liberty provided by the articular complex of the upper limb (Fig. 322): three degrees at the shoulder, one degree at the elbow and three degrees at the forearm and the wrist. The loss of any of these degrees of freedom, as, for example, the loss of elbow flexion, will prevent the hand from being carried to the mouth, thus compromising its function in feeding.

- Mobility per se is not enough, since also needed is the stable support provided by the upper limb, which depends on the functionality of its joints and the efficiency of the motor muscles that control them.
- The upper limb provides the supply of energy via its arterio-venous network (Fig. 323: only the arterial network is shown here).
- It also carries messages and transmits signals in its motor and sensory nerves (Fig. 324: the brachial plexus is not shown here).

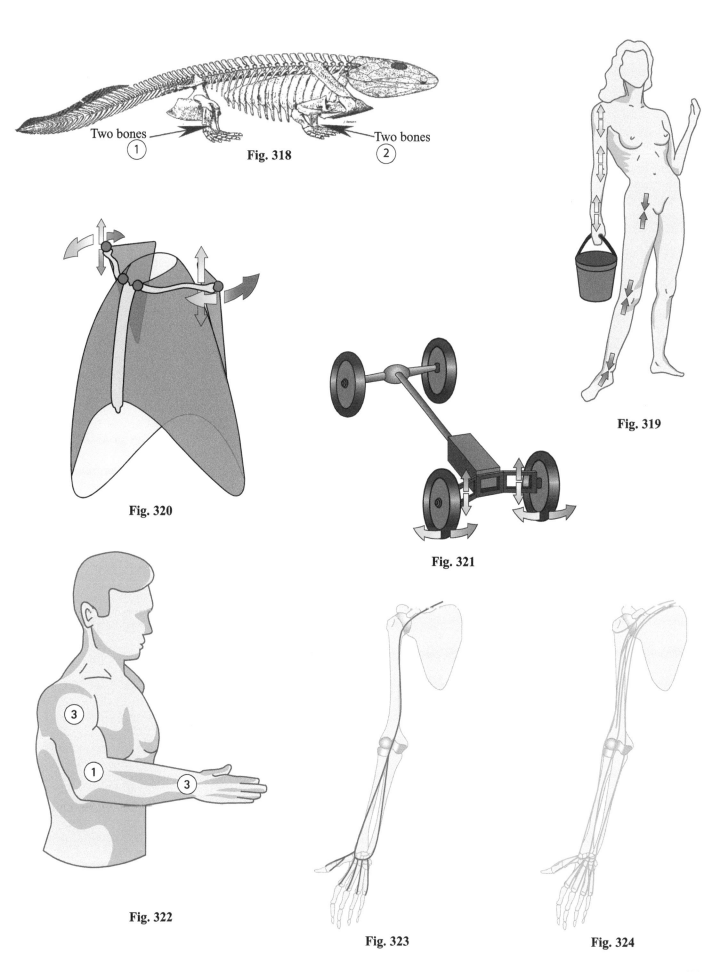

Two bones ① **Fig. 318** Two bones ②

Fig. 319

Fig. 320

Fig. 321

Fig. 322

Fig. 323

Fig. 324

The Automatic Swinging Of The Upper Limbs

The normal gait of Homo Sapiens includes the automatic swinging of the upper limbs. It is an obvious fact, and the question arises: why and how is it useful?

During normal walking (Fig. 325) the left hand moves forward while the right leg is carried forward to prevent a forward fall. In the next phase of the gait cycle the opposite occurs. This is the **diagonal sequence gait** of the majority of quadrupeds, such as the horse (Fig. 326). The odd quadruped, however, e.g., the giraffe (Fig. 327), shows a different walk with both moving limbs being on the same side; this is known as the amble. Since humans descend from quadrupeds that use the diagonal sequence gait, it is easy to find a phylogenetic explanation: all the mechanisms are in place; they only need to be adapted.

For two million years humans have walked on their two legs while swinging their two arms. Had there been no evolutionary advantage, this gait pattern would have disappeared a long time ago. On the contrary, the musculature of the scapular girdle and of the upper limbs is highly developed because it plays an essential role in walking.

Walking **without swinging the upper limbs** (Fig. 328) is slow and tiring, because the line joining the partial centres of gravity of the upper limbs (green square) and of the lower limbs (red square) projects on to the global centre of gravity of the body (green star). Thus there is no additional forward propulsive force. The only propulsive force comes from the extension of the ankle of the posterior limb.

During a walk with **normal swinging of the upper limbs** (Fig. 329) the same representation of the centres of gravity shows that the line joining the centres of gravity of the upper limbs and of the lower limbs projects **in front** of the global centre of gravity of the body. Thus the swinging of the upper limbs generates an additional driving force that **accentuates the forward disequilibrium of the body** by blending with that produced by the posterior foot.

It is possible to increase the efficiency of the swinging of the upper limbs by flexing the elbow (Fig. 330), which 'raises' the partial centres of gravity of the upper limbs and causes the line of the centres of gravity to project farther forward and thus increase the driving force on the global centre of gravity of the body.

Other forms of **augmented swinging of the upper limbs** can further increase the forward driving force.

Thus the swinging of the upper limbs is useful but may not always be available, for example **when both hands carry bags or suitcases** (Fig. 331). Then walking becomes painful and cannot be sustained for long. Some African populations have solved the problem by **carrying their loads on their heads** (Fig. 332), but a strong and healthy cervical spinal column is needed. One can also carry a child **on one's back**, using a harness or an ordinary piece of cloth.

The gait of marching soldiers, which varies from country to country, can also be thus evaluated. Walking with swinging of the upper limbs (Fig. 333) is the least tiring. Walking while carrying a weapon (Fig. 334) is already less comfortable, but even less comfortable is **goose-stepping** (Fig. 335), which is used in marches past the VIP stands.

In the long jump (Fig. 336) the propulsion generated by the upper limbs is directed upwards, as can be seen clearly with the use of **stroboscopy** (Fig. 337). Finally, the Nordic walk, using two poles, belies the riddle of the Sphinx and, according to its adherents, is very well balanced, but it is only a throwback to bipedalism.

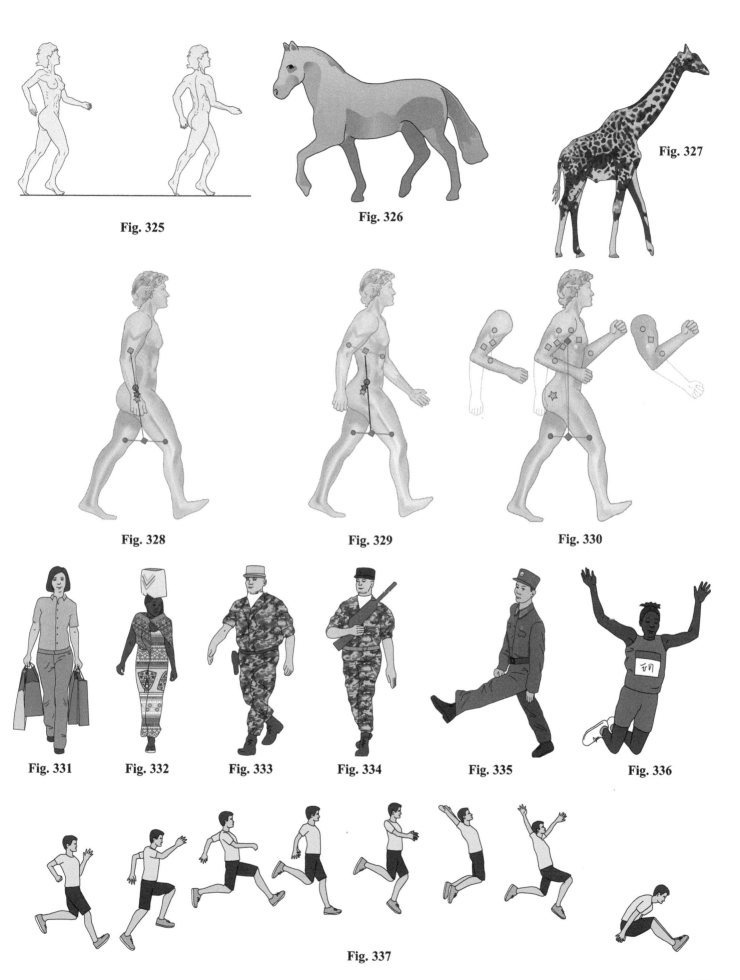

Fig. 325

Fig. 326

Fig. 327

Fig. 328

Fig. 329

Fig. 330

Fig. 331

Fig. 332

Fig. 333

Fig. 334

Fig. 335

Fig. 336

Fig. 337

Extension of the Body Image Thanks to the Hand

The body image is the **image of oneself**, which is carried in one's subconscious mind and which consists of two parts inside the brain:

- **a purely physical component**, i.e. the body schema, strictly speaking, which is the awareness of one's body and of its structural basis, i.e., the locomotor system
- **a purely moral component**, i.e., the image that one has of one's own personality. It exists because one can see it in 'somebody else' and it corresponds to what some philosophies or religions call the **soul**. This exclusively moral aspect is part of one's perception of the soul, without pronouncing on the definition or the existence of the soul. This aspect of the body schema of another person allows one to appreciate fully his or her moral character.

The body schema is the cerebral representation of the portion of space occupied by the body of the individual. It is a virtual image (Fig. 338: the *transparent man of the Mayo Clinic) of the body as a whole and of each of its parts. It can be **static**, but most of the time it is **dynamic** (Fig. 339) as it interacts with the environment.

The skin surface is the frontier between the inside of the individual and the outside world, i.e., a portion of space containing the individual. The **skin**, containing the sensory receptors, is thus the **frontier of the individual with respect to the rest of the universe. The makeup and the retention of the body schema are among the basic functions of the central nervous system.** This body schema is related to the environment via the **sensory receptors** for direct contacts (Fig. 340) and via binocular **stereoscopic vision** (Fig. 341) for the immediate surroundings. This continuous confrontation between our dynamic body schema and the environment allows us not only to move about and practise sports (Fig. 342: high jump) but also to **act upon our environment** in many ways, e.g., feeding ourselves, defending ourselves and especially modifying our body schema by **doing work**. This occurs when the **body schema is extended by the use of a tool or an instrument**. A very common event can shed light on this phenomenon, as when one drives a brand-new car for the first time and unexpectedly dents the bodywork because of a wrong appreciation of the size of the vehicle (Fig. 343: green outline). But after some time the size becomes integrated into the driver's body schema, and it is then easy to drive through congested areas without damaging the bodywork. This applies to all tools and instruments. For example, the blacksmith's hammer becomes an **extension of his hand** (Fig. 344); (hence 'smithing makes a smith', i.e., practice makes perfect). Likewise for any tool a training period of variable duration is needed. The workman's hand is the site of attachment of the tool **destined to be integrated into his body schema**; at this point he becomes a qualified workman.

Musicians also need a period of training: a **concert violinist** (Fig. 345) has spent many years of her youth integrating her violin into her body schema and now, without thinking of her hands or looking at them, she can accurately place her fingers to play the right note. Neither does the **pianist** (Fig. 346) look at his piano: the keyboard, now integrated into his hands, forms an integral part of his body schema. The same applies to the **flautist** (Fig. 347). As for the **blind man** (Fig. 348), his white stick is now simply the extension of his hand for the detection of obstacles. **Surgeons** (Fig. 349), who now perform endoscopy, must also undergo a period of training in order to integrate their instruments using the screen. Likewise for **drone pilots** (Fig. 350), who must guide their unmanned planes from many thousands of kilometres away. The violinist in figure 351 is happy to have recovered his stolen Stradivarius – an example of **'emotional' integration**.

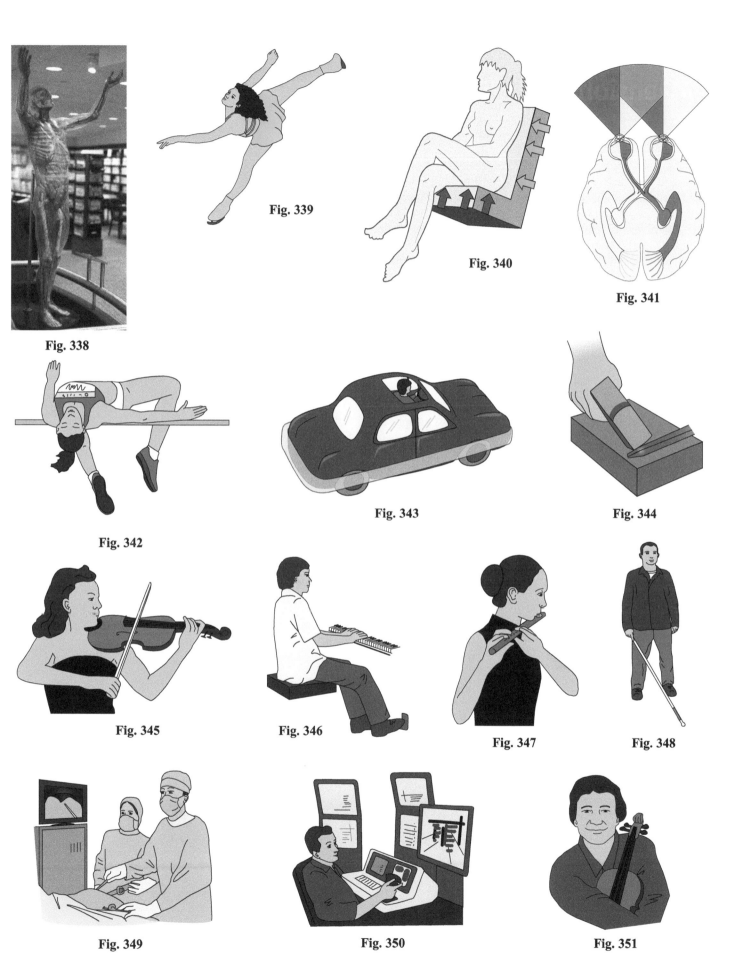

Fig. 338

Fig. 339

Fig. 340

Fig. 341

Fig. 342

Fig. 343

Fig. 344

Fig. 345

Fig. 346

Fig. 347

Fig. 348

Fig. 349

Fig. 350

Fig. 351

Prehension during evolution

Prehension is **taking possession of something**, in particular of food. It is an activity that appeared many million years ago for unicellular animals like the **amoeba** (Fig. 352), which gets hold of its food by **phagocytosis**, i.e., the engulfing of its prey. Even carnivorous plants like the **Drosera Rotundifolia** (Fig. 353) or the **Nepenthes Ventricosa** (Fig. 354) can catch insects as food. A similar mechanism is seen among aquatic animals. The **Actinia** (Fig. 355) is a sac-shaped creature that closes its belly around its prey like a **snare**. Land animals have also been provided by Nature with extraordinary and very efficient instruments of prehension, e.g., the **sticky tongue**, which **chameleons** (Fig. 356) can stick out so far, or the **long tongue** of the **anteater**, which it projects into the anthill to secure its daily food. Finally, readers of Jules Verne will remember the **giant octopus**, which gets its prey by using its numerous **tentacles** fitted with **suction pads** (Fig. 357). It is also in the sea that the most efficient prehensile instrument makes its appearance, i.e., the **pincer** in the **crab** (Fig. 358), which consists of two branches jointed at one end and capable of closing on its prey. We must not, however, forget how the elephant uses the **coiling mechanism of its trunk for prehension** (Fig. 359), and how the spider monkey (not shown), whose hands have no thumbs, uses its long tail to catch hold of branches.

Finally we come to the **mandibular grip** used by the **mouth** or the **beak** as an instrument of prehension, e.g., by the parrot (Fig. 360) or the eagle (Fig. 361), both of which also use their **powerful talons**. This grip **formed by the tightly closed mandibles** is used by many terrestrial mammals like the **dog** (Fig. 362) or the **bear** (not shown), even to **carry their young**. Among the terrestrial mammals a major revolution is in store, i.e., the appearance of the **hand**. For the **squirrel** (Fig. 363) one hand on its own is useless and a **bimanual grip** is needed. In contrast, among our distant ancestors, the **lemurs** (Fig. 365), the hand has **five fingers including a thumb**, which was already there 'in reserve' in the skeleton of the paw of our first terrestrial ancestor, the **Ichthyosega** (Fig. 364), where the two phalanges of the thumb are already seen on the radial side. Manual prehension became generalized among our **simian cousins** (Fig. 366: the pollici-digital pincer), which used it also to get hold of branches as they **moved from tree to tree**. **In Homo Sapiens** it went beyond the thumb-index grip (Fig. 367) and the **hand-grip** (Fig. 368) to include the **'action grips'** and contribute to body language. For humans the hand is an extension of the brain and, with Aristotle, we can call the hand the instrument of instruments.

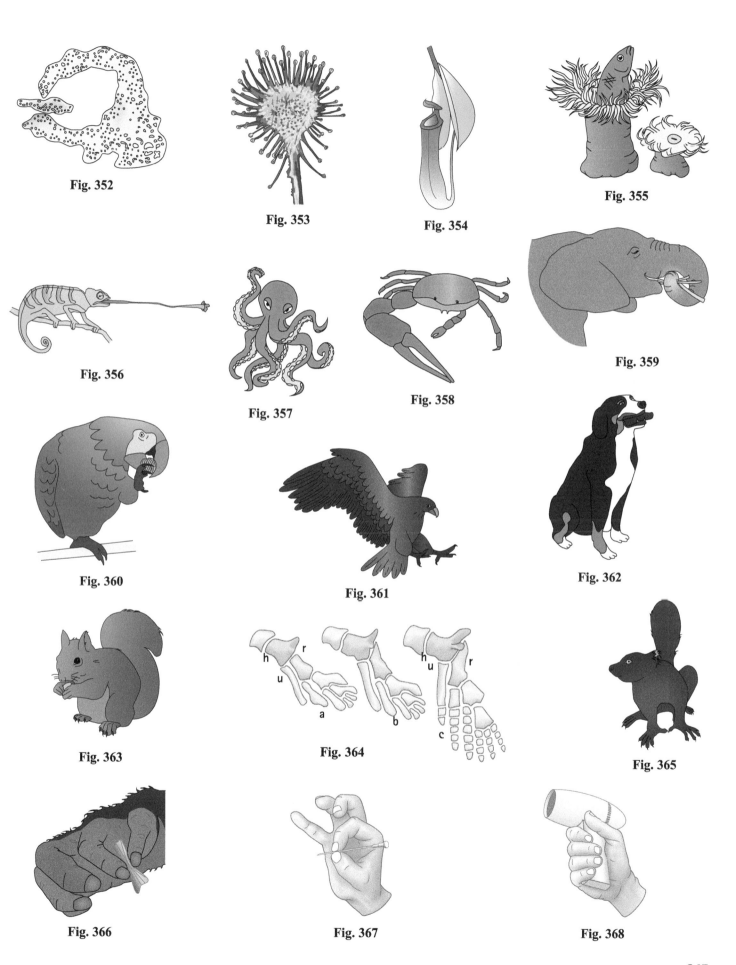

Fig. 352

Fig. 353

Fig. 354

Fig. 355

Fig. 356

Fig. 357

Fig. 358

Fig. 359

Fig. 360

Fig. 361

Fig. 362

Fig. 363

Fig. 364

Fig. 365

Fig. 366

Fig. 367

Fig. 368

The human hand

The human hand has not changed since prehistoric times, as attested by this negative imprint of a hand, which was undoubtedly left behind as a signature by one of our distant ancestors, a cave artist.

Monkeys also have a similar hand, with an opposable thumb, but the difference lies in the way the hand is used, as a result of a tight coupling between hand and brain.

This **hand-brain couple** is bidirectional with reciprocal interaction. The human brain has been able to progress thanks to the capabilities of the hand. Thus the complex architecture of the hand is perfectly logical and adapted to its different functions. It is an example of *Occam's razor, or the principle of universal economy. It is one of the most beautiful examples of **creative evolution**.

Human beings, driven by their **Promethean ambitions, have already created robots able to grip and manipulate, but they are still a long way from achieving the perfection of the original.

---

* William of Occam (1285-1349) is famous for his aphorism known as Occam's razor, i.e. *entia non sunt multiplicanda sine necessitate*, which means that entities should not be multiplied needlessly. In other words, the beauty of a theory is measured by its simplicity. He was a philosopher and a Franciscan theologian working in Oxford and Paris. He was excommunicated and died during the Plague.

** In Greek mythology, **Prometheus** was one of the 12 Titans. His excessive ambition to become the equal of Zeus prompted him to create humans and to give them fire. For this inexpiable crime, called hubris, Zeus chained him to a rock in the Caucasus Mountains, where every day the royal eagle of Zeus fed on the Titan's liver, which – alas! – kept regenerating. Thus was the sin of overweening pride punished in the time of the Greeks.

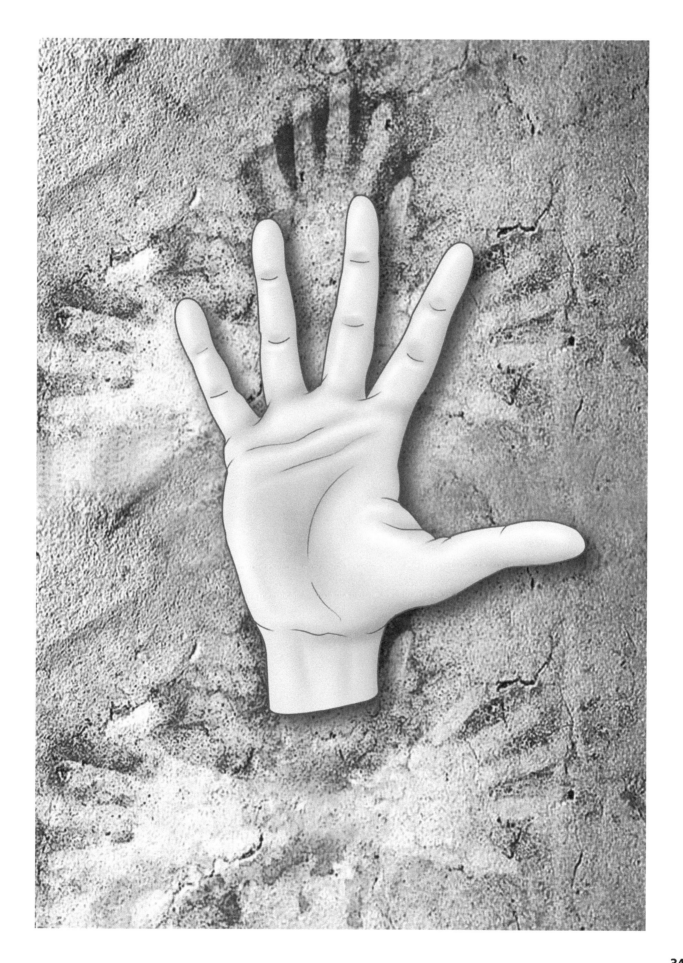

APPENDICES

Bibliography

Barnett CH, Davies DV, MacConaill MA 1961 *Synovial joints. Their structure and mechanics.* CC Thomas, Springfield

Barnier L 1950 *L'Analyse des mouvements.* PUF, Paris

Basmajian JV 1962 *Muscles alive. Their function revealed by electromyography.* Williams & Wilkins, Baltimore

Bausenhardt 1949 Über das Carpometacarpalgelenk des Daumens. *Zeitschr Anat Entw Gesch Bd:* 114-251

Berger RA, Blair WF, Crowninshield PD, Flatt EA 1982 The scapholunate ligament. *J Hand Surg Am* 7(1):87

Bonola A, Caroli A, Celle L 1988 *La Main.* Piccin Nova Libraria, Padua (Selle trapézienne, p. 175)

Bridgeman GB 1939 *The human machine. The anatomical structure and mechanism of the human body.* Vol. 1, p. 143. Dover, New York

Bunnell S 1970 *Surgery of the hand,* 5th edn revised by Boyes. Lippincott, Philadelphia (1st edn 1944)

Caffinière J-Y (de la) 1970 L'Articulation trapézo-métacarpienne: approche biomécanique et appareil ligamentaire. *Arch d'Anat Path* 18:277-284

Caffinière J-Y (de la) 1971 Anatomie fonctionnelle de la poulie proximale des doigts. *Arch d'Anat Path* 19:35

Caffinière J-Y (de la), Hamonet C Secteurs d'activité des muscles thénariens. In: Tubiana R *Traité de chirurgie de la main,* Vol. 1

Caffinière J-Y (de la), Mazas F, Mazas Y et al. 1975 *Prothèse total d'épaule, bases expérimentales et premiers résultats cliniques.* Vol. IV, no. 5. INSERM, Paris

Caffinière J-Y (de la), Pineau H 1971 Approche biomécanique et cotation des mouvements du premier métacarpien. *Rev Chir Orthop* 57(1):3-12

Camus EJ, Millot F, Larivière J et al. 2004 Kinematics of the wrist using 2D and 3D analysis: biomechanical and clinical deductions. *Surg Radial Anat* 26:399-410

Cardano, Gerolamo (Italian mathematician, 1501-1576): see the Internet

Chèze L, Doriot N, Eckert M et al. 2001 Etude cinématique in vivo de l'articulation trapézo-métacarpienne. *Chir Main* 20:22-30

Codman E.A. 1934 *The shoulder : rupture of the supraspinatus tendon and other lesions in or about the subacromial bursa.* Thomas Todd Co, Printers, Boston.

Colville J, Callison JR, White WL 1969 Role of mesotendon in tendon blood supply. *Plat Reconstr Surg* 43:53

Comtet J-J, Auffray Y 1970 Physiologie des muscles élévateurs de l'épaule. *Rev Chir Ortho* 56(3):105-117

Cooney WP, Chao EYS 1977 Biomechanical analysis of static forces in the thumb during hand function. *J Bone and Joint Surg* 59A(1): 27-36

Dautry P, Gosset J 1969 A propos de la rupture de la coiffe des rotateurs de l'épaule. *Rev Chir Ortho* 55(2):157

Descamps L 1950 *Le Jeu de la hanche.* Thèse, Paris

Djbay HC 1972 L'humérus dans la prono-supination. *Rev Méd Limoges* 3(3):147-150

Dobyns JH, Linscheid RL, Chao EYS et al. 1975 Traumatic instability of the wrist. *Am Acad Orthop Surgeons Instruction Course* Lect. 24:182

Dubousset J 1971 Les phénomènes de rotation lors de la préhension au niveau des doigts (sauf le pouce). *Ann Chir* 25(19-20) C:935-944

Duchenne (de Boulogne) GBA 1867 *Physiologie des mouvements.* Vol. 1, p. 871. J-B Ballière, Paris (out of print; edited facsimile published by Annales de Médecine Physique, 1967)

Duchenne (de Boulogne) GBA 1949 *Physiology of motion.* Translated by EB Kaplan. WB Saunders, Philadelphia

Duparc J, Caffinière J-Y (de la), Pineau H 1971 Approche biomécanique et cotation des mouvements du premier métacarpien. *Rev Chir Orthop* 57(1):3-12

Essex-Lopresti P 1951 Fractures of the radial head with distal radioulnar dislocation. *J Bone and Joint Surg* 33B:244-247

Eyler DL, Markee JF 1954 The anatomy and function of the intrinsic musculature of the fingers. *J Bone and Joint Surg* 36A:1-9

Fahrer M 1971 Considérations sur l'anatomie fonctionnelle du muscle fléchisseur commun profond des doigts. *Ann Chir* 25:945-950

Fahrer M 1975 Considérations sur les insertions d'origine des muscles lombricaux: les systèmes digastriques de la main. *Ann Chir* 29:979-982

Fick R 1911 *Handbuch der Anatomie und Mechanik der Gelenke.* Vol. 3, Gustav Fischer, Iena

Fischer LP, Carret JP, Gonon GP, Dimmet J 1977 Etude cinématique des mouvements de l'articulation scapulo-humérale. *Rev Chir Orth* Suppl. 11(63):108-112

Fischer LP, Noireclerc JA, Neidart JM et al. 1970 Etude anatomo-radiologique de l'importance des différents ligaments dans la contention verticale de la tête de l'humérus. *Lyon Méd* 223(11):629-633

Fischer O 1907 *Kinematik urhanischer Gelenke.* F Vierweg, Braunschweig

Froment J 1914-1915 La paralysie de l'adducteur du pouce et le signe de la préhension. *Rev Neurol* 28:1236

Froment J 1920 Paralysie des muscles de la main et troubles de la préhension. *J Méd Lyon*

Galeazzi R 1934 Di una particulare sindrome traumatica dello scheletro dell'avambraccio. *Atti Mem Soc Lombardi Chir* 2:12

Gauss Karl Friedrich (German mathematician, 1777-1855) *La géometrie non euclidienne* (on Codman's paradox): see the Internet

Ghyka Matila C 1978 *Le Nombre d'or.* Vol. 1, p. 190. Gallimard, Paris

Gilula LA, Weeks PM 1978 Post-traumatic ligamentous instability of the wrist. *Radiology* 126:641

Gilula LA, Yin Y 1996 *Imaging of the wrist and the hand.* WB Saunders, Philadelphia

Hamonet C, de la Caffinière J-Y, Opsomer G 1972 Mouvements du pouce: détermination électromyographique des secteurs d'activité des muscles thénariens. *Arch Anat Path* 20(4):363-367

Hamonet C, Valentin P 1970 Etude électromyographique du rôle de l'opposant du pouce *(opponens pollicis)* et de l'adducteur du pouce *(adductor pollicis). Rev Chir Ortho* 56(2): 165-176

Henke J 1859 Die Bewegungen der Handwurzel. *Zeitschrift für rationelle Medezine* 7:27

Henke W 1863 *Handbuch der Anatomie und Mechanik der Gelenke.* CF Wintersche, Heidelberg

Hume MC, Grellman H, McKellop H, Brumfield RH Jr 1990 Functional range of motion of the joint of the hand. *J Hand Surg* 15A:240-243

Inman-Vernet T et al. 1944 Observations on the function of the shoulder joint. *J Bone Joint Surg* 26(1):30

Kapandji AI 1981 Anatomie fonctionnelle et biomécanique de la méta-carpophalangienne du pouce. *Ann Chir* 35(4):261-267

Kapandji AI 1986 Cotation clinique de l'opposition et de la contre opposition du pouce. *Ann Chir Main* 5(1):67-73

Kapandji AI 1987 La Biomécanique 'Patate'. *Ann Chir Main* 5:260-263

Kapandji AI 1987 Biomécanique du carpe et du poignet. *Ann Chir Main* 6:147-169

Kapandji AI 1987 Proposition pour une cotation clinique de la flexion-extension des doigts longs. *Ann Chir Main* 6:288-294

Kapandji AI 1989 La Préhension dans la main humaine. *Ann Chir Main* 8:234-241

Kapandji AI 1996 De la Phylogénèse à la fonction du membre supérieur de l'Homme (Conference paper, Saint-Maurice). *Sport Med* March-April 80-81:4-9

Kapandji AI 1997 Vous avez dit Biomécanique? La Mécanique 'Floue' ou 'Patate'. *Maitrise Orthopédique* 64:1, 4, 5, 6, 7, 8, 9, 10, 11

Kapandji AI 1999 La Défaillance du crochet ulnaire ou encore 'signe de la lime à ongles', signe peu connu d'atteinte du nerf ulnaire. *Ann Chir Main* 18(4):295-298

Kapandji AI 1980 La Main dans l'art main. In: Tubiana R *Traité de chirurgie de la main.* Masson, Paris

Kapandji AI, Kapandji TG 1993 Nouvelles Données radiologiques sur la trapézo-métacarpienne. Résultats sur 330 dossiers. *Ann Chir Main* 4:263-274

Kapandji AI, Martin-Boyer Y, Verdeille S 1991 Etude du carpe au scanner à trois dimensions sous contrainte de prono-supination. *Ann Chir Main* 10:36-47

Kapandji IA 1972 La rotation du pouce sur son axe longitudinal lors de l'opposition. Etude géométrique et mécanique de la trapézo-métacarpienne. Modèle mécanique de la main. *Rev Chir Orthop* 58(4):273-289

Kapandji IA 1975 Pourquoi l'avant-bras comporte-t-il deux os? *Ann Chir* 29(5):463-470

Kapandji IA 1976 La flexion-pronation de l'interphalangienne du pouce. *Ann Chir* 30(11-12):855-857

Kapandji IA 1977 Le membre supérieur, support logistique de la main. *Ann Chir* 31(12):1021-1030

Kapandji IA 1977 La radio-cubitale inférieure vue sous l'angle de la prono-supination. *Ann Chir* 31(12):1031-1039

Kapandji IA, Moatti E 1980 La Radiographie spécifique de la trapézo-métacarpienne, sa technique, son intérêt. *Ann Chir* 34:719-726

Kaplan EB 1965 *Functional and surgical anatomy of the hand*, 2nd edn (1st edn 1953). Lippincott, Philadelphia

Kauer JMG 1974 The interdependence of the carpal articulation chains. *Acta Anat* 88:481

Kauer JMG 1980 Functional anatomy of the wrist. *Clin Orthop* 149:9

Kuckzinski K 1968 *The upper limb*. In: Passmore R, Robson JS *A companion to medical studies*, Vol. 1, Ch. 22. Blackwell Scientific, Oxford

Kuckzinski K 1974 Carpometacarpal joint of the human thumb. *J Anat* 118(1):119-126

Kuhlmann N 1979 Les Mécanismes de l'articulation du poignet. *Ann Chir* 33:711-719

Kuhlmann N, Gallaire M, Pineau H 1978 Déplacements du scaphoïde et du semi-lunaire au cours des mouvements du poignet. *Ann Chir* 38:543-553

Landsmeer JMF 1949 The anatomy of the dorsal aponeurosis of the human finger and its functional significance. *Anat Rec* 104:31

Landsmeer JMF 1955 Anatomical and functional investigations on the articulations of the human fingers. *Acta Anat* Suppl. 24

Landsmeer JMF 1953 A report on the co-ordination of the interphalangeal joints of the human finger and its disturbances. *Acta Morph Neerl Scand* 2:59-84

Landsmeer JMF 1961 Studies in the anatomy of articulations: (1) The equilibrium of the intercalated bone; (2) Patterns of movements of bimuscular, biarticular systems. *Acta Morph Neerl Scand* 32(3-4):287-321

Landsmeer JMF 1976 *Atlas of anatomy of the hand*. Churchill Livingstone, Edinburgh

Lin GT, Amadio PC, An KN, Cooney WP 1989 Functional anatomy of the human digital flexor pulley system. *Hand Surg* 14A:949-956

Linscheid RW, Dobyns JH 1971 Rheumatoid arthritis of the wrist. *Ortho Clin of North America* 2:649

Linscheid RW, Dobyns JH, Beabout JW, Bryan RS 1972 Traumatic instability of the wrist: diagnosis, classification and pathomechanics. *J Bone Joint Surg (Am)* 54:1612-1632

Littler JW 1960 Les Principes architecturaux et fonctionnels de l'anatomie de la main. *Rev Chir Orthop* 46:131-138

Littler JW 1960 The physiology and dynamic function of the hand. *Surg Clin N Amer* 40:256

Long C, Brown E 1962 Electromyographic kinesiology of the hand. Part III Lumbricalis and flexor digitorum profundus to the long finger. *Arch Phys Med* 43:450-460

Long C, Brown E 1964 Electromyographic kinesiology of the hand muscle moving the long finger. *J Bone and Joint Surg Am* 46A:1683

Long C, Brown E, Weiss G 1960 Electromyographic study of the extrinsic-intrinsic kinesiology of the hand. Preliminary report. *Arch Phys Med* 41:175-181

Lundborg G, Myrhage E, Rydevik B 1977 Vascularisation des tendons fléchisseurs dans la gaine digitale. *J Hand Surg* 2(6):417-427

MacConaill MA 1946 Studies in the mechanics of the synovial joints: displacement on articular surfaces and significance of saddle joints. *Irish J M Sci*: 223-235

MacConaill MA 1946 Studies in the mechanics of the synovial joints: hinge joints and nature of intra-articular displacements. *Irish J M Sci* Sept:620

MacConaill MA 1953 Movements of bone and joints: significance of shape. *J Bone and Joint Surg* 35B:290

MacConaill MA 1966 The geometry and algebra of articular kinematics. *Bio Med Eng* 1:205-212

MacConaill MA 1966 *Studies on the anatomy and function of bone and joints*. F. Gaynor Evans, New York

MacConaill MA, Barnett CH, Dvics DV 1962 *Synovial joints*. Longman, London

MacConaill MA, Basmajian JV 1969 *Muscle and movements: a basis for human kinesiology*. Williams & Wilkins, Baltimore

Marey J 1891 *La Machine animale*. Vol. 1. Alcan, Paris

Moreaux A 1959 *Anatomie artistique de l'Homme*. Vol. 1. Maloine, Paris

Occam (or Ockham), William of (English Franciscan monk and scholastic philosopher, 1280-1349) *The principle of economy*: see the Internet

Palmer AK, Glisson RR, Werner FW 1982 Ulnar variance determination. *J Hand Surg* 7:376

Palmer AK, Werner FW 1981 The triangular fibrocartilage complex of the wrist: anatomy and function. *J Hand Surg Am* 6:153

Pieron AP 1973 The mechanism of the first carpo-metacarpal joint. Anatomic and mechanical analysis. *Acta Orthop Scand* Suppl. 148

Poirier P, Charpy A 1926 *Traité d'anatomie humaine*. Masson, Paris

Poitevin HC 2001 Anatomy and biomechanics of the interosseous membrane: its importance in the longitudinal stability of the forearm. *Hand Clinics* 17:97-109

Rabischong P 1963 Innervation proprioceptive des muscles lombricaux chez l'homme. *Rev Chir Orth* 8:234

Rasch PJ, Burke RK 1971 *Kinesiology and applied anatomy. The science of human movement*. Vol. 1, p. 589. Lea & Febiger, Philadelphia

Ricmann, Georg Friedrich Bernhard (German mathematician, 1826-1866) *La géometrie non euclidienne* (on Codmann's paradox): see the Internet

Roud A 1913 *Mécanique des articulations et des muscles de l'homme*. F. Rouge, Librairie de l'Université, Lausanne

Rouvière H 1948 *Anatomie humaine descriptive et topographique*, 4th edn. Masson, Paris

Sauvé L, Kapandji M 1936 Une nouvelle technique de traitement chirurgical des luxations récidivantes isolées de l'extrémité cubitale inférieure. *J Chir* 47:4

Schuind F, Garcia Elias M, Cooney WP III, An KN 1992 Flexor tendon force: in vivo measurements. *L Hand Surg* 17A:291-298

Steindler A 1964 *Kinesiology of the human body*. Vol. 1, p. 708. Thomas, Springfield

Strasser H 1917 *Lehrbuch der Muskel und Gelenkemechanik*. Vol. IV. J Springer, Berlin

Taleisnik J 1976 The ligaments of the wrist. *J Hand Surg* 1-2:110

Taleisnik J 1980 Post-traumatic carpal instability. *Clin Orthop* 149:73-82

Taleisnik J 1985 *The wrist*. p. 441. Churchill Livingstone, New York

Testut L 1893 *Traité d'anatomie humaine*. Doin, Paris

Thieffry S 1973 *La main de l'Homme*. Hachette, Paris

Thomine J-M 1980 Examen clinique de la main. In: Tubiana R *Traité de chirurgie de la main*. Masson, Paris

Tubiana R 1969 Mécanisme des déformations des doigts liées à un déséquilibre tendineux. *La main rhumatoïde*. L'Expansion, Paris

Tubiana R 1973 Les positions d'immobilisation de la main. *Ann Chir* 27(5):459-466

Tubiana R, Fahrer M 1981 Le rôle du ligament annulaire postérieur du carpe dans la stabilité du poignet. *Rev Chir Orthop* 67:231

Tubiana R, Hakstian R 1969 *Les déviations cubitales normales et pathologiques des doigts. Etude de l'architecture des articulations métacarpo-phalangiennes des doigts. La main rhumatoïde*. Monograph, GEM, Expansion scientifique, Paris

Tubiana R, Hakstian R 1969 *Le rôle des facteurs anatomiques dans les déviations cubitales normales et pathologiques des doigts. La Main rhumatismale*. pp. 11-21. L'Expansion, Paris

Tubiana R, Valentin P 1963 L'extension des doigts. *Rev Chir Orthop* T49:543-562

Tubiana R, Valentin P 1964 Anatomy of the extension apparatus. Physiology of the finger extension. *Surg Clin N America* 44:897-906, 907-918

Valentin P 1962 *Contribution à l'étude anatomique, physiologique et clinique de l'appareil extenseur des doigts*. Thèse, Paris

Valentin P, Hamonet C 1970 Etude électromyographique de l'opposant du pouce et de l'adducteur du pouce. *Rev Chir Orth* 56:65

Vandervael F 1956 Analyse des mouvements du corps humain. Maloine, Paris

Van Linge B, Mulder JD 1963 Fonction du muscle sus-épineux et sa relation avec le syndrome sus-épineux. Etude expérimental chez l'homme. *J Bone Joint Surg* 45 B(4):750-754

Verdan C 1960 Syndrome of the Quadriga. *Surg Clin N Amer* 40:425-426

Von Recklinghausen H 1920 *Gliedermechanik und Lühmungsprostesen.* Vol. 1. Julius Springer, Berlin

Watson HK, Ballet FL 1948 The SLAC wrist: scapholunate advanced collapse. Pattern of degenerative arthritis. *J Hand Surg* 9A:358-385

Winckler G 1976 Anatomie normale des tendons fléchisseurs et extenseurs de la main, leur vascularisation macroscopique. In: *Chirurgie des tendons de la main.* Monograph GEM, Expansion Scientifique, Paris, pp. 14-21

Zancolli EA 1979 *Structural and dynamic basis of hand surgery*, 2nd end (1st edn 1968). Lippincott, Philadelphia

Zancolli EA, Zaidenberg C, Zancolli ER 1987 Biomechanics of the trapeziometacarpal joint. *Clin Orthop* 220

Index

Working model of the hand for cutout and assembly

The models presented in these volumes are meant to be cut out, folded and assembled in order to give concrete expression in space to the ideas discussed in the text. They are three-dimensional diagrams that can be manipulated. In building these models you can use your own awareness of muscular activity and gain insights that are otherwise difficult to acquire. The author therefore strongly urges the reader to have the patience to spend some time on this project, which will prove rewarding.

Before starting it is essential to read all the instructions carefully.

This model contains four pieces (A-D) shown in plates I and II. At the bottom of plate II assembly diagrams (a-c) are included.

For editorial reasons the pages containing the drawings are not thick enough to give the model stability. Thus you must first use a sheet of carbon paper to copy these drawings exactly onto a piece of cardboard at least 1 mm thick.

Cutout procedure

First use scissors to cut out the four pieces along their margins, as indicated by the thick lines. Some of these pieces contain the following lines, which need to be cut with a craft knife or a scalpel:

- piece A: the lines between tabs h, j and k
- piece D: the long sides of the rectangle and the two remaining sides of each of the two flattened isosceles triangles near m′ and n′.

Next scoop out the cardboard as follows:

- through the strip of coarse hatching to the right of k′ in A and the horizontal central cleft in D
- along the parallel strokes in A and C, making narrow slits between the two closely set strokes to accommodate the pulleys for the tendons (see diagram c).

Finally make the following circular holes:

- through the circles in D intended for the passage of the tendons, which are numbered in accordance with diagram c
- through the crossed circles for the insertions of the tendons
- through the simple crosses meant for the attachment of the elastic bands.

Folding

First cut into the cardboard with a razor blade to a depth of one-third or one-half of the thickness of the cardboard on the side opposite to the fold. These incisions are made:

- on the front of the cardboard along the dashed lines
- on the back of the cardboard along the dot-dash lines. (To achieve this with precision, you will find it useful to mark

the ends of these lines by piercing through the cardboard with a fine needle or the point of a compass.)

After the incisions are made, you will be able to fold the cardboard easily and precisely on the side opposite to the incisions. In folding the cardboard, do not at first exceed 45°. The two longitudinal folds in A are very shallow and correspond to the hollowing of the palm. The folds marked axis 1 on A and axis 2 on C form a 90° angle, and the two converging folds starting from the end of axis 1 and the folds of tabs j and h can exceed 90°. Piece B has no folds.

Note in C the obliquity of the flexion folds for the inter-phalangeal (IP) and metacarpo-phalangeal (MP) joints, in keeping with their unusual mode of flexion. For the MP joint only one of the three axes is used, i.e. the one that allows flexion-pronation-radial deviation to occur during thumb opposition.

Assembly

Diagram a shows how the components are assembled:

- The base (piece D) is formed by bringing m and m′ and n and n′ closer together until they coincide. Then either glue strips m and n on the dark-shaded surfaces of m′ and n′ or, if you wish to disassemble the model afterwards, fit paper fasteners through the holes marked on m, m′, n and n′.
- After marking the creases for the fingers and the palm on the hand (piece A), construct the trapezo-metacarpal (TM) joint as follows:

1) Fold the semicircular surface g backwards through 90°.
2) Fold the two triangles forwards to form a pyramid with its base lying on top.
3) Keep the pyramid in place by:
   - either gluing tabs h and j over the surfaces of h′ and j′ (for the definitive model)
   - or securing tab k by pushing it through the slot between h′ and j′ and fastening it on the back of k′ with a paper fastener through the circular holes in k and k′.

- Fold C (the thumb) backwards (arrow 1) and glue it (arrow 2) to the front of B so that f lies on top of f and all the holes and the lines representing axis 2 are properly matched. Then glue this composite structure to the pyramid supporting the thumb by applying g′ on the back of B to g on the front of A so that the holes and the lines representing axis 1 are properly matched.

You have thus constructed the biaxial universal joint corresponding to the TM joint.

Diagram b shows how you can attach the hand by sliding it into the central cleft of D.

Use

Passive mobilization of the model will now allow you to understand the three basic characteristic features of the hand:

1) **Hollowing of the palm** by flexion along the longitudinal folds, which simulates the movements of opposition of M4 and, above all, of M5.
2) **Oblique flexion of the fingers**, which makes them converge towards the base of the thenar eminence. This results from the increasing degree of obliquity of the axes of the IP joints and MP joints from the index to the little finger (an example of conical rotation) and is enhanced by the movement of opposition of the medial metacarpals (M4 and especially M5).
3) **Thumb opposition.** You can verify the occurrence of plane rotation, conical rotation and cylindrical rotation presented in the text by making axis 1 (axis xx' in c) the main axis and axis 2 (axis yy' in c) the secondary axis. You can check that flexion taking place successively in the other joints of the thumb (the MP and the IP joints) gives rise to cylindrical rotation of the distal phalanx of the thumb, which changes its orientation without any major flexion at the TM joint and any significant axial rotation of M1. You will be able to observe that there is no mechanical play in the joints of the thumb and yet the thumb can move along the 'short and long paths' of opposition from index to little finger simply by a change in the orientation of its pulp, as occurs in real life.

Flexion-pronation of the IP and MP joints is the result of the obliquity of the folds.

Setting up the 'tendons'

You can activate this model by putting in the 'tendons' (diagram c). They consist of thin cords fixed by knots at their phalangeal insertions (circular holes each marked with a cross) and run freely through the 'pulleys' located on the phalanges and the holes made in the base.

You can easily make these pulleys from small strips of cardboard 6 mm wide and soft enough to be bent to form a tunnel. Thread the ends of these strips from front to back through the narrow slits made in A and C and glue them on the backs of A and C after folding them backwards in the shape of a capital omega.

The double pulley 2-7 (C) is different; it is glued on the front for 2 and on the back for 7, forming two reciprocally inverted capital omegas.

The course of the tendons

Each tendon is labelled with a number that refers to its entire course.

1) *Abductor pollicis longus* (1) is inserted into B and mobilizes the TM joint around its main axis (axis 1).
2) *Flexor pollicis longus* (2) is inserted into P2 of the thumb after passing through the pulley (2) on P1. It flexes both phalanges.

3) This transversely running 'tendon' (3) is reflected at the pulley in the palm and is the combined equivalent of the *adductor* and the *flexor pollicis brevis* combined.
4) The tendon of the *flexor digitorum profundus* for the index (4) is inserted into P3 after passing through three pulleys. It flexes the index as a whole.
5) This transversely running 'tendon' is the counterpart of tendon 3 and is inserted into a wedge 6-7 mm thick corresponding to the darkly shaded trapezium 5 (A). It is reflected in the palm at pulley 5 and is the equivalent of the *opponens digiti minimi*.
6) The tendon of the *flexor digitorum profundus* for the little finger has the same course and action as tendon 4. N.B. For simplicity's sake the flexors of the third and fourth fingers have not been included, but they could easily be included.
7) Tendon (7) is not seen in the diagram but corresponds to the *extensor pollicis longus*. It is inserted on the dorsal surface of P2 in the same hole as the *flexor pollicis longus* (with the two knots facing each other) and passes through the pulley on the dorsal surface of P1 and then through a hole in B.

At the free ends of the 'tendons' you can attach buckles or rings to hold your fingers and allow you to mobilize the tendons more easily.

To stabilize the thumb in a functional position you can use elastic bands to keep axes 1 and 2 in an intermediate position.

For axis 1 the elastic band starts at one of the holes e_1 in B, is reflected through the hole e_1 in the base of A and comes back to be attached to the other hole e_1 in B. The intermediate position is found when the band is allowed to slide in hole e_1 in A. The band is fixed by being glued on either side. The same applies to stabilizing axis 2; the elastic band starts at one of the holes e_2 in B, slides through hole e_2 in C and comes back to be attached to the other hole e_2 in B. To ensure that the index and the little finger can go back into extension you can attach an elastic band to their dorsal surfaces between holes 4 and 4 (for the index) and holes 6 and 6 (for the little finger) located on the palmar surface of A. You can again use glue for stabilization.

Mobilization of the model

With the help of these tendons you can make almost all the movements of the hand:

- **hollowing of the hand** by pulling on tendon 5 (The efficiency of this movement depends on the height of wedge 5 in A.)
- **flexion of the index and little fingers** by pulling on tendons 4 and 6
- **mobilization of the thumb:**
  - **bringing the thumb into the plane of the palm** (i.e. a flat hand corresponding to the initial position of Sterling Bunnell's experiment) by pulling in a balanced fashion on tendons 7 and 3

- **thumb-index opposition** by flexing the index and at the same time pulling on tendons 1, 3 and 7
- **thumb-little finger opposition** by flexing the little finger and at the same time pulling on tendons 1, 3 and 6
- **thumb-base of the little finger opposition** by pulling on tendons 1 and 2 and if necessary on tendon 3

- **termino-lateral (tip-to-side) thumb-index opposition**: same as for b, but with a greater degree of flexion of the index.

Plate I

Plate II